Vision Models for Target Detection and Recognition

SERIES ON INFORMATION DISPLAY

Editor-in-Chief: Hiap L. Ong

Vol. 1: Electroluminescent Displays
     Y. A. Ono

Vol. 2: Vision Models for Target Detection and Recognition
     ed. E. Peli

Series on Information Display – Volume 2

Vision Models for Target Detection and Recognition

In Memory of Arthur Menendez

Editor

Eli Peli

The Schepens Eye Res. Inst., Harvard Medical School

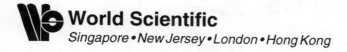 **World Scientific**
Singapore • New Jersey • London • Hong Kong

Published by

World Scientific Publishing Co. Pte. Ltd.

P O Box 128, Farrer Road, Singapore 9128

USA office: Suite 1B, 1060 Main Street, River Edge, NJ 07661

UK office: 57 Shelton Street, Covent Garden, London WC2H 9HE

VISION MODELS FOR TARGET DETECTION AND RECOGNITION

ISBN   981-02-2149-5

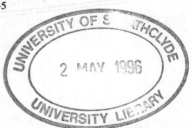

Printed in Singapore.

IN MEMORY OF ARTHUR R. MENENDEZ (1953–1992)

Arthur R. Menendez, a major contributor to research in applied vision, laser safety and aircrew vision, disappeared while scuba diving off the Dutch Antilles on July 5, 1992. Dutch authorities were unable to locate him after an extensive air and underwater search.

At the time of his disappearance, Dr. Menendez was a senior vision scientist at the Armstrong Laboratory, Brooks Air Force Base, Texas. He received his BA, MA, and PhD from Southern Illinois University under the direction of Dr. Fred Lit. Art completed a post-doctoral fellowship at Vanderbilt University. He entered government service in 1986 after working several years in private industry.

Art devoted his professional life to the study of vision and its application to visual problems in aviation. His particular interest was in understanding the visual processes that underlie target detection and recognition. He advanced our knowledge of the visual system's response to intense light, particularly the effects of light adaptation on target detection and the ways that pilots adapt to sudden changes in ambient brightness. The complexity of the visual world of pilots drove Art's interest toward visual modeling. He felt strongly that computational models of light adaptation and spatial vision could be invaluable tools for addressing applied problems in aviation, medicine, and defense.

While trained in visual psychophysics, Art did not limit his research to that field. He was an avid reader of journals across many scientific disciplines, and consequently, was an invaluable source of knowledge to his colleagues. He co-authored a paper applying a probability-summation model to derive quantitative formulation of the cumulative tissue damage associated with repeated laser exposures. Art was instrumental in writing a military medical handbook on laser-induced ocular injuries; the handbook was used by American and Allied medical personnel during Desert Storm. One of his last projects was to investigate the visual consequences of lens fluorescence induced by ultraviolet radiation.

Research pursuits were only one part of his life. He was devoted to his wife, Lisa, his parents, and his brothers. He decided to start scuba diving only a few years prior to his disappearance. Diving, perhaps, was an extension of his larger interests in marine life and aquariums. He read constantly, fueling many lively good-natured debates, which were his trademark, with his colleagues. Art could be as tenacious as a bulldog in advocating his ideas, but he never lost his appreciation for the value of another person's point of view.

In his memory, the Armstrong Laboratory has established the Arthur R. Menendez Memorial Lecture series. The series commemorates Art's devotion to visual science and its application to occupational safety and national defense. On behalf of Art's family, colleagues, and friends, we extend our heartfelt appreciation to Dr. Eli Peli and all of the contributors for this lasting tribute to Art. The book is as much a celebration of Art's professionalism as it is an advancement in vision modeling. For those who knew him, this book is most appropriate, for once again, Art has the last word.

Robert M. Cartledge, D.V.M., M.S.
and many of Art's friends

PREFACE

In May of 1991, Dr. Arthur Menendez, a vision scientist working for the US Air Force, convened a conference titled "Applied Spatial Vision Models for Target Detection and Recognition" in San Antonio, Texas. The conference was organized as the first meeting of an Advisory Group for the Laser Branch, Directed Energy Division, Occupational and Environmental Health Directorate at the Armstrong Laboratory. The meeting was judged by all the participants to be extremely successful. It was a unique opportunity for researchers from the academic ivory towers to meet and discuss issues of common interest with colleagues from industry and the Armed Services. The meeting format, which included pre-assigned discussants and ample discussion time for each presentation, encouraged a free and uninhibited exchange of ideas. Dr. Menendez intended to publish the edited transcriptions of the meeting as a report. The project was well underway when it was interrupted by a tragic diving accident. The spirit of scientific camaraderie fostered by Dr. Menendez at the meeting and the fond memories we all shared were the reasons for my decision to try and publish this book in his memory.

The book is based to a large extent on presentations made at the Armstrong Laboratory Advisory Group Conference. More than two years passed before the decision was made to publish this book. I therefore asked the contributing authors to update and significantly upgrade their respective chapters to represent progress in the area in the passing years. I have also asked a few scientists who did not participate at the original meeting, and whose work I found highly relevant to the subject, to contribute chapters to the book.

This book addresses Spatial Vision Models and their application to the understanding, prediction, and evaluation of the tasks of target detection and recognition. Although the discussion in many of the chapters is framed in terms of military targets and military vision aids, the techniques, analyses, and problems are by no means limited to this area of application. The detection and recognition of an armored vehicle from a reconnaissance image is performed by the same visual system used to detect and recognize a tumor in an X-ray. The analysis of the interaction of the human visual system with night vision devices is not different from the analysis needed in the case of an operator examining underwater structures using a remote camera, etc.

I have organized the book into three general sections. The first covers basic modeling of central (foveal) vision and its theoretical background. The second section is centered on the evaluation of model performance in applications, while the third section is dedicated to aspects of peripheral vision modeling and the expansion of peripheral modeling to include visual search.

The chapter by Wilson opens the first section with a résumé of his well-known discrete model and examples of its performance. This is one of the first models to represent the visual system as a bank of a few filters distributed to provide sufficient coverage in both the space and spatial frequency domains. Wilson describes how such a model can be used to predict target detection and how the same formalism can be extended to the task of target discrimination without a change in the underlying model.

García-Pérez and Sierra-Vázquez provide a formal presentation of a model that is continuous rather than discrete in both the space and spatial frequency domains. They illustrate that representation in the joint domain alone is sufficient to provide adequate explanations to many and varied visual phenomena and illusions.

The chapter by Peli treats simulation as visual modeling. It provides a framework for simulations based on the definition of local band-limited contrast in images that permits consideration of various nonlinearities in the visual system. Both simulation of foveal and peripheral vision are possible using the corresponding contrast sensitivity function. The chapter also illustrates that this type of modeling may be tested in both the foveal and peripheral cases.

Most models address the threshold behavior of vision. In considering the fact that most daily vision is performed with highly supra threshold levels of contrast, Cannon's chapter is aimed at integrating both domains in one model. Once again a discrete model is developed. However, this model explicitly addresses the supra threshold and threshold ranges of contrast and the transition zone between them. Cannon also demonstrates how the expansion into the supra threshold range can be useful in evaluating image sharpness or other image quality measures.

No model can perform better than is permitted by the information available in the signal it processes. This realization has led a number of investigator to examine the performance of the visual system in comparison with that of an ideal observer. Geisler, who has applied ideal observer theory in many domains, examines in his chapter the relative amounts of intensity and chromatic information available for discriminating pairs of natural objects. His investigation led to the finding that most chromatic information available in the natural samples is lost between the cornea and the retina. This leaves, at the level of the photoreceptor, only negligible chromatic information as compared with intensity information, which may be used for pattern discrimination. These results may justify the almost uniform use of luminance rather than color information in the other chapters.

The second section begins with a chapter written by Cooke, Stanley and Hinton. Their discussion of the ORACLE, a long-standing model used to predict target detection and recognition, addresses almost all aspects covered in this book. The ORACLE in its current status predicts target detection in the fovea and in the retinal periphery, under bright and very dim illuminations, with and without optical or electro-optical aids. The ORACLE covers target motion and temporal characteristics of noise, as well as the issue of search. Evolving from older models of the visual system, the analysis is framed in terms of retinal and photoreceptor responses to simple uniform targets. Over time, the ORACLE has been updated to address emerging issues such as multi-scale decomposition and contrast sensitivity to grating patterns. It is interesting to realize the similarity between this model and its retinal base approach and more recent models and their cortical emphasis.

van Meeteren's presentation at the conference is reproduced here in its original transcript format. This chapter represents a review of one of the seminal projects incorporating basic/simple visual modeling concepts to the analysis of complicated performance using night vision devices. It is interesting to see that performance in tasks such as recognition of a set of military targets can be modeled by the detection of a simple contrasting disk on a uniform background. The merits and limitations of such a simple model were discussed by the group following the presentation. This discussion is included in the chapter.

O'Kane takes on the difficult issue of "model validation". In addition to discussing the merit of this concept in general, this chapter provides real-life examples of the multitude of difficulties, obstacles, and pitfalls awaiting those who try to test visual models against human performance in various modes and arenas.

Kosnik has investigated the performance of observers searching for an aircraft target embedded in static and dynamic backgrounds of varying complexity. Using a contrast metric that can treat target and background contrast separately, he was able to find a monotonic relationship between observer performance and target or background contrast. However, his findings demonstrate that other factors have to be included if the performance in these tasks is to be modeled accurately.

Thomas and Barsalou have evaluated the ability of Wilson's model to predict the spatial information content of real images required for target detection and identification. They used images containing only the energy represented by a small subset of filters in Wilson's model. Their study shows that the three highest response filters may suffice to represent the airplane images they used as well as the original images.

Lubin describes the implementation, calibration, and testing of the Sarnoff Visual Discrimination Model developed with the support of NASA and the National Information Display Laboratory. This model was designed to function as part of a design tool for display devices and display systems. The model includes many of the ideas presented in the first section of this book, while maintaining sufficient flexibility to remain a useful engineering tool. In addition to the clear presentation of the various concepts involved in using a visual model in physical system design, the chapter provides examples of successful applications of the model. The same model is shown to be effective in designing compression/decompression algorithms, assessing the optimal CRT spot size, and alphanumeric legibility with noise. The validity of the model is demonstrated using a wide range of prediction data from numerous studies in various laboratories.

The chapter by Ben-Arie and Rao is of special interest as it comes from a different discipline and represents a different approach. In fact, what is interesting about this chapter is that the authors did not try to model the visual system at all. They have developed a new method for template recognition in computer vision that is based on the optimization of a new similarity measure called the Discriminative Signal-to-Noise Ratio. Starting with a few reasonable constraints on the task at hand, they arrive at what is clearly a novel development of a vision system model. It will take little imagination to realize how their approach could be the seed for a new wave of vision models easily integrated with current concepts and knowledge on the structure of the human visual system. It will require some more work to design experiments to test the applicability of this attractive model to human vision.

The third section of the book is centered on considerations of peripheral vision. Although some of the chapters in the preceding sections included some discussion of peripheral vision, the emphasis was clearly on central foveal vision. In this section we turn our attention to the fact that more than 90% of the visual field is processed by the peripheral retina and requires different considerations.

Bradley and Thibos deal first with the optical consequences of off-axis imaging that takes place with peripheral vision or with a decentered electro-optical device. Their analysis and the computational model they develop account for the majority of the effects of off-axis vision on contrast sensitivity and resolution. This model should prove useful to anyone designing a wide field optical or display system or modeling peripheral vision.

Thibos and Bradley, in their second chapter, address the neural aspects of spatial filtering and sampling on off-axis vision. They show that optical quality, which is the limiting factor in central vision, is replaced by neural limits in the periphery. The aliasing effects of neural under-sampling and their effects on practical applications of vision models are discussed.

The last chapter is by Doll *et al.* It represents an attempt to integrate previous retinal based models with modern concepts of cortical image processing. More important is the bolder effort to go beyond just modeling single glimpse detection into the more complex probabilistic area of search and the improvement of performance with training. This is the only direct effort in this collection to touch on the difficult but inevitable problem of top down flow and its role in target detection.

It is my hope that the next book on vision models, which someone else will edit, will move us on from the low level emphasis of this collection at least to the realm of mid level vision. As much as we are tempted to stay within the relative simplicity of low level vision models, and despite their effectiveness as demonstrated here, it is clear to me that the intellectual and computational challenges presented by higher level models are bound to be more scientifically rewarding and possibly even more effective in application.

Art Menendez said that the more we learn about each other's work the more respectful we become. I know this has been true for me in working on this book, and it is my wish that this book will help carry this vision of Art to others in our scientific community.

Eli Peli
Boston, December, 1994

ACKNOWLEDGMENTS

Every book is the product of the efforts of many. In an edited collection such as this one, the contributions of the authors and the editor are visible. However, many others contributed their valuable time and talents, frequently with little or no compensation. I would like to thank and acknowledge every one of the many who made such contributions (at least those I know about).

All the chapters underwent a peer review process. We were lucky to obtain the services of many reviewers who generously gave from time and expertise to provide the authors with constructive criticisms. The reviewers were asked to make recommendations and suggestions aimed toward helping the authors improve the presentation and content of their chapters. We received, with great appreciation, many detailed and elaborate reviews that I am confident, have substantially improved the clarity and scientific accuracy of this book. I would like to thank all of the reviewers for their time and thoughtful comments. The reviewers were: Albert. J. Ahumada, Ray Applegate, Larry Arend, Michael Brill, Stephen Burns, Mark Cannon, Elisabeth M. Fine, Miguel A. García-Pérez, Wilson Geisler, Robert Goldstein, Celeste Howard, William Kosnik, Vasudevan Lakshminarayanan, Leon McLin, Barbara O'Kane, Aart van Meeteren, Robert Webb, Jeremey Wolfe, and Jian Yang.

This book is an outgrowth of a scientific conference on the same subject that was organized by Dr. Arthur Menendez in July 1991. Although most of the responsibility for the organization of the conference fell on Art's shoulders, he was supported by his colleagues at the Armstrong Laboratory. I wish to thank in particular Lt. Col. Frank Cheney, Major Leon McLin, Lt. Col. Robert Cartledge, for helping to organize this outstanding meeting and for all the support and encouragement they gave me when I embarked on the task of editing this book. The conference and the book were sponsored by the US Air Force Office of Scientific Research, and I wish to thank Dr. John Tangney for supporting Art in organizing the meeting and the encouragement and direct help he provided me.

Editing a multi-authored volume is obviously easier than writing a book. It appears, however, that the reduction in writing effort is amply compensated for by the increased administrative demands. My administrative assistant at the Schepens Eye Research Institute, Rose Davis, shared this load with me. However, we would not have been able to accomplish our task without the outstanding help from my student, Elisabeth M. Fine. Her experience in editorial work and control of the various word processing programs made the production of the camera-ready manuscripts possible. The many hours she spent on this project must have delayed her thesis completion by at least a few weeks. I hope that the benefit she got from reading the various chapters (over and over) can somehow compensate for that delay.

Last but not least, I want to thank my wife Tami, and my kids Ben and Dana, who saw this project as one more demand on my already limited time with them.

CONTENTS

Memorial to Arthur R. Menendez — v

Preface — vii

Acknowledgments — xi

Spatial Vision Models — 1

Chapter 1   Quantitative Models for Pattern Detection and Discrimination — 3
H. R. Wilson

Chapter 2   Visual Processing in the Joint Spatial/Spatial-Frequency Domain — 16
M. A. García-Pérez and V. Sierra-Vázquez

Chapter 3   Simulating Normal and Low Vision — 63
E. Peli

Chapter 4   A Multiple Spatial Filter Model for Suprathreshold Contrast Perception — 88
M. W. Cannon

Chapter 5   Discrimination Information in Natural Radiance Spectra — 117
W. S. Geisler

Models Applications and Evaluation — 133

Chapter 6   The Oracle Approach to Target Acquisition and Search Modelling — 135
K. J. Cooke, P. A. Stanley, and J. L. Hinton

Chapter 7   Characterization of Task Performance with Viewing Instruments — 172
A. van Meeteren

Chapter 8   Validation of Prediction Models for Target Acquisition
             with Electro-Optical Sensors   192
             B. L. O'Kane

Chapter 9   Applying Human Spatial Vision Models to Real-World Target
             Detection and Identification: A Test of the Wilson Model   219
             S. R. Thomas and N. Barsalou

Chapter 10   A Visual Discrimination Model for Imaging System Design
             and Evaluation   245
             J. Lubin

Chapter 11   Template Recognition Based on Expansion Matching
             with Neural Lattice Implementation   284
             J. Ben-Arie and K. R. Rao

Peripheral Vision and Search   **311**

Chapter 12   Modeling Off-axis Vision I: The Optical Effects of
             Decentering Visual Targets or the Eye's Entrance Pupil   313
             A. Bradley and L. N. Thibos

Chapter 13   Modeling Off-axis Vision II: The Effect of Spatial
             Filtering and Sampling by Retinal Neurons   338
             L. N. Thibos and A. Bradley

Chapter 14   Quantifying Target Contrast in Target Acquisition Research   380
             W. Kosnik

Chapter 15   Simulation of Selective Attention and Training Effects in
             Visual Search and Detection   396
             T. J. Doll, S. W. McWhorter, D. E. Schmieder,
             and A. A. Wasilewski

Spatial Vision Models

QUANTITATIVE MODELS FOR PATTERN DETECTION AND DISCRIMINATION

HUGH R. WILSON
Visual Sciences Center
University of Chicago
939 E. 57th Street
Chicago, IL 60637, USA

Psychophysical research has resulted in the development of a quantitative model of human spatial vision that accurately predicts both threshold detection and discrimination of localized visual patterns in the fovea. This model incorporates both oriented filters and response nonlinearities characteristic of cortical simple cells. With appropriate modifications, this model is applicable to peripheral vision as well. Extension of such models to include nonlinear (non-Fourier) processing enables them to predict aspects of texture discrimination and illusory contour perception as well.

1. Introduction

Under optimal conditions the human visual system can detect targets differing in luminance from the background by less than 0.5%, and it can discriminate objects that differ in the location of their features by only 5 arc seconds. This latter figures corresponds to a shift of 0.10 inch viewed at a distance of 115 yards! Over the past decade we have developed a quantitative model that is capable of explaining and predicting this detection and discrimination performance both in foveal and peripheral vision. As detailed descriptions of this work have already been published[29-31,39], the goal of this chapter will be to provide an overview of this work along with comments on appropriate extensions occasioned by recent experimental advances.

Before proceeding, the relationship of pattern recognition to detection and discrimination must be discussed. Among these three concepts the central one is clearly pattern *discrimination*. Two visual stimuli are said to be discriminable if a subject can reliably report which of the two has been presented on a given trial. As chance performance with two alternatives is 50% (guessing), the threshold for pattern discrimination is conventionally defined to be the 75% correct point, i.e. half way between chance and certainty. Pattern *detection* is really just a particular case of pattern discrimination in which one must discriminate between a background image, however simple or complex, and the same background with a superimposed target. Pattern *recognition* is closely related to pattern discrimination,

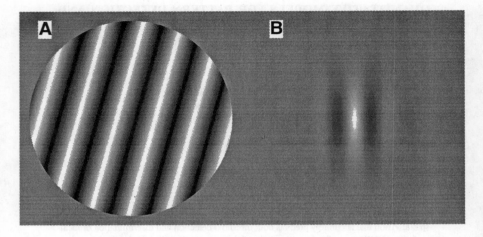

Figure 1. Mask (A) and test (B) patterns used in visual masking studies. The mask is a cosine grating oriented at 15° relative to the vertical test pattern. The luminance profile of the test pattern is defined by a sixth spatial derivative of a Gaussian function (D6) in the horizontal direction multiplied by a single vertical Gaussian. These patterns have a 1.0 octave spatial frequency bandwidth at half amplitude. In masking experiments the test D6 was superimposed on the mask, and the D6 contrast threshold was measured. In orientation masking experiments, D6 thresholds were measured as a function of cosine mask orientation.

as a pattern clearly cannot be recognized unless it can first be discriminated from other similar patterns. Thus, pattern recognition requires pattern discrimination plus a memory record for the particular constellation of features detected and discriminated. In the following, I shall restrict attention to pattern detection and discrimination.

2. Spatial Filters

We have developed a psychophysical technique for measuring the spatial characteristics of the mechanisms that filter the image falling on the human retina[40]. The key to this technique is visual masking. In a visual masking experiment the subject must detect a low contrast test stimulus that is superimposed on a high contrast masking pattern.[a] In our experiments the masks were spatial cosine gratings oriented at 15° to the vertical (Fig. 1A), and the test stimuli were defined by the sixth spatial derivative of a Gaussian function (D6),

---

a. The contrast of a pattern is described as follows. Let L_{Mean} be the mean luminance averaged over the image, and let ΔL_{Max} be the maximum deviation of image luminance from L. Contrast is just $\Delta L_{Max}/L_{Mean}$.

as shown in Fig. 1B. The D6 stimulus has the advantage of being spatially localized as well as having a 1.0 octave spatial frequency bandwidth. When thresholds were measured for the D6 test in the presence of a cosine mask, it was found that the mask raised thresholds by as much as 600% when the bars of the test and mask were of similar width, i.e. when they were of similar spatial frequency. Masks of higher or lower spatial frequency, however, produced progressively less masking. The qualitative explanation for these results is that test thresholds are elevated only when the high contrast mask stimulates the same visual mechanisms that are detecting the test pattern. Therefore, the masking function provides a measure of the spatial frequency sensitivity (i.e. sensitivity to cosine gratings) of the underlying visual mechanisms. The results clearly demonstrate that these mechanisms have a bandpass spatial frequency tuning curve and that there are several distinct spatial frequency tuned mechanisms in human foveal vision. Phillips and Wilson[20] subsequently measured masking as a function of the orientation of the mask relative to the test and demonstrated that masking was reduced as the orientation difference between test and mask increased.

In essence, these masking experiments give us a measure of the Fourier transform of a visual filter expressed in the polar coordinate variables of spatial frequency and orientation. Before this can be inverse transformed to obtain a spatial representation, however, it is necessary to measure and compensate for any nonlinearities in the system. Masking experiments in which mask contrast was varied show that the visual response is a compressive, power law function of contrast with an exponent of about 0.5 at intermediate and higher contrasts[40]. Once the data have been corrected for this nonlinearity, it is possible to inverse transform them. The resulting spatial filters can be described by a function of the following form:

$$RF(x,y) = A\left\{\exp\left(-\frac{x^2}{\sigma_1^2}\right) - B\exp\left(-\frac{x^2}{\sigma_2^2}\right) - C\exp\left(-\frac{x^2}{\sigma_3^2}\right)\right\}\exp\left(\frac{y^2}{\sigma_y^2}\right) . \tag{1}$$

This function describes a vertically oriented filter, but other orientations can be generated using the familiar equations for coordinate rotation. For foveal vision it was discovered that just six of these visual filters varying in peak spatial frequency from 0.8 to 16.0 cycles per degree (cpd) were sufficient to quantitatively fit all of the masking data. Parameter values for these filters have been published elsewhere[29]. The spatial frequency bandwidths of these varied from 2.5 octaves at 0.8 cpd to 1.25 octaves at 8.0 and 16.0 cpd.[b] Likewise, orientation bandwidths were broadest at 0.8 cpd (±30° at half amplitude) and narrowed to ±15° at 8.0 and 16.0 cpd. The spatial sensitivity profile of the smallest of these foveal filters is illustrated in Fig. 2. It is worth mentioning that the characteristics of these human visual filters are in excellent quantitative agreement with recordings from single cells in macaque monkey visual cortex[7].

---

b. Spatial frequency bandwidths are reported as full bandwidth in octaves at half of maximum amplitude. Orientation bandwidths are also reported at half amplitude.

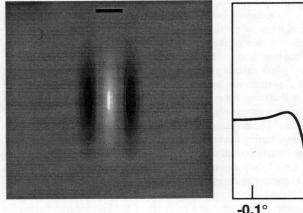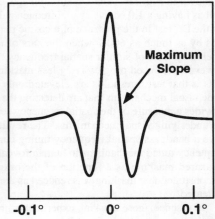

Figure 2. Sensitivity plots of the smallest foveal receptive field or filter measured by masking. This filter has a peak spatial frequency of 16.0 cpd and an orientation bandwidth of ±15 deg at half amplitude. Excitatory (lighter than background) and inhibitory (darker than background) zones are plotted in two dimensions on the left. The entire image is 0.25 deg square, and the small black bar at the top subtends 2.0 arc min, the approximate width of the excitatory zone. A sensitivity profile across the center of the pattern is plotted on the right. The arrow indicates the point at which the slope is maximal, and this is the location where very small (e.g. vernier) stimulus shifts produce a significant change in the filter's response (see Fig. 3B).

3. Pattern Discrimination

Masking studies have provided quantitative measurements of the visual mechanisms or filters subserving human foveal and peripheral (see below) vision. Furthermore, as these filters agree with the characteristics of visual cortical cells in primates, they presumably reflect processing capabilities of simple cells in human visual cortex. We are therefore in a position to compute the representation of any visual pattern in terms of human cortical unit responses. The process is simple. First, the pattern $P(x,y)$ is convolved with each of the six spatial mechanisms at each of 6-12 orientations.[c] If a filter of peak frequency ω and

---

c. The number of orientations is dependent on the orientation bandwidth of each mechanism. At 0.8 cpd, for example, the bandwidth is ±30°, and mechanisms are spaced 30° apart for a total of 6. At 8.0 and 16.0 cpd bandwidths are ±15°, and there are 12 different orientations.

preferred orientation θ is designated by $RF_{\omega,\theta}(x,y)$, then the local sensitivity $S_{\omega,\theta}$ of a cortical filter at point (x,y) will be:

$$S_{\omega,\theta}(x,y) = \int\int_{-\infty}^{\infty} RF_{\omega,\theta}(x-x',y-y')P(x',y')dx'dy' \quad . \tag{2}$$

These responses must then be passed through the compressive, power law nonlinearity that has been measured by masking. As noted above, this is roughly a square root law at suprathreshold contrasts, and the full expression is:

$$R_{\omega,\theta} = \frac{S_{\omega,\theta}^2 + KS_{\omega,\theta}^{3-\varepsilon}}{K + S_{\omega,\theta}^2} \quad . \tag{3}$$

In this equation, K and ε are empirical constants, with ε being about 0.5. Values of K vary somewhat from mechanism to mechanism[36], with the average begin about 2.0.

We may now consider any second pattern $P_2(x,y)$ and compute the cortical response to it. As each of these responses may be thought of as a point in a multi-dimensional cortical unit response space, the distance between the two representations will provide a measure of the degree to which these two patterns can be discriminated. If the difference in response of a single unit to the two patterns as calculated from Eqs. (2) and (3) is $\Delta R_{\omega,\theta}$, then their discriminability will depend on the distance measure ΔR according to the equation:

$$\Delta R = \sqrt{\sum_{\omega}\sum_{\theta}\left(R_{\omega,\theta}\right)^2} \quad . \tag{4}$$

It should be mentioned that the summation is also taken over spatial nearest neighbors rather than over all of space. This is because the human visual system is apparently unable to integrate pattern information over large spatial distances[12,36]. This may be due to cumulative positional uncertainty in the photoreceptor mosaic[11,30].

This distance measure can be converted into a probability of correct discrimination, Ψ, in a two alternative forced choice experiment using the formula:

$$\Psi = 1 - 2^{-(1+k\Delta R)^3} \quad . \tag{5}$$

The constant k is assigned the value 0.2599 so that $\Delta R = 1$ by convention at the threshold value of 75% correct for Ψ[36].

This approach to pattern discrimination has been shown to accurately predict thresholds for vernier acuity, two line separation acuity, spatial frequency discrimination, orientation discrimination, and curvature discrimination[32,33,36,42]. A surprising example is that of vernier acuity. Here the target is a pair of vertical bars, and the subject must judge whether the top bar is to the left or right of the bottom bar (Fig. 3A). Although the central excitatory zone of the smallest foveal filter is about 2.0 min. arc wide (Fig. 2), the discrimination model predicts a vernier threshold of about 6.0 sec. arc (5 to 6 times smaller than the smallest foveal cone diameter). As shown in Fig. 3C, this prediction agrees well with human psychophysical data[26]. An explanation of this model performance may be obtained by referring to Fig. 3B. Although the central excitatory zone is about 2.0 min. arc in width, the sensitivity changes very rapidly near the transition between the excitatory zone (+) and the inhibitory zone (gray). As illustrated in Fig. 3B, when the vernier target bars fall at about this position relative to a filter (as they will for some filters, given the convolution in Eq. (2)), a very small change in bar location will produce a significant change in filter response. This is because one bar will then impinge on the inhibitory zone of the receptive field. Model calculations substantiate this qualitative explanation. The rise in threshold data and predictions for short line lengths in Fig. 3C is due to the decrease in response when the lines are shorter than the receptive field.

Further details of this psychophysically grounded approach to pattern discrimination can be found in the references. As this model has proven accurate at predicting curvature, orientation, and relative position discrimination in the laboratory, it should also prove suc-

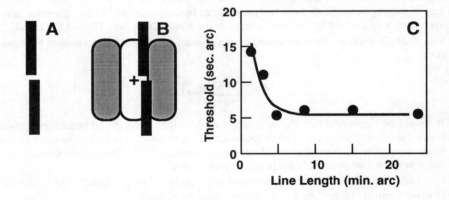

Figure 3. Stimuli and data on vernier acuity. A vernier stimulus is depicted in A, where the top line has been shifted slightly to the left. In an experiment, the subject's task would be to determine the direction of this shift. B shows that when the stimulus falls near the transition point between excitatory (+) and inhibitory (gray) regions of a receptive field (arrow in Fig. 2), this small shift will produce a significant change in response due to the encroachment of one bar into the inhibitory zone. As the fovea contains many such receptive fields at adjacent locations (note convolution in Eq. (2)), the stimulus will always fall near the optimal position for some receptive field. The solid curve in C plots model predictions for vernier acuity as a function of line length. When the individual vernier lines are shorter than about 6.0 min. of arc each, thresholds rise rapidly. This reflects the finite length of the visual filters (see Fig. 2). Solid curves are averaged data from a study by Westheimer and McKee[26].

cessful in discrimination of natural objects as well (see for example, Thomas and Barsalou, this volume).

This has been described as a model for visual pattern discrimination, but it must be emphasized that it is also a model for pattern detection. This becomes apparent once one recalls that the model mechanisms were characterized by masking experiments, as masking is nothing more than detection of a target (e.g. Fig. 1B) superimposed on a background pattern (e.g. Fig. 1A). From the perspective of computation, target detection is nothing more than discrimination of a background from target plus background. Thus, background and target plus background are the two patterns that would be used to compute ΔR in Eqs. (3) and (4) if one wished to predict target detection.

4. Peripheral Vision

Discussion thus far has focused on foveal vision, where detection and discrimination of stationary or slowly moving patterns are most acute. To model pattern detection and discrimination in the periphery one must incorporate the physiological limitations of peripheral vision. First, however, it must be emphasized that the visual system cannot be sharply divided into a central fovea and a surrounding periphery. Rather, almost all psychophysically measured visual functions vary smoothly and continuously from central vision into the far periphery. Let us consider grating acuity as the most salient example. The maximum spatial frequency, ω_{Max}, that can be detected varies with retinal eccentricity E according to the formula:

$$\omega_{\text{Max}} = \frac{\omega_F}{1 + E/E_2} .$$

(6)

In this equation ω_F is the foveal grating acuity, typically 30–50 cpd in young adults, and E_2 is the eccentricity at which ω_{Max} has decreased to half its foveal value. Psychophysical measurements indicate that E_2 is about 4.0° along the horizontal meridian and about 2.0° along the vertical meridian[39]. This means that iso-acuity contours are not circular but rather elliptical with the long axis aligned with the horizon. Thus, humans have a slight visual streak as do cats, rabbits, and various other species.

Given the continuous variation of grating acuity and other visual properties, pattern discrimination models must be scaled for the eccentricity of interest. This is done by multiplying the space constants, σ_1, σ_2, σ_3 and σ_y, in Eq. (1) by the factor $(1 + E/E_2)$, which is just the ratio of foveal to peripheral grating acuities at eccentricity E (see Eq. (6)). At the same time, the gain, A, in Eq. (1) must be divided by $(1 + E/E_2)^2$. Mathematically, these two scaling operations are equivalent to shifting mechanism sensitivity curves towards lower spatial frequencies while maintaining the same maximum sensitivity to the (lower) peak frequency in the periphery. Anatomically, the two operations reflect increased cone spacing and the accompanying decreased cone density per unit area[21,39].

If the foveal model is scaled as just outlined to reflect decreasing cone density with increasing eccentricity[6], the resulting model will accurately predict grating acuity and sensitivity to cosine gratings as a function of eccentricity[21]. However, this is not the entire story of peripheral spatial vision. It has now been well established that other measures of acuity, such as vernier acuity, degrade much more rapidly with eccentricity than does grating acuity[16,25]. This implies that additional factors must vary from fovea to periphery. I have recently shown that peripheral pattern discrimination data can be accurately predicted given two additional assumptions[30,31]. First, peripheral visual filters are not uniformly spaced as in the fovea, but rather are irregularly spaced, thus introducing statistical uncertainty into their positioning. Second, there are too few spatial filters in peripheral vision to capture all of the information in the optical image. That is, the periphery is spatially under sampled relative to the Nyquist sampling rate. In support of these hypotheses, it has been demonstrated that cone spacing becomes much more irregular in the periphery[11,13]. In addition, there is compelling psychophysical evidence that the peripheral retina is indeed spatially under sampled[5,22] (see also, Thibos and Bradley, this volume).

Calculation of the effects of spatial irregularity and under sampling on pattern discrimination is too complex and tedious to be readily summarized here, and the interested reader is referred to Wilson[31] for details. However, it is easy to appreciate that aliasing due to spatial under sampling will produce distortions in peripheral vision, and these in turn will degrade pattern discrimination. Similarly, discrimination tasks that depend on precise spatial localization, such as vernier acuity (see Fig. 3), will be disrupted by the positional uncertainty in the location of the visual filters themselves.

5. Nonlinear Analysis of Visual Textures

The model described above employs oriented filters that have an excitatory central zone flanked on either side by parallel inhibitory zones (see Fig. 2 and Eq. (1)). These filters thus have the properties described by Hubel and Wiesel[14] for simple cell receptive fields in primary visual cortex. Although these psychophysically measured filters accurately predict many aspects of visual pattern discrimination, they do not function well for discriminations involving textured patterns. As a simple example, consider the texture on the left in Fig. 4. Subjects readily perceive a V-shaped contour across the middle of the pattern where the parallel black bars at the top terminate and those at the bottom begin. Yet this "illusory contour" does not exist in the image, as the white background of the pattern is continuous from top to bottom of the pattern. The illusory contour is but one example of a texture boundary.

Vertically oriented on-center filters at locations such as A in Fig. 4 will respond very strongly, as the excitatory zone (white ellipse) is filled with light, while the inhibitory flanks (gray ellipses) fall on the black bars, thus generating little inhibition. Similarly, off-center receptive fields will respond well when centered on a black bar. However, consider the receptive field at location B. As it is centered on the texture boundary, black bars protrude half way through both the excitatory and inhibitory zones regardless of whether it is on- or off-centered. In consequence, the stimulus will generate equal levels of excitation and inhibition here, so these receptive fields will simply not respond to the pattern. Similarly, one can show that horizontally oriented filters will fail to respond to either the

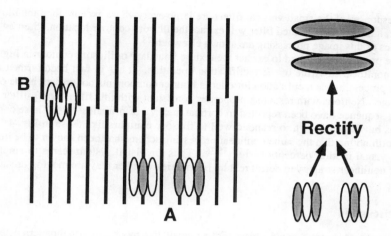

Figure 4. Illusory contours and texture boundaries. A shallow V-shaped texture boundary, defined by the locus of the black line terminations, is clearly visible across the center of the pattern on the left. This boundary is illusory, as the white regions of the pattern are continuous from top to bottom. the simple cell receptive fields (white excitatory zones and gray inhibitory zones) located as shown at A will respond vigorously to the top and bottom of the pattern. However, receptive fields located along the boundary such as at B will receive a balance of excitation and inhibition and therefore will fail to respond. As discussed in the text and illustrated on the right, the sequence of oriented filtering, rectification (pooling of on- and off-center responses), and subsequent oriented filtering with larger receptive fields at a different orientation accurately extracts the texture boundary in such figures.

texture border as well as to the parallel vertical bars. Thus, we are faced with a puzzle: the texture boundary is dramatically visible, yet simple visual receptive fields do not respond to it at all!

How, then, does the visual system extract texture boundary information from images? A number of studies have converged on a common explanation that is both simple and powerful[1,8,15,17,41]. Consider the scheme depicted on the right in Fig. 4. First, the image is processed by the small vertically oriented filters at the bottom. As indicated above, these will respond very well to the vertical bars in the top and bottom halves of the texture on the left, but they will fail to respond along the texture boundary. Half of the units are presumed to have inhibitory centers (gray central region at bottom), so they will respond best at a different relative position on the texture as shown in A. Next, the neural activity generated by these on- and off-center neurons is pooled or summed at each point. Due to the existence of neural thresholds (see Eq. (3)), only positive responses from each type of unit will be non-zero, and it can be shown that the result is a full-wave rectification of the oriented neural responses to the grating. Finally, this rectified result is processed by a larger oriented filter at a different orientation (horizontal in this case). Due to the fact that the rectified responses of the small vertical filters are large everywhere except along the illusory contour, a final larger oriented filter will extract the illusory contour location. Step by step examples of this image processing are shown elsewhere[28].

The processing required to extract the texture boundary or illusory contour in Fig. 4 is highly nonlinear in virtue of the rectification operation. It has in fact been termed non-Fourier processing, as rectification introduces Fourier components not present in the original image. Neurons with response properties consistent with this filter-rectify-filter processing sequence have been reported in cortical area V2 of primates[23,24]. These cortical neurons have been shown to respond well to illusory contours like those in Fig. 4. It is also worth noting that the same nonlinear processing scheme has been shown to be important in visual motion perception[3,4,27,35,38]. Thus the visual system seems to employ a similar nonlinear strategy to detect texture boundaries whether they are moving or stationary.

6. Discussion

This chapter has presented a résumé of a quantitative model for visual pattern detection and discrimination. The model is based on psychophysical masking data[20,40], and it has been successfully applied to a wide range of pattern discrimination tasks including vernier acuity, orientation discrimination, and curvature discrimination[32,33,36,42]. The model has also been used successfully to predict peripheral pattern discrimination by incorporating three modifications: (1) filters must be shifted towards lower spatial frequencies by the ratio of foveal to peripheral acuity (Eq. (6)); (2) spatial irregularity in the positioning of individual filters must be incorporated; and (3) the peripheral image must be spatially under sampled[21,30,31]. Finally, converging evidence from several laboratories indicates that a nonlinear scheme involving filtering, rectification, and subsequent filtering is required to extract texture boundaries and illusory contours[1,8,15,17,41].

The masking studies from which the model receptive fields were derived are experiments measuring the degree to which a background interferes with the visibility of a target. As such, they may be thought of as systematic studies of visual camouflage. Inherent in the model approach presented here is the assumption that the retinal image is processed in parallel by units tuned for various orientations and spatial frequency ranges. Recent research indicates that these units do not operate independently as had been assumed. Rather, the units interact via gain controls that employ divisive inhibition to normalize neural responses and prevent response saturation[9,10,18,19,28,37]. As these gain control interactions have yet to be incorporated into the pattern discrimination models discussed above, it is important to ask how significant this omission might be. Our unpublished data indicate that divisive gain controls have their major effects during the transient period of about 150 msec after a stimulus is presented. During this transient phase a full implementation of gain control dynamics would be necessary for accurate prediction of pattern discrimination. After the gain controls come to equilibrium, however, the assumption of independent, parallel processing by different units provides an accurate approximation for computation of most discrimination thresholds.

One final issue related to the practical employment of this model is that of real time computation. The model as developed was designed to provide as accurate a description of human vision as possible given the available data, and considerations of computational speed were therefore irrelevant. For many purposes, however, it is possible to dramatically speed up model computations without significantly reducing the accuracy of the predictions. To mention but one example, various pyramid schemes (e.g. Burt and Adelson[2]) have been developed that permit computation of the convolution integrals for all six different sized mechanisms with maximum efficiency. The main requirement is that each filter must be a factor of four (in area) scaled version of the next smaller filter. This is a reasonable approximation to the actual filters measured psychophysically.

In closing, it should be emphasized that these models represent a contemporary stage in the evolution of our understanding of human spatial vision. Future studies will doubtless build on this foundation and will therefore permit even more accurate prediction of human visual function not only for pattern discrimination but also for stereoscopic vision and motion perception.

Acknowledgment

This research was supported in part by NIH grant #EY02158 to the author.

References

1. J. R. Bergen and M. S. Landy, "Computational modeling of visual texture segregation," in *Computational Models of Visual Processing*, ed. M. Landy and J. A. Movshon (MIT Press, Cambridge, MA, 1991), pp. 253-271.
2. P. J. Burt and E. H. Adelson, "The Laplacian pyramid as a compact image code," *IEEE Transactions on Communications* **COM-31** (1983) 532-540.
3. C. Chubb and G. Sperling, "Drift-balanced random stimuli: A general basis for studying non-Fourier motion perception," *J. Opt. Soc. Am. [A]* **5** (1988) 1986-2007.
4. C. Chubb and G. Sperling, "Two motion perception mechanisms revealed through distance-driven reversal of apparent motion," *Proc. Natl. Acad. Sci.* **86** (1989) 2985-2989.
5. N. J. Coletta and D. R. Williams, "Psychophysical estimate of extrafoveal cone spacing," *J. Opt. Soc. Am. [A]* (1987) 1503-1513.
6. C. A. Curcio, K. R. Sloan, O. Packer, A. E. Hendrickson, and R. E. Kalina, "Distribution of cones in human and monkey retina: Individual variability and radial asymmetry," *Science* **236** (1987) 579-582.
7. R. L. DeValois, D. G. Albrecht, and L. G. Thorell, "Spatial frequency selectivity of cells in macaque visual cortex," *Vision Res.* **22** (1982) 545-559.
8. N. Graham, J. Beck, and A. Sutter, "Nonlinear processes in spatial frequency channel models of perceived texture segregation: effects of sign and amount of contrast," *Vision Res.* **32** (1992) 719-743.

14

9. D. J. Heeger, "Normalization of cell responses in cat striate cortex," *Vis. Neurosci.* **9** (1992) 181-197.

10. D. J. Heeger, "Nonlinear model of neural responses in cat visual cortex," in *Computational Models of Visual Processing*, eds. M. Landy and J. A. Movshon (MIT Press, Cambridge, MA, 1991), pp. 119-133.

11. J. Hirsch, J. and C. A. Curcio, "The spatial resolution capacity of human foveal retina," *Vision Res.* **29** (1989) 1095-1101.

12. J. Hirsch and R. Hilton, "Limits of spatial frequency discrimination as evidence of neural interpolation," *J. Opt. Soc. Am.* **72** (1982) 1367-1374.

13. J. Hirsch, J. and W. H. Miller, "Does cone positional disorder limit resolution?," *J. Opt. Soc. Am. [A]* **4** (1987) 1481-1492.

14. D. H. Hubel and T. N. Wiesel, "Receptive fields and functional architecture of monkey striate cortex," *J. Physiol.* **195** (1968) 215-243.

15. M. S. Landy and J. R. Bergen, "Texture segregation and orientation gradient," *Vision Res.* **31** (1991) 679-691.

16. D. M. Levi, S. A. Klein, and A. P. Aitsebaomo, "Vernier acuity, crowding and cortical magnification," *Vision Res.* **25** (1985) 963-977.

17. J. Malik and P. Perona, "Preattentive texture discrimination with early vision mechanisms," *J. Opt. Soc. Am. [A]* **7** (1990) 923-932.

18. L. A. Olzak and J. P. Thomas, "Configural effects constrain Fourier models of pattern discrimination," *Vision Res.* **32** (1992) 1885-1898.

19. L. A. Olzak and J. P. Thomas, "When orthogonal orientations are not processed independently," *Vision Res.* **31** (1991) 51-57.

20. G. C. Phillips and H. R. Wilson, "Orientation bandwidths of spatial mechanisms measured by masking," *J. Opt. Soc. Am. [A]* **1** (1984) 226-232.

21. W. H. Swanson and H. R. Wilson, "Eccentricity dependence of contrast matching and oblique masking," *Vision Res.* **25** (1985) 1285-1295.

22. L. N. Thibos, F. E. Cheney, and D. J. Walsh, "Retinal limits to the detection and resolution of gratings," *J. Opt. Soc. Am. [A]* **4** (1987) 1524-1529.

23. R. von der Heydt and E. Peterhans, "Mechanisms of contour perception in monkey visual cortex. I. Lines of pattern discontinuity," *J. Neurosci.* **9** (1989) 1731-1748.

24. R. von der Heydt, E. Peterhans, and G. Baumgartner, "Illusory contours and cortical neuron responses," *Science* **224** (1984) 1260-1262.

25. G. Westheimer, "The spatial grain of the perifoveal visual field," *Vision Res.* **22** (1982) 157-162.

26. G. Westheimer and S. P. McKee, "Spatial configurations for visual hyperacuity," *Vision Res.* **17** (1977) 941-947.

27. H. R. Wilson, "The role of second-order motion signals in coherence and transparency," in *Higher Order Processing in the Visual System*, ed. J. Goode (CIBA Foundation, John Wiley, New York, 1994) pp. 227-244.

28. H. R. Wilson, "Nonlinear processes in visual pattern discrimination," *Proc. Nat. Acad. Sci.* **90** (1993) 9785-9790.

29. H. R. Wilson, "Psychophysical models of spatial vision and hyperacuity," in, *Spatial Form Vision*, ed. D. Regan (MacMillan, London, 1991a), pp. 64-86.

30. H. R. Wilson, "Pattern discrimination, visual filters, and spatial sampling irregularity," in *Computational Models of Visual Processing*, ed. M. Landy and J. A. Movshon (MIT Press, Cambridge, MA, 1991b), pp. 153-168.

31. H. R. Wilson, "Model of peripheral and amblyopic hyperacuity," *Vision Res.* **31** (1991c) 967-982.

32. H. R. Wilson, "Responses of spatial mechanisms can explain hyperacuity," *Vision Res.* **26** (1986) 453-469.

33. H. R. Wilson, "Discrimination of contour curvature: Data and theory," *J. Opt. Soc. Am. [A]* **2** (1985) 1191-1199.

34. H. R. Wilson and J. R. Bergen, "A four mechanism model for threshold spatial vision," *Vision Res.* **19** (1979) 19-32.

35. H. R. Wilson, V. P. Ferrera, and C. Yo, "Psychophysically motivated model for two-dimensional motion perception," *Vis. Neurosci.* **9** (1992) 79-97.

36. H. R. Wilson and D. J. Gelb, "Modified line element theory for spatial frequency and width discrimination," *J. Opt. Soc. Am. [A]* **1** (1984) 124-131.

37. H. R. Wilson and R. Humanski, "Spatial frequency adaptation and contrast gain control," *Vision Res.* **33** (1993) 1133-1149.

38. H. R. Wilson and J. Kim, "A model for motion coherence and transparency," *Vis. Neurosci.* **11** (1994) 1205-1220.

39. H. R. Wilson, D. Levi, L. Maffei, J. Rovamo, and R. L. DeValois, "The perception of form: Retina to striate cortex," in *The Neurophysiological Foundations of Visual Perception*, ed. L. Spillmann and J. S. Werner (Academic Press, New York, 1990), pp. 231-272.

40. H. R. Wilson, D. K. McFarlane, and G. C. Phillips, "Spatial frequency tuning of orientation selective units estimated by oblique masking," *Vision Res.* **23** (1983) 873-882.

41. H. R. Wilson and W. A. Richards, "Curvature and separation discrimination at texture boundaries," *J. Opt. Soc. Am. [A]* **9** (1992) 1653-1662.

42. H. R. Wilson and W. A. Richards, "Mechanisms of contour curvature discrimination," *J. Opt. Soc. Am. [A]* **6** (1989) 106-115.

VISUAL PROCESSING IN THE JOINT
SPATIAL/SPATIAL-FREQUENCY DOMAIN

MIGUEL A. GARCÍA-PÉREZ

Dep. de Metodología, Facultad de Psicología, Universidad Complutense,
28223 Madrid, Spain

and

VICENTE SIERRA-VÁZQUEZ

Dep. de Psicología Básica, Facultad de Psicología, Universidad Complutense,
28223 Madrid, Spain

Vision can be understood as the application of decision processes to the visual representation of a stimulus. This contention implies at least two processing stages: the creation of the visual representation (*early visual processing*) and the subsequent use of that representation in order to achieve visual tasks (*late visual processing*). By assuming that the visual system comprises a number of linear visual channels, we show that early visual processing results in the creation of a joint spatial/spatial-frequency representation whose characteristics are determined by the shape of the channel transfer functions. We specifically consider two plausible choices for these transfer functions which respectively give rise to a *windowed Fourier representation* and a *wavelet representation*. Subsequent processing of each type of representation for the achievement of the late visual processing tasks of detection and identification shows that empirical data on performance in these tasks are consistent with the wavelet representation.

1. Introduction

Visual processing involves, at least, two major stages: the coding of the input image for the creation of a visual representation, and the subsequent use of that representation in order to achieve visual tasks. Building models of these stages, loosely referred to as early and late visual processing, is a challenging way to understand vision. An early visual processing model must specify the characteristics of the mechanisms obtaining the representation, and must also express the visual representation as a transformation of the input image as processed by those mechanisms. A late visual processing model for the achievement of a certain visual task must specify rules or further mechanisms operating on the visual representation to achieve the task.

During the past three decades of experimental vision research, the search for psychophysical data describing the functional characteristics of the front-end mechanisms responsible for early visual processing has been overwhelming. Ever since the seminal work of Campbell and Robson,[1] the notion has evolved that the initial psychophysical coding of the retinal image is accomplished by a set of linear bandpass filters (loosely referred to as visual channels) with spatially localized receptive fields which are also selectively sensitive to narrow ranges of spatial frequencies and orientations. The past three decades have also been prolific in gathering parametric data on visual perform-ance in simple visual tasks such as detection, discrimination and identification under a variety of experimental conditions.

Despite this wealth of data, the present state of visual modeling is rather unsatis-factory. We feel that this is the result of a fragmentary approach to modeling. Early visual processing is a subject rarely deemed worthy of precise modeling, let alone close scrutiny. In fact, most modeling efforts have focused on late visual processing for the achievement of specific tasks, each considering only a rather narrow class of data.[2] Further, each model assumes a somewhat peculiar architecture for early visual processing that is often described in passing without any further considerations. As a consequence, this literature is rather diverse, somewhat dispersed and lacks cohesive-ness, with many authors failing to acknowledge the work of others.

Our main goal in this paper is to describe a unified and congruent approach to modeling early and late visual processing. This amounts to specifying the characteris-tics of early visual processing and the visual representations that it produces, and de-fining further processing stages that operate on visual representations to achieve visual tasks. We provide a unified and general description of early visual processing by con-sideration of a family of joint spatial/spatial-frequency representations. A joint spa-tial/spatial-frequency representation is a transformation of the input image which is ex-pressible as a function of the spatial and the spatial frequency variables simultaneous-ly. Justification for them as the result of early visual processing arises naturally from the fact that the various visual channels consist of localized sensors distributed across the visual field, with the receptive fields from the various channels stacked at every visual field location. The acknowledgement that psychophysical coding involves the creation of a joint representation has been commonplace in auditory research,[3-5] but only recently has this idea succeeded in settling with the vision research community. Some early suggestions of joint representations in spatial vision, although not fully developing the idea, can be found in the work of Stromeyer and Klein,[6] Robson,[7] Cowan,[8] and Marčelja.[9] More recently, complete approaches can be found in Daug-man,[10] Watson,[11] and Porat and Zeevi.[12] Also, and although often not stated explicitly, the idea of visual processing in the joint spatial/spatial-frequency domain underlies many of the spatial vision models proposed in the past few years. These models can be classified into two main categories: those implying *discrete representations*, in which either the spatial variable or the spatial frequency variable or both are regarded as dis-crete and, thus, assume a finite number of channels whose sensors are centered at each of a finite number of spatial locations,[13,14] and those implying *continuous representa-tions*, in which both variables are regarded as continuous and, thus, assume an unlim-ited number of channels whose sensors exist at every spatial location.[15] Formally, any discrete representation can be regarded as the result of sampling a thoroughly equivalent continuous representation at specific frequencies and locations. Yet, discrete representations lack some of the properties of their continuous counterparts, and they may have different implications for the achievement of visual tasks.

The family of joint representations that we will consider is that arising from channels with sensors whose line-weighting functions are described by Gabor functions in complex analytic form.[16] Bearing in mind the distinction between early and late visual processing, we also analyze how visual tasks might be achieved by further processing the visual representations. We show how specific choices for the several parameters of the Gabor function affect the processing characteristics of the system, thus resulting in representations which are or are not compatible with psychophysical data on visual performance.

For clarity of presentation, only the one-dimensional (1D) case is considered here. Thus, all of our analyses involve non-moving 1D patterns, whose luminance varies across one of the spatial dimensions and is constant across the other, orthogonal dimension, and is also constant over time. Also for simplicity, we will only consider the case of space-invariant representations, and we will defer to the final section the discussion of joint representations in the space-variant case.

2. Space-Invariant Joint Spatial/Spatial-Frequency Representations

Joint spatial/spatial-frequency representations, distributions and transforms are well-known tools in signal analysis. Their description as well as an analysis of their characteristics and properties is the subject of a number of papers and books.[17-24] This literature describes joint representations rather technically from the perspective of signal analysis, which obviously has different goals from the modeling of human visual processing. Therefore, an introduction to joint representations from the perspective of visual modeling seems necessary.

A representation for a signal aims at describing its characteristics, and different types of representations make explicit different characteristics of the signal. Thus, a 1D real-valued spatial signal (e.g., a luminance profile) can be described by its spatial representation as a 1D real-valued function which expresses the luminance at each spatial location. Alternatively, the signal can be represented in the spatial-frequency domain through its Fourier transform. The Fourier transform of a signal is a pure spatial-frequency representation which makes explicit its frequency content, and permits a description of the frequency distribution of energy in the signal. Thus, the Fourier transform is useful for describing stationary signals[a] in the alternate spatial-frequency domain. A good number of signals, however, are non-stationary, implying that their frequency content and/or some of their local features (such as discontinuities and sin-

---

[a] In this context, stationarity does not refer to the absence of temporal modulation, but to the property that the local behavior of a signal does not change across its spatial extent. See Flandrin[25] for a formal definition of stationarity in stochastic and deterministic signals.

gularities) are different at different spatial locations (e.g., a spatial signal such as the luminance of a scene with objects of different sizes or textures). For these signals, pure spatial-frequency representations like the Fourier transform fail to provide information about either the frequency distribution of energy at different locations or the spatial distribution of energy at different frequencies. This incapability motivated the development of signal representation methods in which a signal is described as a joint function of space and spatial frequency. Application of these methods provides what is generally referred to as a *joint spatial/spatial-frequency representation*[19] or a *space/scale representation*,[26] each of which is a two-dimensional (2D) function defined in the joint domain where space and frequency (or scale) are orthogonal dimensions.

In general, a joint spatial/spatial-frequency representation describes a signal simultaneously in space and spatial frequency. A subclass of joint representations, called distributions, specifically describe the energy density in the joint domain.[20] Perhaps the most popular joint distribution is the Wigner distribution function,[27] from which a local spatial-frequency spectrum, which indicates the frequency content of the signal in localized regions of the spatial domain, can be obtained.[28] However, there is an infinite number of joint distributions each of which is a particular case of the general class introduced by Cohen.[29] On the other hand, since the seminal work of Gabor,[30] a number of methods to obtain joint representations have been developed. A joint representation is obtained as a transformation of the signal through a 2D kernel, and is subject to the uncertainty principle in signal analysis.[30] Because of this transformation, joint representations are also referred to as joint transforms. For purposes of signal analysis, the choice of a kernel for the transformation is guided by its properties and the signal characteristics that the representation is meant to make explicit. To serve as realistic models of early visual processing, however, these transformations must imply an operation that can be implemented by biological or psychophysical mechanisms. Two of the existing joint representations fulfill this requirement and, thus, are relevant to the modeling of early visual processing. These are the windowed Fourier transform and the wavelet transform. Both of them are briefly described and compared next.

2.1. *Windowed Fourier Transform (WFT)*

The continuous windowed Fourier transform (also referred to as short-time Fourier transform or finite-support Fourier transform) of a 1D signal f, WFT_f, is a 2D complex-valued function given by

$$WFT_f(x',u') = \int_{-\infty}^{\infty} f(x)w^*(x-x')e^{-i2\pi u'x}dx, \qquad x',u' \in \mathbb{R}, \qquad (1)$$

where w is a fixed window, the asterisk denotes complex conjugation, and x' and u' are, respectively, the spatial and spatial-frequency dimensions of the joint domain. Thus, the WFT belongs in the category of spatial/spatial-frequency representations.

The window w can be either a complex- or a real-valued function, and is usually chosen to be compactly supported and centered around $x=0$. Yet, real-valued windows which are not strictly compactly supported (like gaussian windows) are often used. Owing to the replaceability of the window, the WFT representation of a signal is not unique, and its characteristics depend on the choice for this window.

As a complex-valued function, the WFT can be expressed by its real and imaginary parts or, alternatively, by its modulus and argument. The squared modulus of the WFT defines a joint distribution known as *spectrogram* in acoustics and speech analysis,[31] which is a smoothed Wigner distribution function[19] and, as such, the spectrogram can be interpreted as a local spatial-frequency spectrum.

2.2. Wavelet Transform (WT)

The continuous wavelet transform of a 1D signal f with respect to the analyzing (or mother) wavelet g, WT_f, is a 2D complex-valued function given by[32,33]

$$WT_f(b,a) = \frac{1}{\sqrt{|a|}} \int_{-\infty}^{\infty} f(x) g^* \left(\frac{x-b}{a} \right) dx, \qquad a,b \in \mathbb{R}, \quad a \neq 0, \qquad (2)$$

where a and b are, respectively, the scale and spatial dimensions of the joint domain. Thus, the WT belongs in the category of space/scale representations. Yet, for any given analyzing wavelet, a relationship exists between scale and spatial frequency, and the WT can also be expressed as a spatial/spatial-frequency representation. For this reason, we will refer to the the dimensions of the joint domain for the WT as space and spatial frequency whenever the latter is more appropriate than scale to our discussion.

The mother wavelet g can be either a complex- or a real-valued function, and is usually chosen to be regular and centered around $x=0$. The WT can be inverted if g also fulfills the admissibility condition,[34] which implies that its spatial integral be zero. However, this constraint is often relaxed, and analyzing wavelets are regarded as admissible if their spatial integral is negligible. In any case, the possibility of inverting the WT is not a criterion to limit the choice of a mother wavelet for purposes of modeling early visual processing. Owing to the freedom of choice of the analyzing wavelet, the WT representation of a signal is not unique, and its characteristics obviously depend on the mathematical form of the analyzing wavelet.

As a complex-valued function, the WT can also be expressed by its real and imaginary parts or, alternatively, by its modulus and argument. The squared modulus of the WT defines an energy density function known as *scalogram*.[35] The interpretation of the WT as a local spatial-frequency spectrum, however, is not straightforward.

2.3. Comparison of the Windowed Fourier Transform and the Wavelet Transform

Besides the obvious differences between the WFT and the WT in their definitions, some similarities and further differences exist between them. A thorough comparison of the two transforms can be found in Daubechies,[36] but some issues that are relevant to this paper are described next.

In principle, both are cases of square integrable representations, and both provide an exact decomposition of the signal in terms of the window function or the analyzing wavelet, as applicable. Also, both representations are computed as the inner products of the signal with a continuous family of coherent states, i.e., a continuous family of square integrable functions generated from a single square integrable function by translations in the joint domain. In the case of the WFT, the family of (canonical) coherent states, $w^{(x',u')}$, is generated from the window function w by

$$w^{(x',u')}(x) = w(x-x')e^{i2\pi u'x}, \tag{3}$$

whereas in the case of the WT, the family of (affine) coherent states, $g^{(b,a)}$, is generated from the mother wavelet g by

$$g^{(b,a)}(x) = \frac{1}{\sqrt{|a|}} g\left(\frac{x-b}{a}\right). \tag{4}$$

Thus, both representations can be interpreted as the result of filtering the signal with a continuous bank of bandpass filters whose overall shape depends on the mathematical form of the function generating the family of coherent states, and whose tuning characteristics are determined by the scale or frequency dimension of the joint domain.[b] It is this interpretation that highlights the differences between the WFT and the WT.

Note that the window w in the WFT is a fixed function of constant spatial spread, and that the spatial spread of the coherent states is independent of u'. Then, as x' and u' change, the coherent states $w^{(x',u')}$ differ in their spatial location and in the spatial frequency of the complex harmonic oscillation, but their spatial spread and their peak amplitude remains constant. Thus, the WFT involves an analysis of the signal with elementary functions of constant absolute bandwidth, and a 1D cut of the WFT at any given u' represents a bandpass filtered version of the signal, where the actual bandwidth of the filters depends on the precise mathematical form of the window w.

On the other hand, and although the analyzing wavelet, g, is a fixed function of constant spatial spread too, the spatial spread of the coherent states depends on the scale dimension a. Then, as a and b change, the coherent states $g^{(b,a)}$ differ in their spatial location, peak amplitude and spatial spread. As a consequence, the coherent states in the case of the WT are a family of elementary functions of the same shape whose members are displaced in spatial location, dilated or compressed in size, and amplified or attenuated in peak amplitude. Thus, the WT involves an analysis with elementary functions of constant shape ratio[32,33] and, therefore, constant relative bandwidth, and a 1D cut of the WT at any given a represents a bandpass filtered version of the signal, where the bandwidth of the filters depends on the precise mathematical

---

[b] It is important to note, however, that the integrals in Eqs. (1) and (2) define inner products with the coherent states and, therefore, in terms of linear systems analysis, the filtering is explicitly expressed as cross-correlations with line-weighting functions rather than convolutions with line-spread functions.

form of the mother wavelet g. As described by Holschneider,[37] wavelet analysis is the equivalent of a mathematical microscope whose global magnification is $1/a$, whose position is b, and whose optics is determined by the shape of the mother wavelet.

If the energy of a 1D real-valued signal is essentially localized in the spatial interval $[X_1,X_2]$ and the spatial-frequency interval $[-U_2,-U_1]\cup[U_1,U_2]$, both its WFT and its WT representations have two mirror-symmetric parts which are localized around the centers of the two regions $[X_1,X_2]\times[U_1,U_2]$ and $[X_1,X_2]\times[-U_2,-U_1]$ in the joint domain. However, each representation embodies a different stance at balancing the conflicting goals of describing a signal in both the spatial and the spatial-frequency domains. In principle, in both the WFT and the WT, the individual spreads of the representation in the spatial and spatial-frequency dimensions of the joint domain are inversely related, and depend on the bandwidth of the filters (the narrower the bandwidth, the larger the spread of the representation in the x' dimension and the smaller its spread in the u' dimension). However, in the WFT, these spreads are only determined by the bandwidth of the filters, and are independent of the frequency content of the signal. In contradistinction, the spreads of the WT representation in the x' and u' dimensions are not independent of the (bounded) frequency content of the signal: the spread in the x' dimension decreases and that in the u' dimension increases as the interval of frequency components comprising the signal moves towards higher spatial frequencies.

Therefore, in the WFT, a representation that is biased towards resolving either the spatial location or the frequency content of the signal can be customized through the choice of an appropriate spatial spread for the window w, as an accurate description of both the spatial location and the frequency content of a signal is not possible simultaneously. In the WT, on the other hand, a representation of a given sharpness in space or frequency cannot be customized through the choice of an appropriate spatial spread for the mother wavelet *unless* the frequency content of the signal is known beforehand.

Despite these differences, the WT and WFT representations can look very much alike. This point is well illustrated in the WFT and the WT representations of

$$f(x) = \Lambda(x-x_1)\cos(2\pi u_1 x) + \Lambda(x-x_2)\cos(2\pi u_2 x), \tag{5}$$

where $x_1=-3$, $x_2=3$, $u_1=1$, $u_2=4$, and

$$\Lambda(x) = \begin{cases} 0 & \Leftrightarrow & x<-2 \\ 1 & \Leftrightarrow & -2\leq x<0 \\ \exp\left[-x^2/1.44\right] & \Leftrightarrow & 0\leq x \end{cases} \tag{6}$$

As shown in Fig. 1, this signal consists of two separate and localized quasi-sinebursts of different spatial frequency, each with an abrupt discontinuity on the left and a gaussian decay on the right. Also shown in Fig. 1 are the moduli of WFT representations obtained using the window in Eq. (23) below with $s_x=0.265$ and $s_x=1.06$, and the

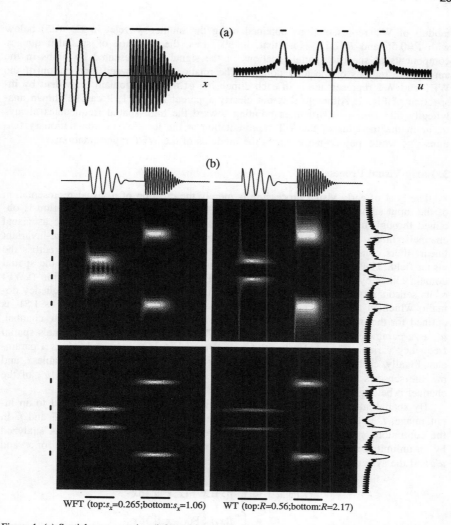

WFT (top:s_x=0.265;bottom:s_x=1.06)   WT (top:R=0.56;bottom:R=2.17)

Figure 1. (a) Spatial representation (left) and log-amplitude spectrum (right) of the signal in Eq. (5). The horizontal segments at the top of each graph represent the spreads at half height of each separate quasi-sineburst in each domain. (b) Moduli of the WFT (left column; top: s_x=0.265; bottom: s_x=1.06) and WT (right column; top: R=0.56; bottom: R=2.17) representations of the signal. In each image, the spatial dimension, x', of the joint domain runs horizontally from x'=-8 on the left to x'=8 on the right, and the spatial-frequency dimension, u', runs vertically from u'=-8 at the bottom to u'=8 at the top. For reference, the spatial profile of the signal is replotted at the top of each column of images, and its log-amplitude spectrum is replotted on the right of each row. The spatial and spatial-frequency spreads are replotted to scale from (a) at the bottom of each column and on the left of each row, respectively.

moduli of WT representations obtained using the mother wavelet in Eq. (25) below with $R=0.56$ and $R=2.17$. Note that, in all cases, the presence of spatial-frequency components at specific spatial locations in the signal is represented by blobs in the appropriate regions of the joint domain. The relationships between localization of the WFT and WT representations in each dimension of the joint domain is evident by inspection of Fig. 1. Although it is not clearly apparent in Fig. 1, it can be shown analytically that cone-like structures pointing toward the high spatial frequencies always occur in the modulus of the WT representation at the location of non-stationary features,[38,39] while they do not occur in the modulus of the WFT representation.

3. Early Visual Processing

The goal of early visual processing is merely the creation of a visual representation of the input signal. Empirical evidence seems to suggest that this representation is obtained through functionally independent mechanisms customarily referred to as visual channels. In this paper, visual channels will be assumed to behave as space-invariant linear filters consisting of a bank of identical sensors uniformly distributed across the visual field. Thus, the behavior of a channel is completely characterized in the spatial domain either by its line-spread function (LSF) or the line-weighting function (LWF) of its sensors or, alternatively, by its transfer function (TF) in the spatial-frequency domain, which is the Fourier transform of the channel's LSF. Each channel's LSF is defined for the output plane's variable x', and has the tuning frequency of the channel, u', as a parameter. Similarly, each channel's TF is defined for the input plane's spatial frequency variable u, and also has the tuning frequency of the channel, u', as a parameter. Finally, each sensor's LWF is defined for the input plane's spatial variable x, and has the sensor's location on the output plane, x', and the tuning frequency, u', of the channel it belongs to as its parameters.

By spatial summation, the response of a given sensor in a given channel to an input image, f, is the integral over space of the product of the sensor's LWF and f. In the continuous space-invariant case, where every point in the visual field is analyzed by an unlimited number of visual channels, a response exists at every value for x' and u', and the system's response to f can be expressed as

$$
\begin{aligned}
G_f(x',u') &= \int_{-\infty}^{\infty} f(x)\,\mathrm{LWF}(x;x',u')\,\mathrm{d}x \\
&= \int_{-\infty}^{\infty} f(x)\,\mathrm{LSF}(x'-x;u')\,\mathrm{d}x \\
&= \int_{-\infty}^{\infty} F(u)\,\mathrm{TF}(u;u')\,\mathrm{e}^{i2\pi ux'}\,\mathrm{d}u ,
\end{aligned}
\tag{7}
$$

where G_f is the 2D function of spatial location and spatial frequency which embodies the visual representation of f, and F is the Fourier transform of f. Note that the first integral in Eq. (7) implies the cross-correlation of f with the sensors' LWFs, while the second integral implies the convolution of f with the channels' LSFs.

The characteristics, properties and perceptual implications of this representation depend on the form of the LWFs, LSFs or TFs, interchangeably. Neither the sensors' LWFs nor the channels' LSFs or TFs can be observed directly. Their mathematical form has occasionally been estimated by indirect methods that have never been certified (by way of a formal proof) to actually recover them.[2] More often, a reasonable choice for these functions has been adopted in spatial vision models. We will follow this latter approach. In doing so, it has some mechanistic appeal to define the sensor LWFs at the outset, thus characterizing their receptive field profiles.

Various functions have been used to describe receptive fields, including some linear combination of a varying number of gaussians,[13,40] some derivative of a gaussian,[41] Cauchy functions,[42] or Gabor functions.[14] We will restrict ourselves to considering the latter case, and describe the LWF of the sensor at spatial location x' (in deg) within the channel tuned to spatial frequency u' (in c/deg) by the complex conjugate of a generalized Gabor elementary signal, ψ^*,

$$\psi^*(x;x',u',s_x,p,\phi) = \frac{1}{\sqrt{2\pi}\,s_x}\exp\left[-\frac{(x-p-x')^2}{2s_x^2}\right]e^{-i(2\pi u'(x-x')+\phi)}, \tag{8}$$

where s_x (in deg) is the spread of the gaussian envelope, and the additional parameters p (in deg) and ϕ (in rad) represent, respectively, the horizontal shift for the gaussian envelope and the initial phase of the complex harmonic oscillation. Note that the initial phase ϕ was present in Gabor's definition, while addition of the extra parameter p, which does not change the properties of the elementary signal as described by Gabor,[30] generalizes its definition.

This LWF is a complex-valued function, implying that each sensor's LWF has two parts. The real part of ψ^* is

$$\mathrm{Re}\left[\psi^*(x;x',u',s_x,p,\phi)\right] = \frac{1}{\sqrt{2\pi}\,s_x}\exp\left[-\frac{(x-p-x')^2}{2s_x^2}\right]\cos(2\pi u'(x-x')+\phi) \tag{9}$$

and its imaginary part is

$$\mathrm{Im}\left[\psi^*(x;x',u',s_x,p,\phi)\right] = -\frac{1}{\sqrt{2\pi}\,s_x}\exp\left[-\frac{(x-p-x')^2}{2s_x^2}\right]\sin(2\pi u'(x-x')+\phi), \tag{10}$$

respectively representing the well-known even- and odd-symmetric (real) Gabor filters.

As each channel's LSF equals the channel's response to an input Dirac delta function, δ, our choice for ψ^* determines that the LSF, h, of the channel tuned to spatial frequency u' is the generalized Gabor elementary signal

$$h(x';u',s_x,p,\phi) = \int_{-\infty}^{\infty} \delta(x)\psi^*(x;x',u',s_x,p,\phi)\,dx$$

$$= \psi^*(0;x',u',s_x,p,\phi)$$

$$= \frac{1}{\sqrt{2\pi}\,s_x}\exp\left[-\frac{(x'+p)^2}{2s_x^2}\right]e^{i(2\pi u'x'-\phi)}, \tag{11}$$

and the TF, H, of any channel, which is the Fourier transform of its LSF, is

$$H(u;u',s_x,p,\phi) = \exp\left[-2\pi^2 s_x^2(u-u')^2\right]e^{i(2\pi(u-u')p-\phi)}, \tag{12}$$

which implies the modulation transfer function (MTF)

$$\text{MTF}(u;u',s_x) = \left|H(u;u',s_x)\right| = \exp\left[-2\pi^2 s_x^2(u-u')^2\right] \tag{13}$$

and the phase transfer function (PTF)

$$\text{PTF}(u;u',p,\phi) = 2\pi(u-u')p-\phi. \tag{14}$$

Note that a channel's MTF is independent of the shift parameters p and ϕ, while its PTF is independent of the spread parameter s_x. In the sequel, we will refer to the continuous family of MTFs implied in Eq. (13) as Ω, that is,

$$\Omega(u,u') \triangleq \exp\left[-2\pi^2 s_x^2(u-u')^2\right]. \tag{15}$$

It is interesting to note that $\Omega(u,u')>0$ for all u and u'. This characteristic implies that the real and imaginary parts of each channel's LSF cannot form a Hilbert transform pair. Therefore, contrary to common belief, Gabor channels described in complex analytic form cannot be claimed to be quadrature-pair filters. Further, it can be easily seen from Eq. (12) that any channel's TF has a *dc* component,

$$H(0;u',s_x,p,\phi) = \exp\left[-2\pi^2 s_x^2 u'^2\right]e^{-i(2\pi u'p+\phi)} \neq 0+0i. \tag{16}$$

Some consequences of these two characteristics have been described by Fleet and Jepson,[43] and will become apparent below.

An important processing characteristic of the channels thus defined is their bandwidth, which can be measured in a number of ways. The absolute half-amplitude bandwidth (B_u, in c/deg) is the unsigned difference between the two spatial frequencies at which each channel's MTF equals half its maximum value. The relative half-amplitude bandwidth (B_{oct}, in octaves) is the base-2 logarithm of the ratio of the larger to the smaller of those two frequencies. Given the MTF in Eq. (13), it can be shown that

$$B_u = \frac{\sqrt{2\ln2}}{\pi s_x} \tag{17}$$

and

$$B_{oct} = \log_2\left[\frac{2\pi s_x|u'| + \sqrt{2\ln2}}{2\pi s_x|u'| - \sqrt{2\ln2}}\right]. \tag{18}$$

Note that the absolute bandwidth depends only on the spread parameter s_x, while the relative bandwidth depends also on the tuning frequency, u', of the channel.

The foregoing presentation has refrained from assigning values to any of the several parameters in each LWF. Three exemplary cases are now used to illustrate the effects of these parameters on the shapes of the LWFs and TFs, which are displayed in Fig. 2 for the 2 c/deg channel. For simplicity, in the three cases displayed in Fig. 2 the spread parameter s_x has been kept constant and valued so that the channel has a relative half-amplitude bandwidth of an octave. The well-known effect of s_x on the LWFs is to stretch or shrink their gaussian envelopes, thus covering more or less cycles of the complex harmonic oscillation. Similarly, its effects on the TFs is to change their spreads conversely, thus making them narrowly or broadly tuned as measured by their relative or absolute bandwidth. We will come back to this issue later on.

The first, simplest case is the customary one in which $p=0$ deg and $\phi=0$ rad. In this case, the real and imaginary parts of the LWF are, respectively, the conventional even- and odd-symmetric Gabor filters, while the TF is real owing to these symmetries. This implies that the MTF equals the TF and the PTF is identically 0 rad for all u.

In the second case, $p=0$ deg too but $\phi=-\pi/4$ rad. Neither the real nor the imaginary parts of the LWF are symmetric in this case, thus making the TF complex. Nevertheless, as compared to the previous case, the only effect of this parameter is to make the PTF identically $\pi/4$ rad for all u, as the MTF was shown above to be independent of ϕ. As a consequence, as long as $p=0$ deg, the channel's TF lies on a plane rotated an angle $|\phi|$ from the real plane, clockwise if $\phi>0$ rad and counter-clockwise if $\phi<0$ rad.

In the third case, $p=-1/4u'=-1/8$ deg and $\phi=0$ rad. Also in this case, neither the real nor the imaginary parts of the LWF are symmetric, thus making the TF complex. As the MTF is independent of p too, the only effect of this parameter is to make the PTF a linear function of u. This linear function has positive slope when $p>0$ deg, negative slope when $p<0$ deg and evaluates to 0 rad at $u=u'$. As a consequence, as long as $\phi=0$ rad, the channel's TF winds about the real plane, the curliness and sign of its twist depending on p.

The effects of other combinations for the values of p and ϕ on the channel's TF can be easily pictured from their separate effects shown in Fig. 2: the plane on which the TF for the case $p=0$ deg and $\phi=0$ rad lies rotates an angle ϕ around the u axis, and the TF itself winds about that plane as a function of p.

The effects just described illustrate how the processing characteristics of a channel change with the values for the parameters in its sensors' LWFs. A more critical issue

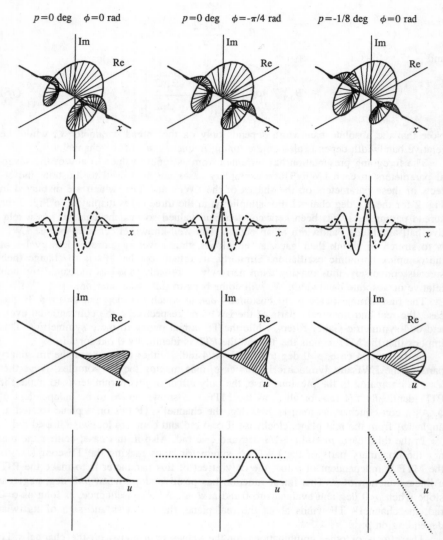

$p=0$ deg $\phi=0$ rad $p=0$ deg $\phi=-\pi/4$ rad $p=-1/8$ deg $\phi=0$ rad

Figure 2. Line-weighting function of the sensors at $x'=0$ deg and transfer functions of a one-octave (relative) bandwidth visual channel tuned to 2 c/deg resulting from each of three different combinations of the parameters p and ϕ. First column: $p=0$ deg and $\phi=0$ rad; Second column: $p=0$ deg and $\phi=-\pi/4$ rad; Third column: $p=-1/8$ deg and $\phi=0$ rad. First row: complex LWFs; Second row: real (continuous curves) and imaginary (dashed curves) parts of the LWFs; Third row: complex TFs; Fourth row: MTFs (continuous curves) and PTFs (dotted curves).

concerns the processing characteristics of the whole system, which determine the properties of the joint representation obtained by the channels. These depend on how the parameters p, ϕ and s_x change across channels. We will now consider the effects of these parameters in two stages, dealing first with the parameters that affect the channels' PTFs (p and ϕ) and, then, with the parameter affecting the channels' MTFs (s_x).

Psychophysical data bearing on the values for p and ϕ for any visual channel are not available owing to the lack of experimental methods to unravel the PTFs of visual channels. Therefore, any assumption as to how these parameters may change with the tuning frequency of the channels will seem rather arbitrary. Nevertheless, in general, these variations may be assumed to be described by some function of the tuning frequency of the channel, say, $p=P(u')$ and $\phi=\Phi(u')$. Although determining the precise mathematical expression that best describes these functions might be considered a theoretically relevant issue, these functions are relatively inconsequential to our understanding of late visual processing, where only rules or processes operating on the visual representation are involved. The reason for this is that the joint representation resulting from any given choice for these functions can be expressed as a transformation of the joint representation resulting from the simpler case where $P(u')=0$ and $\Phi(u')=0$ adopted as our first example. Let $G_f(x',u';p,\phi)$ be the joint representation resulting from any given choice for the functions P and Φ. It can be easily shown that

$$G_f\big(x',u';p,\phi\big) \;=\; G_f\big(x'+p,u';0,0\big)\,\mathrm{e}^{-\mathrm{i}\left(2\pi u'p+\phi\right)}. \tag{19}$$

Thus, as long as late visual processing models only imply rules applied to the joint representation, any such rule expressed for the particular representation for the case $p=0$ deg and $\phi=0$ rad has a functionally equivalent expression for any other conceivable case. For this reason, and to avoid unnecessary complexity, in the sequel we will restrict ourselves to considering the simple case in which $p=0$ deg and $\phi=0$ rad, although we will eventually mention how some properties of the joint representation in this case generalize to the remaining cases.

As for the spread parameter s_x or, equivalently, the relative or absolute channel bandwidths, psychophysical data are too scarce to give a clear-cut picture of the relationship between bandwidth and tuning frequency. Furthermore, the several experimental methods that have been devised to estimate channel bandwidth are known to provide different estimates,[44] probably reflecting that the data obtained thereby are contaminated to some extent by the peculiarities of the visual task posed by each method.[2,45] In contrast, with few exceptions, nearly every spatial vision model proposed so far has assumed channels with constant relative bandwidth, usually valued at around an octave. Rather than committing ourselves here with a single particular choice as to the relationship between s_x and u', we will adopt two extreme cases for this relationship and later analyze the joint representations resulting from them. These are the case of constant absolute bandwidth and the case of constant relative bandwidth.

From Eq. (17), the case of constant absolute bandwidth implies

$$s_x = \frac{\sqrt{2\ln 2}}{\pi B_u}, \tag{20}$$

where B_u is constant and independent of the tuning frequency of the channels. Note that this case is similar to case A of Kulikowski, Marčelja and Bishop,[46] and is also in line with suggestions by Robson.[7]

Similarly, from Eq. (18), the case of constant relative bandwidth implies

$$s_x = \frac{\sqrt{2\ln 2}}{2\pi} \frac{2^{B_{oct}}+1}{2^{B_{oct}}-1} \frac{1}{|u'|} = \frac{R}{|u'|}, \tag{21}$$

where B_{oct} is constant and independent of the tuning frequency of the channels, and R is the shape ratio of the channels.[46] Note also that this case is similar to case B of Kulikowski, Marčelja and Bishop,[46] and has been adopted by Watson.[14]

Each of these cases implies a different pattern of variation of the shapes of the LWFs and TFs with the tuning frequency of the channels. These effects are shown in Fig. 3, which displays the real parts of the LWFs as well as the MTFs of channels tuned to 2, 4, and 8 c/deg when $p=0$ deg and $\phi=0$ rad. Note that constant absolute bandwidth, where s_x is constant across channels, involves LWFs with exactly the same gaussian envelope for all channels, thus covering an increasing number of cycles of the oscillation with increasing tuning frequency. At the same time, on a linear scale, the MTFs are displaced versions of each other, their location on the abscissa depending on the tuning frequency of the channel. On the other hand, constant relative bandwidth, where s_x is inversely related to tuning frequency, involves LWFs whose gaussian envelopes shrink on the abscissa and stretch on the ordinate with increasing frequency, and MTFs which also broaden, on a linear scale, with increasing frequency.

Interestingly, these cases result in joint representations each of which is a transformation of one of the representations introduced in Section 2. Let $G_f(x',u';s_x)$ be the visual joint representation of f in the constant absolute bandwidth case. Then, from Eq. (7) and the LWF in Eq. (8) with $p=0$ deg and $\phi=0$ rad,

$$\begin{aligned} G_f(x',u';s_x) &= \int_{-\infty}^{\infty} f(x)\psi^*(x;x',u',s_x)\,dx \\ &= e^{i2\pi u'x'} \int_{-\infty}^{\infty} f(x)\frac{1}{\sqrt{2\pi}\,s_x}\exp\left[-\frac{(x-x')^2}{2s_x^2}\right]e^{-i2\pi u'x}\,dx \\ &= e^{i2\pi u'x'}\,WFT_f(x',u'), \end{aligned} \tag{22}$$

thus expressing the constant absolute bandwidth representation as a transformation of the particular WFT representation in Eq. (1) which is widely known as *Gabor transform*,[19,35] and implies the gaussian window given by constant absolute bandwidth, B_u=1.33 c/deg   constant relative bandwidth, B_{oct}=1 octave

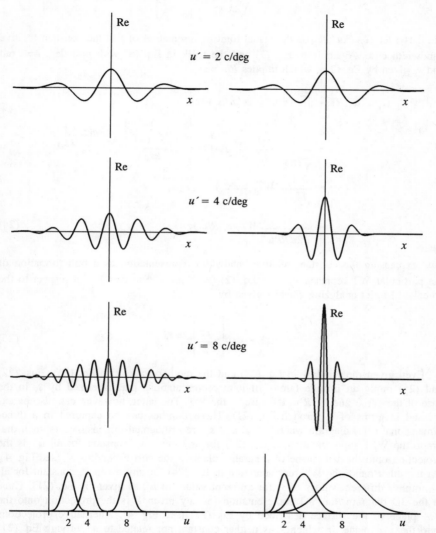

Figure 3. Real parts of the LWFs of the sensors at x'=0 deg of the channels tuned to 2 (first row), 4 (second row), and 8 (third row) c/deg in the constant absolute bandwidth case (s_x=0.28 deg, B_u=1.33 c/deg; left column) and the constant relative bandwidth case (R=0.56, B_{oct}=1 octave; right column). The MTFs of the three channels in each case are displayed on a linear scale at the bottom of each column.

$$w(x) = \frac{1}{\sqrt{2\pi}\, s_x} \exp\left[-\frac{x^2}{2s_x^2}\right]. \tag{23}$$

Similarly, let $G_f(x',u';R)$ be the visual joint representation of f in the constant relative bandwidth case. Again from Eq. (7) and the LWF in Eq. (8) with $p=0$ deg, $\phi=0$ rad and s_x given by Eq. (21), which implies $R/u'=\pm s_x$,

$$
\begin{aligned}
G_f(x',u';R) &= \int_{-\infty}^{\infty} f(x)\,\psi^*(x;x',u',s_x)\,dx \\
&= \frac{1}{\sqrt{2\pi s_x}}\frac{1}{\sqrt{s_x}}\int_{-\infty}^{\infty} f(x)\exp\left[-\frac{1}{2}\left(\frac{x-x'}{\pm s_x}\right)^2\right] e^{-i2\pi R\left(\frac{x-x'}{\pm s_x}\right)}\,dx \\
&= \frac{1}{\sqrt{2\pi s_x}}\, WT_f(x',\pm s_x) \\
&= \frac{1}{\sqrt{2\pi R/|u'|}}\, WT_f(x',R/u'),
\end{aligned} \tag{24}
$$

thus expressing the constant relative bandwidth representation as a transformation of the particular WT representation in Eq. (2) (with $|a|=s_x$ and $b=x'$) with respect to the so-called Morlet analyzing wavelet given by

$$g(x) = \exp\left[-\frac{x^2}{2}\right] e^{i2\pi Rx}. \tag{25}$$

Even given the window in Eq. (23) and the mother wavelet in Eq. (25), Eqs. (22) and (24) imply an infinite family of joint representations parameterized by s_x in the case of the WFT, and by R in the case of the WT. The latter, however, can also be expressed in terms of s_x through Eq. (21). These families can be captured in a three-dimensional (3D) diagram where x', u' and s_x are orthogonal dimensions. In such diagram, the WFT representation in Eq. (22) for any given s_x, constant for all u', is the projection onto the $x'u'$ plane of a parallel plane at the corresponding s_x (see Fig. 4). On the other hand, the WT representation in Eq. (24) for any given R, constant for all u', implies different values of s_x for different values of u', as given by Eq. (21). Thus, in the 3D diagram, the WT representation for any given R is the projection onto the $x'u'$ plane of the surface described by Eq. (21) (see Fig. 4). Alternative projections onto the $x'u'$ plane, in which s_x is neither constant nor related to u' through Eq. (21) define (unnamed) joint representations which might have useful properties and/or describe early visual processing better than either the WFT or the WT representations.[46]

In summary, early visual processing results in the creation of a joint representation which is akin to a WFT if Gabor visual channels have constant absolute bandwidth, or akin to a WT if they have constant relative bandwidth. We will refer to these as *psychophysical WFT representation* and *psychophysical WT representation*, respectively.

4. Measurable Magnitudes of the Psychophysical WFT and WT Representations

In relying on the output of early visual processing for any subsequent processing, visual tasks must be accomplished by applying rules to the joint representation. Different visual tasks may require different rules and, thus, a detection model might state that a pattern is detected whenever some measurable magnitude in its representation exceeds a fixed detection threshold; a discrimination model might state that two patterns are discriminated whenever some measurable magnitudes of their respective representations differ at least by a fixed discrimination threshold; and an identification model might state that a given pattern is identified as what it is as opposed to mistaken for some other pattern whenever the magnitude of some defining property of its representation reaches a fixed identification threshold. This section defines some magnitudes of the visual representation that can be the bases for these rules.

As a visual representation is the continuous collection of filtered images produced by the visual channels, an analysis of the output from any such channel to a 1D image serves to identify some useful magnitudes. This output is a cross-sectional profile of

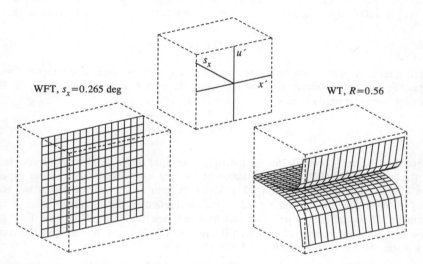

Figure 4. 3D space including the families of WFT and WT representations. The WFT corresponding to s_x=0.265 deg (B_u=1.41 c/deg) is shown on the left as a plane at the appropriate location. The WT corresponding to R=0.56 (B_{oct}=1 octave) is shown on the right as the surface described by Eq. (21). Coordinates are as sketched at the top, with the origin at the intersection of the three orthogonal axes.

the 2D visual representation at the u' of the selected channel. For our illustration, we will use the output from the channel tuned to 8 c/deg in the $R=0.56$ (i.e., $B_{oct}=1$ octave) psychophysical WT representation of the compound quasi-sineburst in Eq. (5). From Eqs. (7) and (8), this channel's output is the complex function

$$G_f(x',8) = \int_{-\infty}^{\infty} f(x) \frac{1}{\sqrt{2\pi} s_x} \exp\left[-\frac{(x-x')^2}{2s_x^2}\right] e^{-i2\pi 8(x-x')} dx, \qquad (26)$$

where, from Eq. (21), $s_x=0.07$ deg and f is the signal described by Eq. (5).

This complex function can also be expressed by its real and imaginary parts ($\text{Re}[G_f]$ and $\text{Im}[G_f]$, respectively) or by its modulus and argument (see Fig. 5), where $\text{Mod}[G_f]=(\text{Re}^2[G_f]+\text{Im}^2[G_f])^{0.5}$ and $\text{Arg}[G_f]=\arctan(\text{Im}[G_f]/\text{Re}[G_f])$. While the real and imaginary parts of the ouptut at any given spatial location are magnitudes directly obtained by the sensors at that location, computation of both the modulus and the argument of the sensors' responses would require further units. Provided that these units exist in the visual system, these four magnitudes are available for use in subsequent processing. Therefore, a more thorough look at their characteristics is worth pursuing.

For a signal whose Fourier transform is null at $u=0$ c/deg (i.e., a signal with no *dc* component), the output from any channel is a sum of complex harmonic oscillations each of which winds about the origin of the complex plane. Actual luminance signals have some positive mean luminance and, as a consequence, their Fourier transform is not null at $u=0$ c/deg. A useful way to describe any luminance signal, f_L, is through

$$f_L(x) = L(1+mf(x)), \qquad (27)$$

which implicitly defines the luminance signal as the superposition of the signal f with amplitude Lm on a uniform field of luminance L, with L and m such that $f_L \geq 0$. By linearity, it can be easily seen that

$$G_{f_L}(x',u') = L\exp[-2\pi^2 R^2] + Lm G_f(x',u'), \qquad (28)$$

where the first and second terms on the right-hand side of Eq. (28) respectively stand for the psychophysical WT representations of the first and second terms in the expansion of the right-hand side of Eq. (27). The first term arises because $\Omega(0,u')\neq0$ [see Eq. (15) with $R^2=(s_x u')^2$ from Eq. (21)] and, in particular, the imaginary part of the channel's TF is null when $p=0$ deg and $\phi=0$ rad [see Eq. (16)]. Note that Eq. (28) represents a scaled version of G_f which is also shifted along the real axis of the complex plane. As a consequence, the real part of Eq. (28),

$$\text{Re}\left[G_{f_L}(x',u')\right] = L\exp[-2\pi^2 R^2]+Lm\text{Re}\left[G_f(x',u')\right], \qquad (29)$$

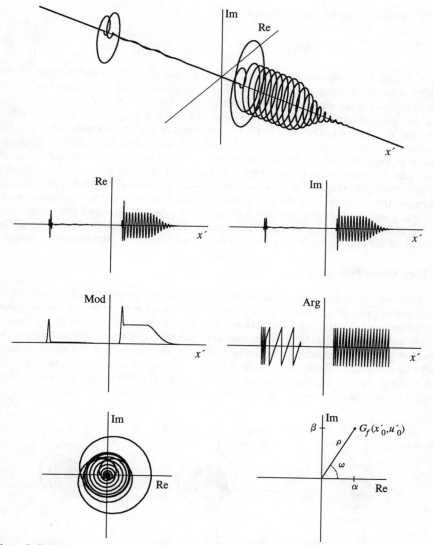

Figure 5. Output from the 8 c/deg channel in the $R=0.56$ psychophysical WT representation of the quasi-sineburst in Eq. (5). Top: Output in the complex plane. Second row: Real and imaginary parts of the output. Third row: Modulus and argument of the output. Fourth row: locus on the complex plane (left) and sketch of the four magnitudes at location (x'_0, u'_0) in the joint domain as defined on the complex plane (right), where $\alpha = \mathrm{Re}[G_f(x'_0, u'_0)]$, $\beta = \mathrm{Im}[G_f(x'_0, u'_0)]$, $\rho = \mathrm{Mod}[G_f(x'_0, u'_0)]$, and $\omega = \mathrm{Arg}[G_f(x'_0, u'_0)]$.

has a pedestal which its imaginary part,

$$\text{Im}\left[G_{f_L}(x',u')\right] = Lm\,\text{Im}\left[G_f(x',u')\right], \tag{30}$$

lacks. Figure 6a illustrates this fact by plotting the locus on the complex plane of the output from the 8 c/deg channel in the $R=0.56$ psychophysical WT representation of the compound quasi-sineburst transformed through Eq. (27) with $L=25$ and $m=0.03$. The foregoing discussion applies to the case $p=0$ deg and $\phi=0$ rad. When the psychophysical WT representation in Eq. (28) is subjected to the transformation in Eq. (19) for the other cases displayed in Fig. 2, the output from the 8 c/deg channel changes as shown in Figs. 6b and 6c. Besides a phase shift, each of these two alternative cases results in different pedestals affecting the real and imaginary parts of the channel's output: when $p=0$ deg and $\phi=-\pi/4$ rad, the real and imaginary pedestals are identical; when $p=-1/4u'$ and $\phi=0$ rad, the real pedestal is null and the imaginary pedestal equals the real pedestal when $p=0$ deg and $\phi=0$ rad. In the three cases, the Pythagorean sum of the real and imaginary pedestals is identical. For cases other than these three, the balance of the two pedestals may change, but their Pythagorean sum remains constant.

5. Late Visual Processing

Because a model of early visual processing is built on assumptions for which direct empirical support is difficult to obtain, the plausibility of a given model can be tested by determining the compatibility between the characteristics of the resulting representation and empirical data on performance in visual tasks. This amounts to determining whether general (i.e., pattern-independent) rules for the achievement of specific visual tasks can be found which, when applied to the postulated joint representation, can account for empirical data on performance in the task. The following subsections illustrate this procedure for the simple visual tasks of detection and identification.

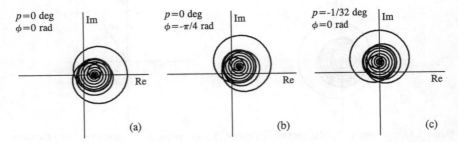

Figure 6. Locus on the complex plane of the output from the 8 c/deg channel in the $R=0.56$ psychophysical WT representation of the quasi-sineburst in Eq. (5) transformed through Eq. (27) with $L=25$ and $m=0.03$ for different combinations of the parameters p and ϕ in the sensors' LWFs. (a) $p=0$ deg and $\phi=0$ rad. (b) $p=0$ deg and $\phi=-\pi/4$ rad. (c) $p=-1/4u'=-1/32$ deg and $\phi=0$ rad.

5.1. Detection

Detection experiments involve determining the minimum contrast that a waveform, f_L, with mean luminance L and contrast m should have for an observer to detect it. In practice, the observer's task is one of discriminating a waveform whose luminance is given by Eq. (27) from a uniform field of luminance L. All visual channels play a role in the detection process, each contributing a real and positive-valued magnitude, $\wp(u')$, which can be expressed by some functional, $\Re$, of the difference between the channel's response to f_L and its response to a uniform field of luminance L, that is,

$$\wp(u') = \Re\Big[G_{f_L}(x',u') - G_L(x',u') \Big] = \Re\Big[Lm G_f(x',u') \Big]. \tag{31}$$

Although the detectability of sine-wave gratings depends on L,[47] we will omit mean luminance from our discussion given its secondary role at photopic levels.

Application of the functional $\Re$ may involve a simple search of the maximum value in the real part, the imaginary part, or the modulus of the channel's difference response (as in peak detection rules), but it may also involve more complicated calculations based on the array of channel responses over space (as in detection rules based on probability summation over space). Further, an additional functional of $\wp$ can be assumed to represent probability summation across channels. Although none of the existing detection rules seems capable of accounting for all of the detection data in the literature,[48] probability summation is generally accepted as the "true" detection rule. Nevertheless, and for illustration purposes, in this paper we will adopt a simple peak-to-mean detection rule that is consistent with a fairly large class of detection data. This specific detection rule implies that a waveform is detected at the minimum contrast necessary for the maximum unsigned difference response over x' within some channel to reach the channel's response threshold, $T(u')$, regardless of the channel, part (real or imaginary), and location where the maximum occurs.[c] Thus, using a method-of-limits analogy, as contrast of the waveform increases from zero detection occurs as soon as

$$m \max\left[\max_{x' \in \mathbf{R}}\left\{ \Big| \Re\big[G_f(x',u') \big] \Big| \right\}, \max_{x' \in \mathbf{R}}\left\{ \Big| \Im\big[G_f(x',u') \big] \Big| \right\} \right] = T(u') \tag{32}$$

for some channel. In Eq. (32), the maxima over x' in the real and imaginary parts of G_f define functions of u' that will be referred to as *real peak profile* and *imaginary peak profile*, respectively. The expression on the left-hand side of Eq. (32) defines the functional $\Re$, and it is also a function of u' that will be referred to as the *peak profile*

---

[c] Incidentally, we have found that the results to be presented below are identical if the rule is based instead on the modulus of the channels' responses. This implies that the real (imaginary) part of a channel's response is null when its imaginary (real) part is maximal. However, we have been unable to prove this as a property of the psychophysical WT and WFT representations of periodic waveforms.

of the visual representation of the corresponding waveform. In order to apply the detection rule in Eq. (32), a mathematical form for the channel threshold function, T, must be assumed. As discussed next, this function can be straightforwardly estimated from sine-wave contrast sensitivity data.

5.1.1. Detection of Sine-Wave Gratings and the Mathematical Form of the Channel Threshold Function

The real and imaginary parts of the visual representation of $f(x)=\sin(2\pi ux)$ are

$$\mathrm{Re}\left[G_f(x',u')\right] = \frac{1}{2}\left[\Omega(-u,u') + \Omega(u,u')\right]\sin(2\pi ux'), \tag{33}$$

and

$$\mathrm{Im}\left[G_f(x',u')\right] = \frac{1}{2}\left[\Omega(-u,u') - \Omega(u,u')\right]\cos(2\pi ux'), \tag{34}$$

with Ω as defined in Eq. (15). From Eqs. (33) and (34), the peak profile of the psychophysical WT representation of a sine-wave grating of frequency u and contrast m is

$$\frac{m}{2}\left[\Omega(-u,u') + \Omega(u,u')\right] = \frac{m}{2}\exp\left[-2\pi^2\left(\frac{R}{u'}\right)^2(-u-u')^2\right] + \frac{m}{2}\exp\left[-2\pi^2\left(\frac{R}{u'}\right)^2(u-u')^2\right]. \tag{35}$$

As shown elsewhere,[49] the channel threshold function can be estimated from Eq. (35) by assuming a mathematical form for the (foveal) sine-wave contrast sensitivity function (CSF). For our purpose here, it suffices to adopt any reasonable function, like

$$\mathrm{CSF}(u) = 168\,u\exp(-0.2\,u). \tag{36}$$

This function is a variant of that proposed by Kelly,[50] peaks at $u=5$ c/deg, has a low-frequency cut-off at $u_{min}=0.006$ c/deg and has a high-frequency cut-off at $u_{max}=44.6$ c/deg. Also, the shape of this function very closely matches that of the function proposed by Wilson[51] to fit the data of Campbell and Robson,[1] which is remarkably less tractable mathematically. Then, given Eq. (35) and the CSF in Eq. (36), the channel threshold function can be shown to be[49]

$$T(u') = \frac{5\pi^2R^2 + 5\pi^2R^2\exp\left[-4\pi^2R^2 - \dfrac{u'+s(u')}{5}\right]}{42u'\left(20\pi^2R^2+u'+s(u')\right)\exp\left[\pi^2R^2 - \dfrac{u'\left(u'+s(u')\right)}{400\pi^2R^2} - \dfrac{2u'+s(u')+10}{20}\right]}, \tag{37}$$

where

$$s(u') = \sqrt{\left(20\pi^2 R^2 + u'\right)^2 - \left(20\pi R\right)^2} \,. \tag{38}$$

As discussed elsewhere,[49] our assumption that channels have equal gains and varying thresholds as described by Eq. (37) is equivalent to the more popular assumption that channels differ in their gains and share a common threshold.[14,15]

Given the way in which it was derived, the channel threshold function in Eq. (37) reproduces the CSF in Eq. (36) through the detection rule in Eq. (32).[d] Yet, some subtleties of this detection rule are worth commenting on. Figure 7 plots the peak profile [Eq. (35)] of the $R=0.56$ psychophysical WT representation of a 16 c/deg sine-wave grating at its contrast threshold, $m=1/CSF(16)=0.0091$. Also displayed in Fig. 7 are the channel threshold function and the inverse of the CSF. Four important characteristics of the shape of the peak profile of the psychophysical WT representation of this 16 c/deg sine-wave grating-at-threshold hold also for that of any other grating-at-threshold: (i) the real peak profile at any u' is always (minimally) greater than the imaginary peak profile, (ii) a maximum in the real and imaginary peak profiles occurs at the channel whose tuning frequency matches the spatial frequency of the sine-wave grating, (iii) the magnitude of the real peak profile at its maximum is half the value of the psychophysically determined contrast threshold for detection of the sine-wave grating, and (iv) this magnitude is still lower than the threshold of the implied channel, but the real peak profile is tangent to the channel threshold function at the tuning frequency of some other channel (at $u'=13.88$ c/deg in Fig. 7), thus determining the detection of the grating. The only exception to (iv) occurs when the spatial frequency of the grating is that to which the visual system is maximally sensitive, in which case detection is mediated precisely by the channel tuned to the spatial frequency of the grating. Indeed, for frequencies below (above) the peak of the CSF, sine-wave gratings are detected by channels tuned to a spatial frequency slightly higher (lower) than that of the grating.[49] On the other hand, (iii) is a direct consequence of the fact that the detection rule in Eq. (32) is based on the peak-to-mean rather than the peak-to-trough amplitude of the channels' responses. Although the criterion used in the detection rule affects the mathematical form of the channel threshold function, any two criteria which are linearly related predict the same sensitivities.[48]

The discussion in this subsection extends straightforwardly to the psychophysical WFT representation, with only replacing R^2 in Eqs. (35), (37) and (38) with $(s_x u')^2$.

---

[d] This assertion needs some qualification. At the very low end of the frequency range, sensitivity is not guaranteed to be precisely reproduced because of a potential incompatibility between the CSF in Eq. (36) and the channel transfer functions given an assumed bandwidth.[49] For the bandwidth considered here in the WT case, it can be shown that this incompatibility manifests itself only for frequencies well below 0.01 c/deg, where our detection rule produces sine-wave sensitivities only minimally higher than those implied by the CSF in Eq. (36). At higher frequencies, sine-wave sensitivity is exactly reproduced. It should be noted, however, that the validity of the CSF in Eq. (36) for frequencies below 0.2 c/deg is dubious, as that is the lowest spatial frequency in the data of Campbell and Robson[1] that this function was adjusted to fit. In any case, this point is irrelevant to our present discussion.

40

Note from Eq. (38) that any assumed value for R determines the lowest spatial-frequency channel that may exist in the visual system. In the WT case, Eq. (38) implies that channels may exist for all $u' \geq 20\pi R(1-\pi R)$ c/deg which implies $u' > 0$ c/deg provided that $R > 1/\pi$;[49] in the WFT case, Eq. (38) implies $u' \geq (\pi s_x)^{-1} - (20\pi^2 s_x^2)^{-1}$. In both cases, the lowest channel turns out to be responsible for the detection of any sinewave grating of spatial frequency lower than its tuning frequency.

5.1.2. Detectability of Periodic Waveforms Compared with That of Sine-Wave Gratings

Campbell and Robson[1] reported extensive measurements on the detectability of square waveforms, and also some measurements for sawtooth and rectangular waveforms. Their main and well-known result is that, for spatial frequencies above a certain value, the detectability of non-sinusoidal waveforms can be explained by assuming that the visual system detects the first harmonic of their Fourier series expansions, while square and rectangular waveforms of lower frequencies seem to be detected in a way that certainly is not related to the detection of their first harmonics. Campbell, Howell and Johnstone[52] provided some further data on the detectability of square waveforms with missing harmonics (either high or low), and Campbell, Johnstone and Ross[53] reported data on the detectability of trapezoidal waveforms, and also attempted an explanation of the results for low spatial frequency waveforms in terms of gradient detectors. Still a different explanation was proposed by Jaschinski-Kruza and Cavo-

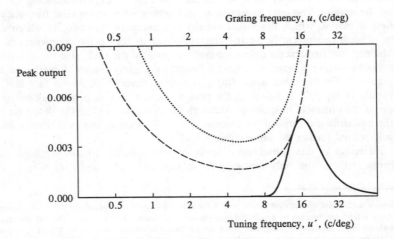

Figure 7. Peak profile of the $R=0.56$ psychophysical WT representation of a 16 c/deg sine-wave grating at its threshold for detection (continuous curve), channel threshold function (dashed curve) and inverse of the CSF (dotted curve). The lower abscissa applies to the peak profile and the channel threshold function. The upper abscissa applies to the inverse of the CSF.

nius,[15] who showed that these results can be accounted for with no need to resort to gradient detectors. The analysis presented next is similar to that in Jaschinski-Kruza and Cavonius,[15] but is somewhat more thorough and highlights a number of issues that were not clearly established in that paper. In addition, our analysis is carried out on both the WT and the WFT representations (they only considered the former), and differs in that we use Gabor channels described in complex analytic form and also in that we do not use interchangeably the channel threshold function and the CSF.

The detection rule in Eq. (32), along with the channel threshold function in Eq. (37), can be used to predict the detectability of arbitrary 1D periodic waveforms. Let f be a 1D periodic waveform of frequency u, whose Fourier series expansion is

$$f(x) = \sum_{n=0}^{\infty} B_n \sin(2\pi nux + \theta_n), \tag{39}$$

where B_n and θ_n are the coefficients of the n-th harmonic of the expansion of f. By linearity of both the WT and the WFT, the real and imaginary parts of the visual representation of f are straightforwardly seen to be

$$\text{Re}\left[G_f(x', u')\right] = \frac{1}{2} \sum_{n=0}^{\infty} \left[\Omega(-nu, u') + \Omega(nu, u')\right] B_n \sin(2\pi nux' + \theta_n), \tag{40}$$

and

$$\text{Im}\left[G_f(x', u')\right] = \frac{1}{2} \sum_{n=0}^{\infty} \left[\Omega(-nu, u') - \Omega(nu, u')\right] B_n \cos(2\pi nux' + \theta_n). \tag{41}$$

Closed-form expressions for the real and imaginary peak profiles of the visual representation of these waveforms cannot be obtained, nor is it guaranteed that the absolute maximum will occur in the real or the imaginary peak profile. Thus, theoretical predictions must be obtained using numerical methods. As an illustration of the procedure used to obtain them, the top panel in Fig. 8 displays the peak profiles of the $R=0.56$ psychophysical WT representation of square waveforms of 0.5, 1.5, 5 and 16 c/deg at their theoretical contrasts for detection. The theoretical threshold contrast was established by evaluating the peak profile numerically and finding the minimum contrast at which this profile is tangent to the channel threshold function at some point. Note that the shape of the peak profile of the psychophysical WT representation of a square waveform is invariant on a logarithmic scale, except for a horizontal shift that places its absolute maximum at the u' of the channel whose tuning frequency matches the fundamental frequency of the square waveform. Note also that the contrast of the square waveform represents a scaling factor for the ordinate of the peak profile.

As contrast increases, detection occurs when the peak profile first touches the channel threshold function, wherever this touching occurs. Given the shapes of the channel threshold function and the WT peak profile for the square waveform, at frequencies above about 0.87 c/deg, this touching occurs for the portion of the peak profile that pertains to the first harmonic of the square waveform. Therefore, consistent with empirical results,[1] in this range of frequencies detection occurs whenever the presence of the first harmonic of the waveform is detected. For spatial frequencies below 0.87 c/deg, however, the first touching no longer occurs within the part of the peak profile associated with the first harmonic of the square waveform. Rather, due to the flat right tail of the peak profile and the U-shaped form of the channel threshold function, this touching always occurs at the u' of the channel with the minimum thres-

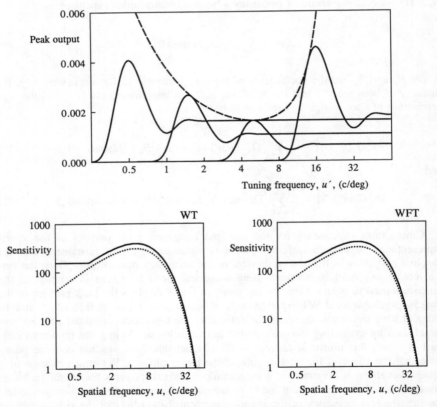

Figure 8. Top: Peak profiles of the R=0.56 psychophysical WT representation of square waveforms of 0.5, 1.5, 5 and 16 c/deg at their contrast thresholds for detection (left to right, continuous curves). The channel threshold function (dashed curve) is also plotted for reference. Bottom: Sensitivity to square waveforms (continuous curve) as predicted by the detection rule applied to the R=0.56 psychophysical WT (left) and s_x=0.265 deg psychophysical WFT (right) representations. The CSF (dotted curve) is also plotted for comparison.

hold regardless of the particular spatial frequency of the square waveform. Therefore, square waveforms of frequency below approximately 0.87 c/deg are detected when the channel tuned to u'=5 c/deg reaches its threshold, something which occurs at a constant contrast of the square waveform regardless of its spatial frequency. This fact accounts for Campbell and Robson's[1] results for low frequency square waveforms.

The bottom panels in Fig. 8 show the theoretical contrast sensitivity to square waveforms arising from the R=0.56 psychophysical WT representation and the s_x=0.265 deg psychophysical WFT representation.[e] In agreement with empirical data,[1] both the WT and the WFT contrast sensitivities to square waveforms are predicted to be $4/\pi$=1.273 times the contrast sensitivity for the first harmonic above approximately 0.87 c/deg, while they are predicted to be constant below that frequency.

It is interesting to note that the source for the flat low end in the predicted WFT sensitivity to square waveforms is different from that in the WT case. Given s_x=0.265 deg, the peak profile of the WFT representation is defined only for u'>1.13 c/deg. In addition, the shape of the WFT peak profile of square waveforms of different frequencies is not invariant. Indeed, at very low waveform frequencies, the WFT peak profile is a negatively-accelerating decreasing function. As frequency increases, the left tail of the peak profile progressively flattens and, for u>1.13 c/deg, it changes its shape to accommodate a local maximum at the channel whose tuning frequency matches the fundamental frequency of the square waveform. At the same time, the right tail of the peak profile grows an increasing number of local maxima which, for sufficiently high waveform frequencies, occur one at the tuning frequency of every channel whose tuning frequency matches the frequency of one of the harmonics comprising the square waveform. The magnitude of each of these maxima is proportional to the amplitude of the corresponding harmonics of the square waveform. However, as the transition between these two extreme shapes occurs, a part of the peak profile remains virtually invariant at low spatial frequencies. And, as it turns out, this is the critical part of the peak profile for the detection of the square waveform, thus producing the flat sensitivity in the low spatial-frequency range.

Thorough contrast sensitivity measurements for trapezoidal waveforms of various ramp widths in the low frequency range (below 1 c/deg) showed that sensitivity to trapezoids in this range of frequencies can sometimes be explained by the assumption that they are detected at the contrast necessary for detection of their fundamental component.[53] The ramp width, $2t$, of a trapezoidal waveform ranges from zero (corresponding to a square waveform) to π (corresponding to a triangular waveform), and the amplitude of its first harmonic equals $4\sin(t)/\pi t$. Empirical data show that low spatial frequency trapezoids with t>$\pi/8$ are detected at the contrast at which their first harmonics become detectable, while sensitivity to low frequency trapezoids of smaller ramp widths increases with decreasing t.[53,15] Figure 9a shows the theoretical contrast sensitivity to trapezoidal waveforms of various ramp widths arising from the R=0.56 psychophysical WT representation and the s_x=0.265 deg psychophysical WFT repre-

---

[e] The value s_x=0.265 deg implies B_u=1.41 c/deg, corresponding to an absolute half-power bandwidth of 1 c/deg.[54]

44

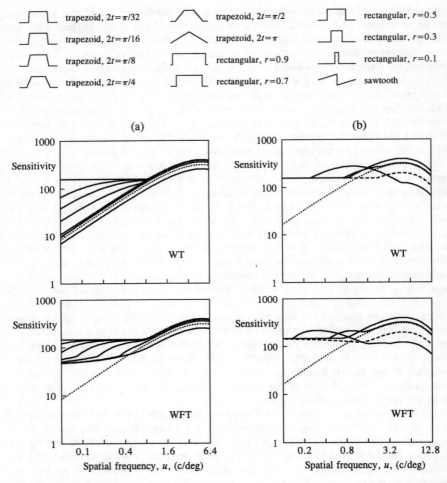

Figure 9. Top: Luminance profiles across one cycle of several waveforms. (a) Theoretical contrast sensitivity to trapezoidal waveforms (continuous curves) arising from the $R=0.56$ psychophysical WT representation (top) and the $s_x=0.265$ deg psychophysical WFT representation (bottom). Top to bottom, the continuous curves correspond to ramp widths of zero (square waveforms), $\pi/32$, $\pi/16$, $\pi/8$, $\pi/4$, $\pi/2$ and π (triangular waveforms). The CSF is also plotted as a dotted curve for comparison. (b) Theoretical contrast sensitivity to rectangular waveforms (continuous curves) and sawtooth waveforms (dashed curve) arising from the $R=0.56$ psychophysical WT representation (top) and the $s_x=0.265$ deg psychophysical WFT representation (bottom). Top to bottom on the right boundary of each graph, the continuous curves correspond to duty cycles of 0.5 (square waveforms), 0.3 and 0.1. The theoretical curves for rectangular waveforms of duty cycles r and $1-r$ are coincident.

sentation. Unlike for square waveforms, the predicted WFT and WT sensitivities are not coincident, and it is the WT curves that are in good agreement with experimental data (compare with Fig. 5 in Jaschinski-Kruza and Cavonius[15]).

Contrast sensitivity data for other periodic waveforms are scarce. A sawtooth waveform of 11 c/deg was found to be detectable at $\pi/2$ times the contrast of a sine-wave grating of the same frequency,[1] and it has also been reported that low frequency sawtooth waveforms have the same detection thresholds as square waveforms.[53] Similarly, the threshold contrast for detection of a number of rectangular waveforms of 11 c/deg and various duty cycles, r ($0<r<1$), was that necessary for detection of their first harmonics at all duty cycles tested, which equals $\pi/4\sin(\pi r)$ times the contrast for detection of their first harmonics when presented alone,[1] and low frequency rectangular waveforms of any duty cycle also have the same detection thresholds as square waveforms.[53] Figure 9b shows the theoretical contrast sensitivity to sawtooth waveforms and rectangular waveforms of various duty cycles arising from the $R=0.56$ psychophysical WT representation and the $s_x=0.265$ deg psychophysical WFT representation. Note that the shapes of the WT and WFT curves, though different, are both consistent with the (scarce) empirical data just mentioned. In any case, the predicted WFT sensitivities to trapezoidal waveforms are in clear disagreement with empirical data and, therefore, the WFT representation can be rejected as the outcome of early visual processing. For this reason, in the sequel we will discontinue consideration of the WFT representation.

The Fourier series expansion of waveforms with missing harmonics is easily obtained from that for the corresponding complete waveforms in Eq. (39), except that some of the harmonics are removed and, therefore, the sums on the right-hand side run for the values of n corresponding to the harmonics retained. Similarly, the expressions for the real and imaginary parts of their visual representations are obtained from Eqs. (40) and (41), with the sums on the right-hand sides also changed accordingly.

The effects of the removal of harmonics from square waveforms on their detectability can be summarized as follows:[52] (i) removal of very high frequency harmonics does not affect significantly the detection threshold, (ii) removal of the fundamental component (and even some of the next higher harmonics) does not affect the detection threshold provided that the frequency of the waveform is sufficiently low, but (iii) if the frequency is higher, the missing-fundamental square waveform is detected at the contrast necessary for the third harmonic to reach its own detection threshold. These results are easily understandable from the shapes of the peak profiles for square waveforms with missing harmonics.

Figure 10a shows the peak profiles of the $R=0.56$ psychophysical WT representation of a complete square waveform and waveforms containing the first (sine-wave grating), three first, five first, nine first and 15 first harmonics of the square waveform, all of them having a spatial frequency of 1 c/deg and the same physical contrast, set below their thresholds for detection. Note that, as more harmonics are present, the range of channels over which the shape of the peak profile matches the peak profile for the complete square waveform grows towards higher frequencies. Since square waveforms of 0.87 c/deg or less are detected by the 5 c/deg channel, if the square

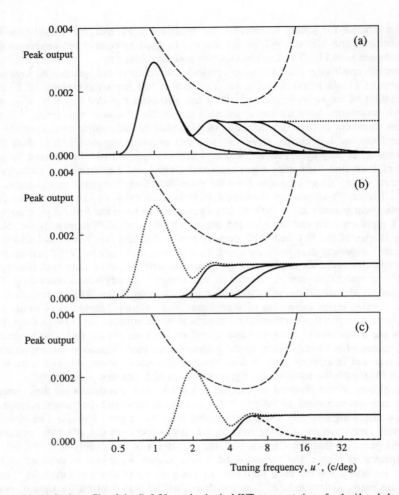

Figure 10. (a) Peak profile of the $R=0.56$ psychophysical WT representation of a 1 c/deg, below thresh-old, square waveform (dotted curve) and peak profiles for waveforms of the same frequency and contrast (continuous curves) but containing only (bottom to top) the first, three first, five first, nine first, and 15 first harmonics of the square waveform. The channel threshold function is plotted as a dashed curve for reference. (b) Peak profiles for a square waveform (dotted curve) and waveforms of the same frequency and contrast (continuous curves) but missing (top to bottom) the first, three first and five first harmonics of the square waveform. (c) Peak profiles for a 2 c/deg square waveform at threshold (dotted curve), a 2 c/deg missing-fundamental square waveform of the same frequency and contrast (continuous curve), and a 6 c/deg sine-wave grating (short-dashed curve) at its contrast as the third harmonic of the square waveform.

waveform missing high frequency harmonics contains enough low frequency components so that its peak profile is still flat at $u'=5$ c/deg, then the threshold for detection of that waveform will coincide with that of a complete square waveform. Then, at low spatial frequencies where detection is not determined by the fundamental component, the effect of the removal of higher harmonics will depend both on the spatial frequency of the waveform and on the number of harmonics that are retained. On the other hand, for waveforms of spatial frequency above 0.87 c/deg, where detection is determined by the part of the peak profile pertaining to the first harmonic, the presence or absence of high frequency harmonics is immaterial as far as detection is concerned.

Figure 10b shows the peak profiles for 1 c/deg square waveforms missing the first, three first and five first harmonics, along with the peak profile for a complete square waveform, all of them at the same physical contrast, set below their detection thresholds. As can be seen, removal of the first harmonic has little effect on the flatness of the right tail of the peak profile, which is the key to detection at low spatial frequencies. As more of the low harmonics are removed, the spatial frequency below which their removal has no effect on the detectability of the waveform becomes lower.

Finally, Fig. 10c shows the peak profile for a 2 c/deg square waveform at its contrast for detection, along with the peak profiles for a missing-fundamental square waveform of the same spatial frequency and contrast and a sine-wave grating of 6 c/deg (third harmonic of the square waveform) at one third the contrast of the fundamental component of the square waveform (its contrast as the third harmonic of the square waveform). Clearly, the missing-fundamental square waveform is not detectable at this contrast, as neither is the 6 c/deg sine-wave grating. For the missing-fundamental square waveform to be detected, its contrast will have to be raised so that its peak profile touches the channel threshold function, exactly to the same extent as the contrast of the 6 c/deg sine-wave grating should have to be raised for it to be detected.

The detectability of other periodic waveforms consisting of arbitrary combinations of a varying number of sine-wave gratings has also been studied.[55,56] At spatial frequencies of 1 and 3 c/deg, a waveform consisting of the first nine harmonics of a square waveform (with their appropriate amplitudes as components of the square waveform) was equally as detectable as a thoroughly analogous waveform differing only by a π rad phase shift of the fifth harmonic, while at 0.2 c/deg the latter waveform was less detectable than the former.[55] Figure 11a shows the peak profiles for these two waveforms at a spatial frequency of 0.5 c/deg and a contrast below their detection thresholds. At relatively high spatial frequencies, the two waveforms should be equally detectable, for the detection of either of them would be determined by the left tail of their peak profiles, which both waveforms share. At lower spatial frequencies, however, the detection of either waveform would be determined by the right tail of their peak profiles. As the right tail of the peak profile for the waveform with the phase-shifted fifth harmonic is lower than that for the other waveform, this waveform is predicted to require a higher contrast to be detected.

On the other hand, a waveform consisting of two sine-wave gratings differing in frequency by a factor of three (with the lower frequency grating in the range between

0.9 and 6.3 c/deg) is equally as detectable when the gratings are added in peaks-add phase as it is when they are added in peaks-substract phase.[56] Figure 11b shows that it is only in the right tails that the peak profiles for these waveforms differ slightly, a difference which is perhaps too small to be noticeable in experimental data.

Given the detection rule in Eq. (32), the empirical data considered in this subsection is consistent with the notion that early visual processing creates a WT representation, while data on the detectability of trapezoidal waveforms clearly rules out the hypothesis of a WFT representation. The foregoing analyses have arbitrarily (however reasonably) assumed $R=0.56$ and $s_x=0.265$ deg. It is interesting at this point to determine the extent to which the specific choices for R and s_x assumed in the analyses affect the results obtained. As an illustration, Fig. 12a shows the predicted contrast sensitivity to square waveforms arising from the $R=0.39$, $R=0.56$ and $R=1.09$ (i.e.,

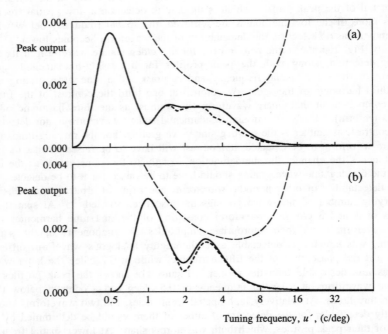

Figure 11. (a) Peak profiles of the $R=0.56$ psychophysical WT representation of a 0.5 c/deg, below threshold waveform consisting of the first nine harmonics of a square waveform (continuous curve) and a thoroughly analogous waveform except for a π rad phase shift of the fifth harmonic (short-dashed curve). The channel threshold function (long-dashed curve) is also displayed for reference. (b) Peak profiles of the $R=0.56$ psychophysical WT representation of the sum of two sine-wave gratings of frequencies 1 and 3 c/deg, each at 0.8 times its individual contrast threshold. The gratings are added in peaks-add phase (continuous curve) or peaks-substract phase (short-dashed curve). The channel threshold function (long-dashed curve) is also displayed for reference.

B_{oct}=1.5, 1 and 0.5 octaves, respectively) psychophysical WT representations. Similarly, Fig. 12b shows the predicted contrast sensitivity to square waveforms arising from the s_x=0.133, s_x=0.265 and s_x=0.53 deg (i.e., B_u=2.828, 1.414 and 0.707 c/deg, respectively) psychophysical WFT representations. In both cases, the theoretical contrast sensitivity to square waveforms always has a flat low frequency end, whose limiting frequency depends on channel bandwidth. A similar effect of bandwidth is also found in the theoretical WFT and WT contrast sensitivities to trapezoidal, rectangular and sawtooth waveforms. Interestingly, the determination of the spatial frequency below which contrast sensitivity to square waveforms is constant provides for a simple and reliable means for the assessment of individual differences in channel bandwidths.

5.2. Identification

The identification of a pattern implies its classification as belonging in a certain, "labeled" category. This does not necessarily mean that the observer will be able to supply the technical name for the pattern but, rather, that he or she can describe the appearance of the pattern or some of its spatial characteristics or features. Strictly speaking, a pattern can be identified as soon as it is detected, although the pattern can be misclassified at this stage: a medium or high spatial frequency square waveform at or slightly above threshold is identified as a sine-wave grating of the same frequency, insofar as those two patterns are indistinguishable from each other.[1]

The identification process can be modeled as the application of a decision rule to the visual representation of the pattern.[57] Data on identification performance are gathered either by having observers describe the appearance of a pattern or report the pres-

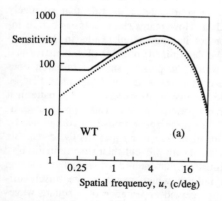 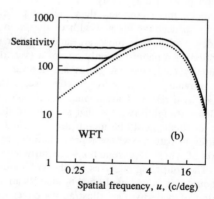

Figure 12. (a) Theoretical contrast sensitivity to square waveforms arising from the R=1.09, R=0.56 and R=0.39 psychophysical WT representations (continuous curves, bottom to top). The CSF is also plotted as a dotted curve for comparison. (b) Theoretical contrast sensitivity to square waveforms arising from the s_x=0.53, s_x=0.265 and s_x=0.133 deg psychophysical WFT representations (continuous curves, bottom to top). The CSF is also plotted as a dotted curve for comparison.

ence of spatial features at specific locations in the pattern, or by measuring the minimum extent to which two patterns must differ along one or more of at least up to 15 dimensions[58] for an observer to be able to discriminate them. The design of the latter type of experiment provides for an objective assessment that the two patterns are classified as belonging in different categories, but the observer's task is one of discrimination and, therefore, data from these experiments bear on discrimination rules (i.e., how different the visual representations of two patterns must be in order for them to be perceptually distinguishable) rather than identification rules (i.e., what "signatures" in the visual representation of a pattern determine its classification). The task posed by the former type of experiment, on the other hand, definitely implies only the application of identification rules. We will restrict ourselves here to considering pure identification tasks in which discrimination processes do not play any significant role.

Models of the identification process fall into two main categories. The simpler type of model involves rules which attempt to account for the perception (or lack thereof) of elementary spatial features (discontinuities and singularities or, in other words, sharp edges and bright or dark bars) at specific locations in a pattern,[59] regardless of what the whole pattern may look like to the observer. The second type of model incorporates rules which permit the building of a spatially complete brightness description of the perceived appearance of the pattern,[41,60] in which the presence or absence of perceived spatial features at specific locations can be noted. In the particular models just referred to, the proposed rules are applied to a discrete visual representation of the pattern which consists of the set of filtered images produced by a finite and small number of visual channels.

Given the diversity of categories into which a pattern can be classified, the identification process may imply the application of a rule whose logical structure is likely to be much more complex than the comparatively simple detection rule that so nicely seems to account for a wealth of detection data. How many statements such rule includes, which ones those are, and whether or not its application results in the classification of a pattern in only one of a (yet to be determined) number of exhaustive and mutually exclusive categories are questions which the present state of research does not provide an answer for. In any case, if the contention is accepted that identification arises as a result of the application of rules to the visual representation of a pattern, it follows straightforwardly that any two (different) patterns whose visual representations are identical should be identically classified.[61] For these above-threshold conditions, by "different patterns whose representations are identical" we mean patterns the detectable parts of whose representations are sufficiently similar to prevent their discrimination.[f]

The following analyses for the WT case illustrate that identity of representation can account for some well-known identification failures which result in the misclassification of patterns. Our illustrations cover the perceived appearance of a square waveform at or slightly above its detection threshold, the appearance of Mach bands, and

---

[f] A more precise definition of identity of representation would obviously require the provision of a discrimination rule.

the Craik-Cornsweet-O'Brien effect.

Figure 13 shows the peak profile of the $R=0.56$ psychophysical WT representation of a 2 c/deg square waveform at 1.3 times its threshold contrast, plus the peak profiles for a sine-wave grating of the same frequency at its contrast as the first harmonic of the square waveform, and a 6 c/deg sine-wave grating at its contrast as the third harmonic of the square waveform. Note that the detectable parts in the representations of the 2 c/deg sine-wave grating and the 2 c/deg square waveform (as illustrated for simplicity through their peak profiles) are identical, thus accounting for the classification of both patterns into the same category. The detectable part in the representation of the square waveform begins to differ from that of the sine-wave grating as soon as contrast is high enough for the right tail of the peak profile for the square waveform to lie above the channel threshold function although, for reasons that must be attributed to the operation of discrimination rules, the two patterns are distinguishable (and, thus, classified into different categories) only at a still higher contrast, that at which the third harmonic of the square waveform reaches its threshold contrast when presented alone.[1] On the other hand, at sufficiently low frequencies, the square waveform can be discriminated at threshold from a sine-wave grating of the same frequency.[1] At those frequencies, the detectable part of the sine-wave grating (which occurs around the tuning frequency of the channel detecting that particular grating) differs from that of the square waveform (which, as discussed in Section 5.1, occurs around the channel tuned to 5 c/deg) by an extent that must hence be understood as large enough to satisfy some discrimination rule. These characteristics apply literally to sawtooth waveforms, and generalize straightforwardly to trapezoidal and rectangular waveforms.

As a preliminary to the upcoming illustrations, Fig. 14 shows the modulus and

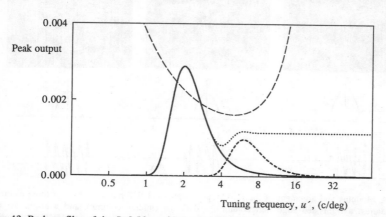

Figure 13. Peak profiles of the $R=0.56$ psychophysical WT representation of a 2 c/deg square waveform at 1.3 times its threshold for detection (dotted curve), a sine-wave grating of the same frequency at its contrast as the first harmonic of the square waveform (continuous curve), and a 6 c/deg sine-wave grating at its contrast as the third harmonic of the square waveform (short-dashed curve). The channel threshold function (long-dashed curve) is also plotted for reference.

argument of the $R=0.56$ psychophysical WT representation of three elementary features: a right step edge, a dark bar and a bright bar. Note that the three moduli are similar in that they show a cone-like structure centered at the location of the discontinuity or singularity in the profile, broader at low spatial frequencies and progressively narrowing as frequency increases. (The moduli of the WT representations of dark and bright bars of the same width but opposite polarity are indeed identical.) In addition, at

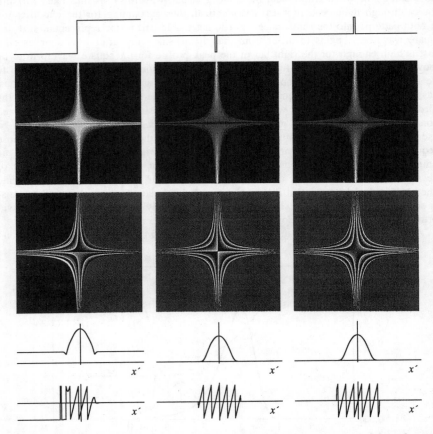

Figure 14. Modulus and argument of the $R=0.56$ psychophysical WT representation of three elementary visual features: a right step edge (left column), a dark bar (middle column), and a bright bar (right column). First row: spatial profile of the feature. Second row: log-modulus of the WT representation. Third row: argument of the WT representation. Fourth row: cross-sectional profile of the log-modulus at $u'=1$ c/deg. Fifth row: cross-sectional profile of the argument at $u'=1$ c/deg. The x' and u' dimensions of the moduli and arguments are as in Fig. 1. The arguments are represented linearly from $-\pi$ rad (black) to π rad (white).

any u' the modulus is maximal at the exact location of the feature. Yet, the argument is clearly different for each type of feature but, importantly, at the location of the feature (where each modulus has a local maximum over space at all frequencies in the joint domain) and for all $u'>0$ c/deg, the argument is identically $-\pi/2$ rad for the right step edge, identically $\pm\pi$ rad for the dark bar, and identically 0 rad for the bright bar, while the argument has opposite sign for all $u'<0$ c/deg.[g] These characteristics are the bases for Morrone and Burr's[59] approach to predicting the perception of features in images. We will refer to the psychophysical WT representation of a feature (expressed through its modulus and argument) as its *spectral signature*. Note that the spectral signature of a bright bar differs from that of a dark bar only by a π rad shift of the argument, while the spectral signature of a left step edge (not shown in Fig. 14) similarly differs from that of a right step edge only by a π rad shift of the argument.

Figure 15a shows the modulus and argument of the $R=0.56$ psychophysical WT representation of a ramp defining a transition between a dark uniform field on its left and a bright uniform field on its right. This luminance profile is known to elicit the perception of Mach bands (illusory dark and bright bars next to the discontinuities in the profile) under a variety of conditions.[62,63] Figure 15a clearly shows that the WT representation of a ramp contains traces of the spectral signatures of dark and bright bars at the locations where they are seen (compare with the spectral signatures of dark and bright bars in Fig. 14, middle and right columns). Interestingly, the WT representation of the smoothed ramp $f(x)=\tanh(\pi x/4)$, a profile in which Mach bands are not seen, does not contain anything remotely approaching the spectral signatures of the bars (see Fig. 15b), and neither are they found in the WT representation of a step edge (see Fig. 14, left column), a profile in which Mach bands are not seen either.[64,65] Therefore, the presence or absence of the spectral signatures of dark and bright bars in the WT representation of a luminance profile can be regarded as the basis for their perception and, as a consequence, for the selective appearance of Mach bands.

Finally, Fig. 15c shows the modulus and argument of the $R=0.56$ psychophysical WT representation of a version of the Craik-Cornsweet-O'Brien profile due to Tolhurst.[66] Note that the spectral signature of a right step edge is found in this representation at the location of the discontinuity in the profile (compare with Fig. 14, left column), possibly sustaining the perception of an edge when an image with this luminance profile is inspected.

The preceding illustrations are consistent with the notion that identification is based on rules, but they only represent a methodological first step towards the identification of those rules. In view of the results presented in this subsection, one might be tempted to conclude that a pattern is identified as the most elementary pattern whose visual representation its is identical to. Thus, perception of a square waveform (and, presumably, other periodic waveforms as well) "defaults" to a sine-wave grating in the absence of compelling evidence as to its identity, perception of a ramp defining a transi-

---

[g] These characteristics hold in the case that $p=0$ deg and $\phi=0$ rad, and are subject to the changes dictated by Eq. (19) when the sensors' LWFs are based on different parameters.

tion between bright and dark uniform fields defaults to bright and dark bars at the appropriate locations, and perception of the Craik-Cornsweet-O'Brien pattern defaults to an edge. Although this rule is consistent with the results presented above, it should be noted that this represents the type of textbook explanation[67] which is inherently devoid

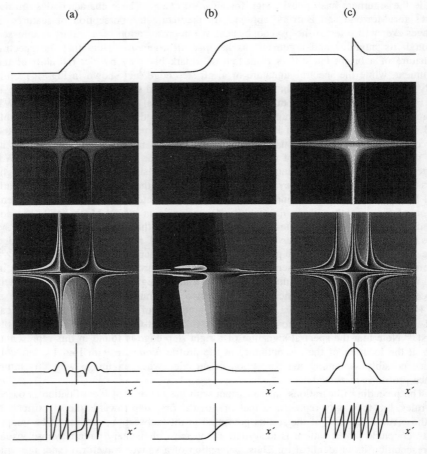

Figure 15. Modulus and argument of the R=0.56 psychophysical WT representation of three luminance profiles: a ramp (a), a smoothed ramp (b), and the Craik-Cornsweet-O'Brien profile (c). First row: spatial profile. Second row: log-modulus of the WT representation. Third row: argument of the WT representation. Fourth row: cross-sectional profile of the log-modulus at u'=1 c/deg. Fifth row: cross-sectional profile of the argument at u'=1 c/deg. Cone-like structures in the moduli of the ramp and the smoothed ramp are only clearly visible after the logarithmic transformation because the large amplitudes at very low spatial frequencies obscure these characteristics. Pictorial conventions are as in Fig. 14.

of content unless the mechanisms for the assimilation of a pattern to a default are explained. We will refrain from dwelling on ecological rationalizations to this effect. A stronger explanation for the identification of patterns must propose explicit rules or processes which transform the visual representation into a perceived brightness description, something for which a systematic study of the conditions under which each of a number of key patterns are correctly classified as opposed to misclassified should be most enlightening. Although a number of studies that may be relevant to this issue have already been carried out,[1,68-70] a thoroughly satisfactory account of identification performance is not as yet available.

6. Discussion

This paper has described and illustrated a unified approach to modeling early and late visual processing. Our main contention is that the mechanisms subserving early visual processing constitute the basic (and fixed) processing architecture, whose operation results in the creation of a visual representation which is subjected to further (late) visual processing for the achievement of visual tasks. Thus, late visual processing can be modeled as the application of task-dependent rules to the task-independent visual representation of a stimulus. From this point of view, vision research has the twofold goal of (i) unraveling the structural and functional characteristics of the mechanisms responsible for early visual processing, and (ii) identifying the rules which operate on the visual representation of a stimulus for the achievement of specific visual tasks.

While it may not be simple to disentangle what experimental data owe to the early versus late visual processing stages, adoption of this framework may be useful for organizing our experimental hypotheses as well as for aiding the interpretation of our results. For instance, the interpretation of the CSF as the MTF of the visual system is at odds with the fact that the perceived contrast of well above-threshold sine-wave gratings is independent of spatial frequency.[71] These conflicting results have led to claims that visual channels have different gains at threshold but equal gains in suprathreshold conditions, thus attributing these results to contrast-dependent differences in the organization of the early stages of the visual processing of a stimulus. It may be more fitting, perhaps, to interpret these results as indicating that the detection of sine-wave gratings and the judgement of their apparent contrast in suprathreshold conditions define two different visual tasks each of which is accomplished by applying a distinct rule to the visual representation of a sine-wave grating of whatever contrast.[72] In the former case, the outcome of the rule is a binary decision, whereas in the latter case application of the rule provides a graded response.

As shown in this paper, early visual processing can be characterized as a stage which creates a joint spatial/spatial-frequency representation of the input image. Further, the type of representation which is thus built depends on the tuning characteristics of visual channels. Our analyses of detection tasks indicate that empirical data support the notion of a wavelet representation based on one-octave wide Gabor channels described in complex analytic form, although these data are also qualitatively in agreement with channels of broader or narrower bandwidths. Analysis of identification tasks, discrimination tasks (including spatial-frequency masking experiments[73]) and adaptation data might be crucial to further support this type of architecture or reject it in favor of some other, although this endeavor is hindered by lack of precise statements for the rules governing pattern identification, pattern discrimination and the functional aspects of channel adaptation or fatigue.

For the sake of simplicity, we have refrained from incorporating into our description a number of well established facts about human visual processing. Firstly, we have restricted ourselves to the space-invariant case, while inhomogeneity is one of the most conspicuous and undebated characteristics of visual processing.[2] Although visual space-variance seems to have a structural basis,[74,75] there are at least two different (but probably functionally equivalent) ways of incorporating this characteristic into the processing scheme presented in this paper.

One of these is to consider that each channel processes a limited, roughly circular area of the visual field, centered at the fovea, and whose radius decreases with increasing tuning frequency of the channel.[h,13,14,76-78] This is a strictly structural account of visual space-variance which, for all practical purposes, is likely to be equivalent to the alternative functional account which assumes a strict space-invariant architecture and places space-variance in the rules that govern late visual processing, e.g., by assuming that the channel response threshold is not unique but varies with the spatial location of the sensors.[79] The former approach could be incorporated into the processing scheme by bounding the joint domain over which the visual representation is defined. The latter could be incorporated by extending the channel threshold function T to represent the response threshold for the sensor at spatial location x' in the channel tuned to frequency u'. In this latter case, estimation of the channel/sensor threshold function would proceed through steps thoroughly analogous to those followed in the derivation of Eq. (37), but using the family of CSFs that hold at different visual field locations.[80]

A second characteristic that has been neglected in this description is probability summation across space and/or among channels. This can be easily incorporated into this processing scheme by assuming a convenient psychometric function relating sensor output to probability of detection and replacing the deterministic detection rule in Eq. (32) with a probabilistic one. A particularly efficient implementation of probability summation across space and/or among channels is the so-called *Quick pooling model*,[81] whose application merely implies a different definition of the functional $\Re$ in Eq. (31) and an additional functional of $\wp$ as defined also in Eq. (31).[48] The combined effects of space-variance and probability summation can account for the asymptotic increase in sensitivity with increasing stimulus size,[77] for regional variations in sensitivity across the visual field,[82-84] as well as for other seemingly stray detection data[85,86] which the simple peak-to-mean detection rule adopted in this paper cannot account for.

---

[h] As discussed in García-Pérez,[77] there are two different versions of this approach, which only differ as to the assignment of sensors to channels.

A final characteristic that has been neglected in this paper is the inherent 2D nature of both the spatial visual stimulus and the channel TFs. A generalization of the analysis presented in this paper to the 2D case faces three distinct problems. The most important one is the empirical problem of determining what is the best fitting 2D function describing the sensor point-weighting functions (PWFs), and what are the relationships between the tuning frequency of the channels and their spatial frequency and orientation bandwidths. Although some work along these lines has been carried out,[73,87-90] the 2D characterization of visual channels is far from complete. A second, theoretical, problem is whether the four-dimensional (4D) visual representations obtained by 2D channels can be regarded as a WT representation (or any other known joint spatial/spatial frequency representation, for that matter), a problem which arises from the lack of a unique definition of continuous wavelet transforms in two or more dimensions.[91] The third problem is computational, and arises when trying to obtain numerical predictions for, e.g., the detectability of non-sinusoidal waveforms as described in Section 5.1.

Besides these problems, the actual extension of the analyses presented in this paper to two dimensions is straightforward. Indeed, it can easily be proved that the results presented in Section 5.1 remain unchanged (except for a scaling factor) if the 2D PWFs are described as 2D Gabor functions with the empirical restrictions described by Daugman.[10]

In closing, it is important to note that the possibility of characterizing the visual joint spatial/spatial-frequency representation as either a WT or a WFT is primarily dependent on the assumed mathematical form for the sensors' LWFs, and not only on the way in which bandwidth changes with tuning frequency. Specifically, for the visual representation to qualify as a WFT representation, it is necessary that the sensor's LWFs be described by the product of a complex harmonic oscillation and an envelope of arbitrary but fixed shape (i.e., described as canonical coherent states). Neither difference or derivatives of gaussians nor Cauchy functions fall in this class. On the other hand, the visual representation can qualify as a WT representation whenever a bandpass LWF is assumed which is also relatively well localized in space and spatial frequency,[92] although the LWFs for the various channels must necessarily be related through Eq. (4) (i.e., they must be described as affine coherent states). Although difference or derivatives of gaussians and Cauchy functions lend themselves to these transformations, models based on those functions[13,41,42] are not built on the assumption that the LWFs for the various channels are related in that way. These considerations aside, early visual processing will create a joint spatial/spatial-frequency representation whose properties should not be very different from those of the WFT or WT representations provided that channel bandwidths vary appropriately, whether or not the shape of their transfer functions meet the requirements for a strict WFT or WT analysis. In any case, there is no *a priori* reason to believe that the visual representation should qualify as a WFT or a WT representation. Justification for any of them is to be sought in their capability to account for empirical data and not in further rationalizations.

Acknowledgements

This work was supported by DGICYT grant PB90-0257 to the authors. We are indebted to John Daugman, Eli Peli and an anonymous reviewer, who generously provided their comments and criticisms of an earlier draft of this chapter.

References

1. F. W. Campbell and J. G. Robson, "Application of Fourier analysis to the visibility of gratings", *J. Physiol. (London)* **197** (1968) 551-566.
2. D. H. Kelly and C. Burbeck, "Critical problems in spatial vision", *CRC Crit. Rev. Biomed. Engng.* **10** (1984) 125-177.
3. J. C. R. Licklider, "Basic correlates of the auditory stimulus", in *Handbook of Experimental Psychology*, ed. S. S. Stevens (Wiley, New York, 1951), pp. 985-1039.
4. J. L. Flanagan, *Speech Analysis, Synthesis and Perception* (Springer, Berlin, 1972).
5. B. C. J. Moore, *Introduction to the Psychology of Hearing* (MacMillan, London, 1977).
6. C. F. Stromeyer and S. Klein, "Evidence against narrow-band spatial frequency channels in human vision: The detectability of frequency modulated gratings", *Vision Res.* **15** (1975) 899-910.
7. J. G. Robson, "Receptive fields: Neural representation of the spatial and intensive attributes of the visual image", in *Handbook of Perception. Vol V. Seeing*, ed. E. C. Carterette and M. P. Friedman (Academic Press, New York, 1975), pp. 81-116.
8. J. D. Cowan, "Some remarks on channel bandwidths for visual contrast detection", *Neurosciences Res. Prog. Bull.* **15** (1977) 492-517.
9. S. Marčelja, "Mathematical description of the responses of simple cortical cells", *J. Opt. Soc. Am.* **70** (1980) 1297-1300.
10. J. G. Daugman, "Complete discrete 2-D Gabor transforms by neural networks for image analysis and compression", *IEEE Trans. Acoust., Speech, Signal Processing* **36** (1988) 1169-1179.
11. A. B. Watson, "Efficiency of a model human image code", *J. Opt. Soc. Am. A* **4** (1987) 2401-2417.
12. M. Porat and Y. Y. Zeevi, "The generalized Gabor scheme of image representation in biological and machine vision", *IEEE Trans. Patt. Anal. Machine Intell.* **10** (1988) 452-468.
13. H. R. Wilson and J. R. Bergen, "A four mechanism model for threshold spatial vision", *Vision Res.* **19** (1979) 19-32.
14. A. B. Watson, "Detection and recognition of simple spatial forms", in *Physical and Biological Processing of Images*, ed. O. J. Braddick and A. C. Sleigh (Springer, Berlin, 1983), pp. 100-114.
15. W. Jaschinski-Kruza and C. R. Cavonius, "A multiple-channel model for grating detection", *Vision Res.* **24** (1984) 933-941.

59

16. J. G. Daugman, "Quadrature-phase simple-cell pairs are appropriately described in complex analytic form", *J. Opt. Soc. Am. A* **10** (1993) 375-377.
17. T. A. C. M. Claasen and W. F. G. Mecklenbräuker, "The Wigner distribution–A tool for time-frequency signal analysis. Part I: Continuous-time signals", *Philips J. Res.* **35** (1980) 217-250.
18. T. A. C. M. Claasen and W. F. G. Mecklenbräuker, "The Wigner distribution–A tool for time-frequency signal analysis. Part III: Relations with other time-frequency signal transformations", *Philips J. Res.* **35** (1980) 372-389.
19. L. D. Jacobson and H. Wechler, "Joint spatial/spatial-frequency representation", *Signal Processing* **14** (1988) 37-68.
20. L. Cohen, "Time-frequency distributions–A review", *Proc. IEEE* **77** (1989) 941-981.
21. G. Strang, "Wavelets and dilation equations: A brief introduction", *SIAM Rev.* **31** (1989) 614-627.
22. J. M. Combes, A. Grossmann and P. Tchamitchian, *Wavelets* (Springer, Berlin, 1989).
23. Y. Meyer, *Ondelettes et Opérateurs* (Hermann, Paris, 1990).
24. *IEEE Trans. Inform. Theory* special issue on Wavelet Transforms and Multiresolution Signal Analysis, **38(2-II)** (1992).
25. P. Flandrin, "Some aspects of non-stationary signal processing with emphasis on time-frequency and time-scale methods", in *Wavelets*, ed. J. M. Combes, A. Grossmann and P. Tchamitchian (Springer, Berlin, 1989), pp. 68-98.
26. A. P. Witkin, "Scale space filtering: A new approach to multi-scale description", in *Image Understanding 1984*, ed. S. Ullman and W. Richards (Ablex, Norwood, 1984), pp. 79-95.
27. E. Wigner, "On the quantum correction for thermodynamic equilibrium", *Phys. Rev.* **40** (1932) 749-759.
28. H. O. Bartelt, K.-H. Brenner and A. W. Lohmann, "The Wigner distribution function and its optical production", *Opt. Commun.* **32** (1980) 32-38.
29. L. Cohen, "Generalized phase-space distribution functions", *J. Math. Phys.* **7** (1966) 781-786.
30. D. Gabor, "Theory of communication", *J. Inst. Elect. Eng. (London)* **93** (1946) 429-457.
31. R. K. Potter, G. Kopp and H. C. Green, *Visible Speech* (Van Nostrand, New York, 1947).
32. J. Morlet, G. Arens, I. Forgeau and D. Giard, "Wave propagation and sampling theory–Part I: Complex signal and scattering in multilayered media", *Geophys.* **47** (1982) 203-221.
33. A. Grossmann and J. Morlet, "Decomposition of Hardy functions into square integrable wavelets of constant shape", *SIAM J. Math. Anal.* **15** (1984) 723-736.
34. I. Daubechies, "Orthonormal bases of wavelets with finite support–Connection with discrete filters", in *Wavelets*, ed. J. M. Combes, A. Grossmann and P. Tchamitchian (Springer, Berlin, 1989), pp. 38-66.

35. N. Delprat, B. Escudie, P. Guillemain, R. Kronland-Martinet, P. Tchamitchian and B. Torresani, "Asymptotic wavelet and Gabor analysis: Extraction of instantaneous frequencies", *IEEE Trans. Inform. Theory* **38** (1992) 644-664.

36. I. Daubechies, "The wavelet transform, time-frequency localization and signal analysis", *IEEE Trans. Inform. Theory* **36** (1990) 961-1005.

37. M. Holschneider, "On the wavelet transformation of fractal objects", *J. Stat. Phys.* **50** (1988) 963-993.

38. A. Grossmann, R. Kronland-Martinet and J. Morlet, "Reading and understanding continuous wavelet transforms", in *Wavelets*, ed. J. M. Combes, A. Grossmann and P. Tchamitchian (Springer, Berlin, 1989), pp. 2-20.

39. F. Argoul, A. Arneodo, G. Grasseau, Y. Gagne, E. J. Hopfinger and U. Frisch, "Wavelet analysis of turbulence reveals the multifractal nature of the Richardson cascade", *Nature (London)* **338** (1989) 51-53.

40. I. D. G. MacLeod and A. Rosenfeld, "The visibility of gratings: Spatial frequency channels or bar-detecting units", *Vision Res.* **14** (1974) 909-915.

41. R. J. Watt and M. J. Morgan, "A theory of the primitive spatial code in human vision", *Vision Res.* **25** (1985) 1661-1674.

42. S. A. Klein and D. M. Levi, "Hyperacuity thresholds of 1 sec: Theoretical predictions and empirical validation", *J. Opt. Soc. Am. A* **2** (1985) 1170-1190.

43. D. J. Fleet and A. D. Jepson, "Stability of phase information", *IEEE Trans. Patt. Anal. Mach. Intell.* **15** (1993) 1253-1268.

44. O. J. Braddick, F. W. Campbell and J. Atkinson, "Channels in vision: Basic aspects", in *Handbook of Sensory Physiology. Vol VIII. Perception*, ed. R. Held, H. W. Leibowitz and H.-L. Teuber (Springer, Berlin, 1978), pp. 3-38.

45. D. W. Williams and H. R. Wilson, "Spatial-frequency adaptation affects spatial-probability summation", *J. Opt. Soc. Am.* **73** (1983) 1367-1371.

46. J. J. Kulikowski, S. Marčelja and P. O. Bishop, "Theory of spatial position and spatial frequency relations in the receptive fields of simple cells in the visual cortex", *Biol. Cybernet.* **43** (1982) 187-198.

47. F. L. van Nes and M. A. Bouman, "Spatial modulation transfer in the human eye", *J. Opt. Soc. Am.* **57** (1967) 401-406.

48. M. A. García-Pérez and V. Sierra-Vázquez, "Some detection rules and their implications on the visibility of periodic and aperiodic patterns", manuscript in preparation.

49. M. A. García-Pérez and V. Sierra-Vázquez, "Deriving channel gains from large-area sine-wave contrast sensitivity data", *Spatial Vision*, in press.

50. D. H. Kelly, "Spatial frequency selectivity in the retina", *Vision Res.* **15** (1975) 665-672.

51. H. R. Wilson, "A synaptic model for spatial frequency adaptation", *J. Theor. Biol.* **50** (1975) 327-352.

52. F. W. Campbell, E. R. Howell and J. R. Johnstone, "A comparison of threshold and suprathreshold appearance of gratings with components in the low and high spatial frequency range", *J. Physiol. (London)* **284** (1978) 193-201.

53. F. W. Campbell, J. R. Johnstone and J. Ross, "An explanation for the visibility of low frequency gratings", *Vision Res.* **21** (1981) 723-730.

54. R. F. Quick and T. A. Reichert, "Spatial-frequency selectivity in contrast detection", *Vision Res.* **15** (1975) 637-643.

55. J. Ross and J. R. Johnstone, "Phase and detection of compound gratings", *Vision Res.* **20** (1980) 189-192.

56. N. Graham and J. Nachmias, "Detection of grating patterns containing two spatial frequencies: A comparison of single-channel and multiple-channel models", *Vision Res.* **11** (1971) 251-259.

57. J. P. Thomas, "Detection and identification: How are they related?", *J. Opt. Soc. Am. A* **2** (1985) 1457-1467.

58. N. Graham, "Detection and identification of near-threshold visual patterns", *J. Opt. Soc. Am. A* **2** (1985) 1468-1482.

59. M. C. Morrone and D. C. Burr, "Feature detection in human vision: A phase-dependent energy model", *Proc. R. Soc. Lond. B* **235** (1988) 221-245.

60. F. Kingdom and B. Moulden, "A multi-channel approach to brightness coding", *Vision Res.* **32** (1992) 1565-1582.

61. G. Brindley, *Physiology of the Retina and Visual Pathways* (Edward Arnold, London, 1960), p. 144.

62. A. Fiorentini, "Mach band phenomena", in *Handbook of Sensory Physiology. Vol VII/4. Visual Psychophysics*, ed. D. Jameson and L. M. Hurvich (Springer, Berlin, 1972), pp. 188-201.

63. J. Ross, M. C. Morrone and D. C. Burr, "The conditions under which Mach bands are visible", *Vision Res.* **29** (1989) 699-715.

64. J. Ross, J. J. Holt and J. R. Johnstone, "High frequency limitations on Mach bands", *Vision Res.* **21** (1981) 1165-1167.

65. F. Ratliff, "Why Mach bands are not seen at the edges of a step", *Vision Res.* **24** (1984) 163-165.

66. D. J. Tolhurst, "On the possible existence of edge detector neurones in the human visual system", *Vision Res.* **12** (1972) 797-804.

67. D. Teller, "Linking propositions", *Vision Res.* **24** (1984) 1233-1246.

68. J. Hirsch, R. Hylton and N. Graham, "Simultaneous recognition of two spatial-frequency components", *Vision Res.* **22** (1982) 365-375.

69. T. Shipley and C. Wier, "Asymmetries in the Machband phenomena", *Kybernetik* **10** (1972) 181-189.

70. C. S. Furchner, J. P. Thomas and F. W. Campbell, "Detection and discrimination of simple and complex patterns at low spatial frequencies", *Vision Res.* **17** (1977) 827-836.

71. M. A. Georgeson and G. D. Sullivan, "Contrast constancy: Deblurring in human vision by spatial frequency channels", *J. Physiol. (London)* **252** (1975) 627-656.

72. M. W. Cannon (1995), chapter in this book.

73. J. G. Daugman, "Spatial visual channels in the Fourier plane", *Vision Res.* **24** (1984) 891-910.

62

74. B. Sakitt and H. B. Barlow, "A model for the economical encoding of the visual image in cerebral cortex", *Biol. Cybernet.* **43** (1982) 97-108.
75. R. E. Kronauer and Y. Y. Zeevi, "Reorganization and diversification of signals in vision", *IEEE Trans. Syst., Man, Cybern.* **15** (1985) 91-101.
76. J. J. Koenderink and A. J. van Doorn, "Visual detection of spatial contrast; Influence of location in the visual field, target extent and illuminance level", *Biol. Cybernet.* **30** (1978) 157-167.
77. M. A. García-Pérez, "Space-variant visual processing: Spatially limited visual channels", *Spatial Vision* **3** (1988) 129-142.
78. H.-J. Fleck, "Measurement and modeling of peripheral detection and discrimination thresholds", *Biol. Cybernet.* **61** (1989) 437-446.
79. E. Peli, J. Yang and R. B. Goldstein, "Image invariance with changes in size: The role of peripheral contrast thresholds", *J. Opt. Soc. Am. A* **8** (1991) 1762-1774.
80. V. Virsu and J. Rovamo, "Visual resolution, contrast sensitivity, and the cortical magnification factor", *Exp. Brain Res.* **37** (1979) 475-494.
81. R. F. Quick, "A vector-magnitude model of contrast detection", *Kybernetik* **16** (1974) 65-67.
82. R. Hilz and C. R. Cavonius, "Functional organization of the peripheral retina: Sensitivity to periodic stimuli", *Vision Res.* **14** (1974) 1333-1337.
83. J. G. Robson and N. Graham, "Probability summation and regional variation in contrast sensitivity across the visual field", *Vision Res.* **21** (1981) 409-418.
84. J. S. Pointer and R. F. Hess, "The contrast sensitivity gradient across the human visual field: With emphasis on the low spatial frequency range", *Vision Res.* **29** (1989) 1133-1151.
85. N. Graham and B. E. Rogowitz, "Spatial pooling properties deduced from the detectability of FM and quasi-AM gratings: A reanalysis", *Vision Res.* **16** (1976) 1021-1026.
86. N. Graham, "Visual detection of aperiodic spatial stimuli by probability summation among narrowband channels", *Vision Res.* **17** (1977) 637-652.
87. T. Caelli, H. Brettel, I. Rentschler and R. Hilz, "Discrimination thresholds in the two-dimensional spatial frequency domain", *Vision Res.* **23** (1983) 129-133.
88. H. R. Wilson, D. K. McFarlane and G. C. Phillips, "Spatial frequency tuning of orientation selective units estimated by oblique masking", *Vision Res.* **23** (1983) 873-882.
89. G. C. Phillips and H. R. Wilson, "Orientation bandwidths of spatial mechanisms measured by masking", *J. Opt. Soc. Am. A* **1** (1984) 226-232.
90. L. O. Harvey and V. V. Doan, "Visual masking at different polar angles in the two-dimensional Fourier plane", *J. Opt. Soc. Am. A* **7** (1990) 116-127.
91. I. Daubechies, *Ten Lectures on Wavelets* (SIAM, Philadelphia, 1992), pp. 33-34.
92. C. K. Chui, *An Introduction to Wavelets* (Academic Press, New York, 1992), pp. 60-62.

SIMULATING NORMAL AND LOW VISION

ELI PELI

*The Schepens Eye Research Institute, Harvard Medical School
and The New England Eye Center, Tufts University School of Medicine
Boston, MA 02114 , USA*

Simulation may provide insights into the factors that control the appearance of images to normal and visually impaired observers. The linear spectral methods that have been useful in interpreting low contrast, threshold phenomena with periodic stimuli are inappropriate for analyzing the local contrast in images. Linear simulations commonly use the normalized contrast sensitivity function (CSF) as a modulation transfer function (MTF) applied to the image amplitude rather than to contrast. Simulations within the linear model are limited by a number of problems discussed here. To achieve a valid simulation, a measure of local band-limited contrast in images is needed. Such a measure was developed and was used to simulate the threshold nonlinear characteristics of the visual system and suprathreshold contrast constancy. This approach was used to simulate both central vision and vision with peripheral retina. In the latter, the simulations were based on CSF measurements across the retina. Methods to test the validity of these simulations were implemented. The results of preliminary testing confirm our ability to evaluate important parameters of the model and point to previously unnoted image dependent characteristics of visual perception.

1. Introduction

Simulations of various environments are frequently created to provide cost effective or less dangerous methods of training or evaluating operational capabilities of machines and their operators. I will discuss here the simulation of the appearance of a scene in the environment to an observer when viewed on a display. Such pictorial representations have been attempted by many over the years in an effort to illustrate the effects on observers of visual disability[5,15,30], changes in observation distance[10], and the use of peripheral vision[34]. More recently, the simulation of human observers has been integrated with the physical simulation of new display systems[16]. This combination should enable visual effects to be considered as part of the display.

Why do we need simulations? After all, the concepts of linear filters and convolution have become common enough in visual perception research to provide most workers with intuitions about the effects of simple filters on various signals. I will try to show that these basic linear system concepts may not be sufficient or appropriate for the analysis of the appearance of complex images. The simulations that I propose overcome some

64

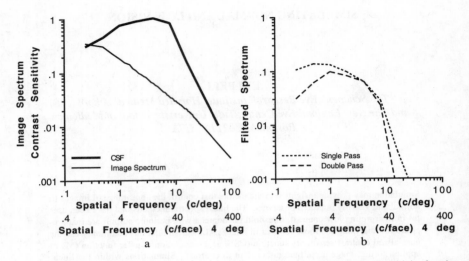

Figure 1. Linear simulation of the appearance of images. a) The normalized contrast sensitivity function (CSF, thick line) used to multiply the Fourier transform of the image. The Fourier transform is illustrated by the radially averaged amplitude spectrum of a face image (thin line). b) The result of the multiplication is illustrated by a dotted line. When the observer examines the simulation it is processed once more by the same contrast sensitivity function (dashed line) leading to the *double-pass* problem.

of these difficulties and thus can provide the required insight. Further, I will demonstrate that the simulated images may be useful for testing the visual system models underlying them and may lead to better, more refined models.

When simulations are intended to illustrate differences among subjects' visual sensitivities, one must be particularly careful about interpreting the resulting images. There are two problems. First, the images must be computed and displayed to the observer in such a way that the observer's spatial sensitivity characteristics do not interact with the phenomena being portrayed. Ginsburg's[10] linear simulations of the appearance of images to normal subjects have been criticized for the *double-pass* effect, resulting when the simulated image is processed again by the reader's visual system[36]. However, by careful design it is possible to present images in which the important details are relatively unaffected by the characteristics of the reader's visual system. For example, the linear systems approach, in which the ratio of the abnormal to the normal contrast sensitivity function (CSF) represents the modulation transfer function (MTF), was used to simulate low vision and represent the appearance of images to amblyopes[15]. When simulating low vision, the double-pass problem is insignificant. The detail loss suffered by the patient and portrayed in the simulation is at a spatial scale and of such a large magnitude that the effects of the normal reader's visual system can be ignored.

The second problem, which arises from treating the CSF as an MTF, is more serious and applies to simulation of both normal and low vision. The linear systems approach to simulation[10,11] ignores many aspects of the nonlinearities of the visual system, at least three of which are important for simulations. First, information that is below threshold is not merely highly attenuated, it is lost and cannot be recovered (the threshold nonlinearity). Second, curves of constant suprathreshold apparent contrast are not multiples of the CSF. Above threshold, apparent contrast is relatively independent of retinal eccentricity and spatial frequency (contrast constancy), while the contrast threshold changes significantly[2]. Third, thresholding should be applied to image contrast, which is a nonlinear function of the local amplitudes in the image (contrast nonlinearity). To be valid, simulations must take these nonlinearities into account.

In the simulations presented here, all three nonlinearities were incorporated. The simulations explicitly applied the threshold nonlinearity, and the processing was done in the nonlinear contrast domain rather than the amplitude domain. This approach has the additional effect of reducing the double-pass problem. When one wishes to portray the loss of details that occurs in viewing an object from a specified distance, the simulations

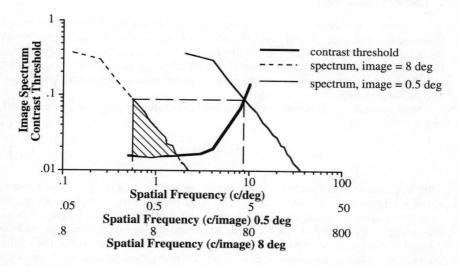

Figure 2. Reducing the double-pass problem within the context of a nonlinear threshold model of the visual system. Assume that the amplitude spectrum (thin solid line) represents a "contrast" spectrum of an image spanning 0.5 deg. Image content beyond the intersection of the observer's contrast detection threshold (thick line) and the spectrum will not be visible to the observer. This could be simulated by removing all image content to the right of the intersection. If the simulated image is then magnified or inspected from a short distance, where it spans 8 deg (dashed line), most of the effects of simulation (shaded area) will be suprathreshold and these effects can be detected by the observer when the simulation is compared to the unprocessed original image.

should remove the details that drop below threshold at that distance with a process that mimics the effect of the visual system[22]. The image then should be magnified (or equivalently, examined from a shorter distance) so that the surviving fine details are large enough to be seen without being affected appreciably by the reader's visual system (Fig. 2). Since the subthreshold information was removed completely, it cannot be altered by the reader's visual system. To use this approach, a method of measuring local contrast in images is required.

In this chapter I will:

1) Define a metric to represent local band-limited contrast in complex images;
2) Discuss the effects of visual nonlinearities on the appearance of images in foveal vision;
3) Illustrate how the simulations can be used to evaluate the contrast thresholds obtained with different psychophysical stimuli;
4) Present a formulation for simulating the appearance of images processed with an inhomogeneous retina.

2. Local Band-limited Contrast

Contrast is a basic perceptual attribute, based on the amplitudes within an image. However, the measurement and evaluation of contrast and contrast variations in arbitrary images are not uniquely defined in the literature. I have proposed a definition of local band-limited contrast in complex images[22] that is more closely aligned to the common definition of contrast in simple test patterns and can better relate measured physical contrast to visual perception.

Most commonly, the contrast of images has been evaluated using the Michelson definition

$$c = \frac{L_{max} - L_{min}}{L_{max} + L_{min}} . \tag{1}$$

With this definition the contrast of the whole image is dependent on only a few points of extreme brightness or darkness. Thus, there is no reference to, or dependency on, the spatial frequency content of the image. In addition, all commonly used measures of contrast assign a single value of contrast to the whole image, ignoring the local variations of contrast within images[18]. The basis of the local band-limited contrast is that the level of the local mean luminance should be considered in defining the contrast at every point and at every frequency band[22].

To define local band-limited contrast for a complex image, a band-limited version of the image in the frequency domain, $A(u,v)$, must first be obtained using a radially symmetric bandpass filter, $G(\rho)$.

$$A(u,v) \equiv A(\rho,\theta) = F(\rho,\theta) \cdot G(\rho) \tag{2}$$

where u and v are the horizontal and vertical spatial frequency coordinates, and ρ and θ represent the polar spatial frequency coordinates:

$$\rho = \sqrt{u^2 + v^2} \tag{3}$$

$$\theta = \tan^{-1}\left(\frac{v}{u}\right); \tag{4}$$

and where $F(\rho,\theta)$ is the Fourier transform of the image $f(x,y)$. We call the spatial frequency support of this bandpass filter the band.

In the space domain, the filtered image $a(x,y)$ can be represented similarly:

$$a(x,y) = f(x,y) * g(x,y) \tag{5}$$

where $(*)$ represents the convolution operator and $g(x,y)$ is the inverse Fourier transform of the bandpass filter $G(\rho)$. We also can define for every $a(x,y)$ the corresponding $l(x,y)$, which is a lowpass filtered image containing all energy below the band of interest. The contrast at the band can be represented as a two-dimensional array $c(x,y)$:

$$c(x,y) = \frac{a(x,y)}{l(x,y)} \tag{6}$$

where $l(x,y) > 0$. This definition provides a local contrast measure for every band that depends not only on the local energy at that band, but also on the local background luminance as it varies from place to place in the image.

The computation of local band-limited contrast as described above is conceptually identical to any of the commonly used pyramids of bandpass-filtered images[38]. Since for the application of the simulation images of equal size are used at all bands, we avoid the common approach of sub sampling the image recursively, filtering, and then upsampling the reduced size images. Instead, all filtering is done in the frequency domain. Thus the content of the final pyramid of image scales is identical to the images that would be calculated by upsampling images obtained on a pyramid of image resolution.

The details of the implementation of this pyramidal image analysis structure in the discrete, digital case have been described elsewhere[22]. Various implications of this definition of contrast, and their relation to the perceived contrast in complex images, were also discussed. The most important implications for the purposes of simulation are the facts that contrast and amplitude differ and cannot simply be interchanged, and that "linear rescaling" of images, which linearly scales amplitudes, results in a nonlinear space-varying change of contrast. Other investigators have recently adopted similar approaches to the calculations of local contrast and the generation of simulations[3,4]. The following section illustrates pictorially the steps involved in calculating the local band-limited contrast for an image and demonstrates the way it is used to generate simulations of image

68

appearance. The same basic method is applied to the simulation of vision with the central retina and the simulation of image appearance with peripheral retina. Preliminary results of psychophysical testing of the validity of these simulations are described as well.

3. Appearance of Images Using Central Retina

The pyramidal image-contrast architecture described above enables the use of non-linear processing to simulate the appearance of centrally fixated images point-by-point

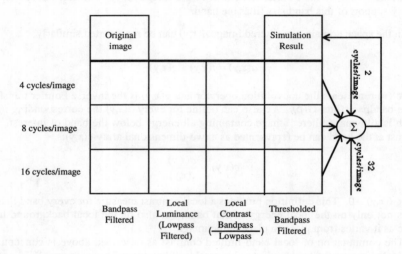

Figure 3a. Schematic illustration of the process of generating the simulations depicted in Fig. 3b. Upper left, the original image; top right, the final simulated appearance of the same image to the observer. The three rows represent processing at different spatial frequencies on the pyramid. The left column in each row represents the bandpass filtered image obtained from the original image. The second column in each row represents the corresponding lowpass filtered version for the same scale, i.e. all the energy below the band represented in the first column. The third column represents the contrast images. The bandpass filtered arrays are bipolar and a DC level of 128 has been added arbitrarily in order to present those arrays as images. Images in the right column represent the thresholded bandpass filtered images. For each image in the third column, each point was tested against the threshold value for the corresponding spatial frequency. If the contrast of the image at that point is above threshold, the corresponding point from the left image is maintained and reproduced in the right column. If the contrast at a point is below threshold, the corresponding point is set to zero (gray) in the right image. The simulated image, top right, is generated by summing all of the images in the right column. Actual processing included two additional rows, one at 2 cycles per image and one at 32 cycles per image, not shown.

Figure 3b (facing page). The process of simulating the appearance of an image (spanning 4 deg of visual angle) to a low vision patient. The rows and columns are explained in the schematic of Fig. 3a.

and for every spatial frequency band in the image. This process is illustrated in Fig. 3 using the CSF of a patient with a central scotoma due to macular disease. (A patient's CSF was used to obtain more noticeable effects than those obtained with a normal observer's CSF.) The images were sectioned in the frequency domain into 1-octave bands.

Contrast at each spatial position was calculated by dividing, for each pixel location, the bandpass filtered pixel value by the lowpass filtered pixel value at the same point. At each pyramid (scale) level, every point was compared with the appropriate observer's contrast threshold for the corresponding spatial frequency. If the contrast at that point was higher than the threshold, the amplitude of that point was not affected. If the contrast at the point was below threshold, the amplitude was set to zero. Thus, the final image in Fig. 3, top right, represents the appearance of the original image to a patient using the

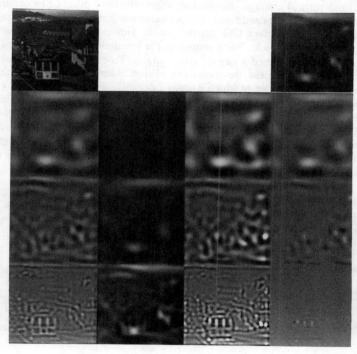

Fig. 3b

same retinal area used to obtain the CSF data. This image was processed with the stipulation that the image span 4 deg of visual angle. On this scale, this patient's visual loss had little effect on information at 4 cycles per image (corresponding to 1 c/deg, top row). A small effect may be noted at 8 cycles per image (middle row), and a substantial effect at 16 cycles per image (corresponding to 4 c/deg, bottom row). The complete processing also included the band at 2 cycles per image and 32 cycles per image, neither of which is shown. The simulated image maintains the full-contrast appearance reported by patients with central visual loss and clear media and is not faded or washed out, as may be the appearance of images simulated with linear filtering.

To simulate the appearance to a normal observer, the mean CSF from 14 normal observers[23] was used. The CSF data were obtained from a task requiring discrimination of horizontal from vertical gratings. Simulations were calculated using CSFs obtained with both 1-octave Gabor patches and fixed-aperture extended gratings. The appearance of an image to a subject with a given CSF depends on the viewing geometry assumed for the modeled observation situation. For example, in the simulations shown in Fig. 4, we assumed that the scene spanned 2 deg of visual angle. To evaluate the simulations and avoid the double-pass problem, the reader should first examine the original image (Fig. 4a) from a distance of 1 meter, at which it spans 2 deg.

This appearance should then be compared with the simulated images examined from a distance of 25 cm. At this distance, the simulations calculated using the patch-CSF (1-octave) (Fig. 4c) should resemble the appearance of the original when viewed from 1 meter. Specifically, the loss of fine details is visible. On the other hand, the simulations based on the fixed-aperture CSF (Fig. 4b) viewed at a distance of 25 cm appear to be al-

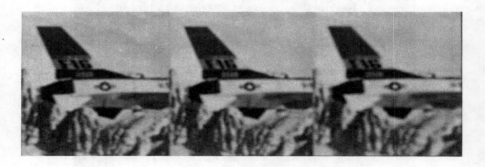

a   b   c

Figure 4. Simulations of the appearance of an image under several viewing conditions. a) Original image. b) Image processed to simulate the original's appearance when it spans 2 deg of visual angle based on the CSF measured with fixed-aperture gratings. c) Same as b, but processed using the CSF measured with the 1-octave patch stimuli. The printed images should span 2 deg at a distance of 1 meter (about 29 times the image width).

most identical to the original image. Thus, the appearance of the patch simulation at 25 cm more closely represents normal perception of the original (2 deg) image, suggesting that the 1-octave bandwidth Gabor patch may be a better stimulus if one wishes to measure a CSF that characterizes the normal appearance of complex images[25].

A second way to view these images is to examine all three of them side by side from different distances. The original image should appear indistinguishable from the simulated image when both are viewed from a distance larger than that assumed in computing the simulation. However, as the two images are moved closer to the observer, the simulation should be easy to discriminate from the original. The reader may verify that these relations appear to hold when the patch simulation is compared to the original image, but the fixed-aperture simulation is not easily distinguished from the original even at short distances. These effects may be difficult to discern in the printed photographs due to problems in obtaining accurate reproduction. However, both effects are visible when observed on a calibrated display. A formal application of this method to test the simulations is described below.

Figure 5 depicts the relationship between the measured contrast thresholds and the amplitude spectra of the image at various viewing distances. The radially averaged amplitude spectrum of the image gives the approximate contrast at each frequency expressed in cycles per face. (It is only approximate because in the simulations we were working with local contrast, not amplitude.)

The same logic applies to both the patch-CSF simulation (Fig. 5, bottom) and the fixed-aperture CSF simulation (Fig. 5, top). The dashed line in each panel represents the radially averaged amplitude spectra of the real (thin line) and simulated (thick dashed line) images when they subtend 2 deg on the retina. The solid curves represent the spectra of the same images when they subtend 4 deg. Any information in the image that falls below the observer's threshold (i.e., to the right of the point at which the contrast threshold curve intersects the image spectrum curve) is not visible to the observer. To illustrate this, the simulation should (as is shown) remove all that information (thick curve). If the original and simulated images are viewed from the simulated distance or farther (subtending 2 deg or less), they should be indistinguishable because the reader's CSF removes the same information from the original that was removed in the simulation. However, if the original and simulation are viewed from a closer distance, the difference in content (shaded area) between the original and the patch simulation should be visible.

Figure 5 is useful only to illustrate the logic of the simulations. The analysis it represents does not provide the information obtainable from the simulations. The effects of contrast threshold on apparent contrast in the image are local, not global. The effective contrast is not represented accurately by the radially averaged amplitude spectrum, and the simulation algorithm is not represented accurately by the filtering.

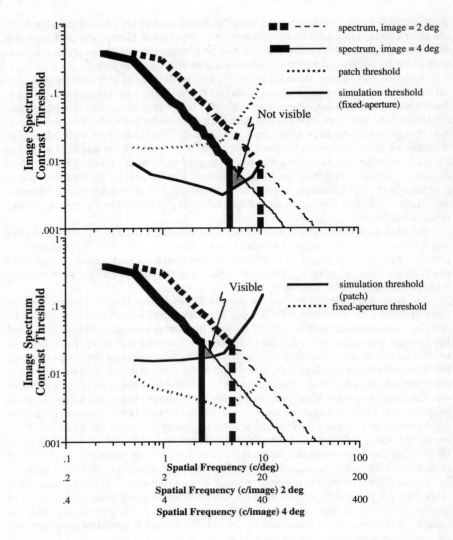

Figure 5. See caption opposite page.

This analysis, used in conjunction with the results of the observations of Fig. 4, described above, lead to the following conclusion: The loss of detail depicted by the shaded area is visible in the case of the patch-CSF simulation (Fig. 5, bottom and Fig. 4c), but not for the fixed-aperture CSF simulation (Fig. 5, top and Fig. 4b), indicating that the simulation-viewer's actual threshold lies above the shaded area in Fig. 5, top and below the shaded area in Fig. 5, bottom. Therefore, the patch-CSF simulation more closely represents the visibility of detail to a normal observer. One can test the validity of the simulations and the CSF data used by formally measuring the observations described above. Preliminary results from such testing are described next.

3.1. Testing the Simulations of Central Vision

The simulations can be tested by presenting the original image side by side with the simulation. If the simulations are valid, the simulated image and the original will be indistinguishable from a distance equal to or larger than the distance assumed in the simulation. The two images should be progressively easier to distinguish at distances shorter than the simulated distance.

Observers viewed image pairs from various distances and were asked to make a forced-choice distinction between the simulated and the original image. In each presentation one of the images was the original and the other was one of the simulations. We used four different images in this experiment. From each image, we calculated three simulated views representing views from three different distances. For the three distances (40, 80, and 160 in) the images spanned visual angles of 4, 2, and 1 deg, respectively. The subjects observed the image pairs from six distances, including shorter (20 in) than the shortest simulated distance and longer (300 in) than the longest simulated distance. From each observation distance the percent correct identification of the processed/simulated image was tabulated. The data for each simulated distance were fitted with a Weibull psychometric function to determine threshold at a 75% correct level of performance (Fig. 6). The CSF data used in the simulations were obtained for each sub-

---

Figure 5. Relationships among spatial frequency spectra of images and contrast thresholds. Spatial frequency is expressed in c/deg and cycles/image for different image sizes. Thin solid-line spectrum: 2 deg image; thin dotted-line spectrum: 4 deg image. Top: Simulation using fixed-aperture CSF. Bottom: Simulation using patch CSF. The medium thickness solid line represents the CSF used for simulation. Contrast below that curve is below the simulated subject's contrast threshold. Therefore, we remove image components to the right of the point where the threshold curve intersects the 2 deg image spectrum (thick dotted line). At the 2 deg distance, the removed components are below threshold and thus the original image and simulation should appear identical. When the original and simulation are moved to the 4 deg distance, a portion of the removed components (shaded area) will be above threshold and visible if the CSF used for the simulation is an accurate description of the viewer's visual system. Viewers can see the difference at 4 deg between the patch simulation and the original (Fig. 4a and c) but cannot see the difference between the fixed-aperture simulation and the original (Fig. 4a and b), indicating that the viewer's threshold curve lies below the shaded area of Fig. 5, bottom and above the shaded area of Fig. 5, top.

ject individually. In the first set of experiments, simulated images were produced with CSFs obtained using 1-octave Gabor patches and the observer's task was to discriminate gratings of horizontal orientation from those of vertical orientation[23]. Three observers participated in this experiment and their results were similar.

Data from one subject (Fig. 6) illustrates that the simulations generated using the CSF obtained with a discrimination of orientation task of 1-octave stimuli did not support our hypothesis. The hypothesis tested is that if the simulations are veridical the fitted curves should cross the 75% correct level at the simulated distance, marked by diamonds at the bottom of the graph. It appears that the observer could detect the changes at greater distances from the screen than the distance assumed in the simulation. The next set of experiments involved simulated images produced with the CSF obtained for the same type of stimuli but using a simple detection task. When we used CSF data obtained using a detection task for the same 1-octave stimuli, the results were much closer to the predictions. The results from one subject are illustrated in Fig. 7. These results illustrate that,

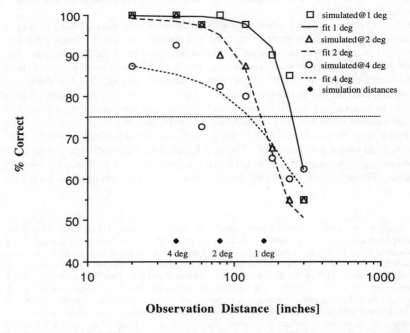

Figure 6. Results of testing central vision simulation using the CSF based on discrimination of orientation of 1- octave Gabor patches. The data and the psychometric function fits indicate that the subject could distinguish the simulation from the original at distances larger than the distances assumed in the simulations (see diamond inserts at bottom of graph).

using this methodology, we can reject the simulations generated using the orientation discrimination threshold but not the simulations using the contrast detection threshold. The differences between the CSFs used in these two modes of testing are illustrated in Fig. 8.

4. Vision with Central Scotoma

Vision with central visual field loss (scotoma) frequently is simulated using a black spot covering a central part of an image. Image details outside the simulated area of the scotoma remain unaltered and thus appear sharp and clear. This simplistic representation is static and does not represent the patient's ability to see details of interest by moving his or her eyes and thus the scotoma. In addition, these simulations, which have been applied to both still print images[5] and video motion picture simulations[30], fail to represent the reduced visual capabilities of the patient's functioning peripheral retina. Patients rarely report their visual experience as that of losing a part of the visual field. Instead they commonly complain of blurred or foggy vision. Experiencing the field loss requires directed

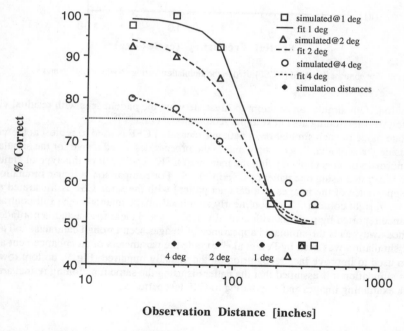

Figure 7. Results of simulation testing using the CSF based on detection of 1-octave Gabor patches. Here the subject could distinguish the simulation from the original approximately at the distance assumed in the simulations (see diamond inserts at bottom of graph).

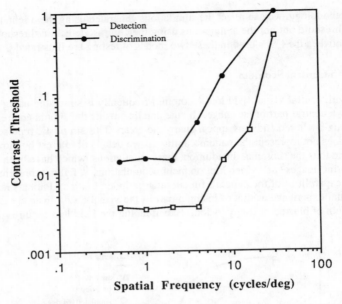

Figure 8. The contrast threshold (1/CSF) used in the simulation testing shown in Figs. 6 and 7.

examination. Our simulations attempt to illustrate what the patient sees with residual vision using the functioning area next to the scotomatous retina[26,28].

In one mode of such simulation, a patient's measured CSF is used to represent the vision outside the scotoma. Processing equal to the process described above for the simulation of normal vision is applied using the measured CSF. The result of this type of simulation is illustrated using one patient's CSF in Fig. 9. For comparison, a linear simulation of the appearance of the images to a cataract patient with the same CSF is illustrated as well (Fig. 9, right column). The nonlinearly simulated image maintains the full-contrast appearance reported by patients with central visual loss and clear media and is not faded or washed away, as is the simulated appearance of images seen through cataracts[27]. This type of simulation was used by Peli et al.[26] to tune the parameters of an enhancement algorithm used to improve face recognition by the visually impaired (Fig. 9, bottom row). For this simulation it is assumed that the patient is using the same functioning retinal area for both examining images and responding to CSF test patterns.

4.1. Vision with Nonuniform Retina

Another way to simulate and understand vision with central scotoma is to include in the simulation the variability in sensitivity across the retina of a normal observer and then examine the consequences of losing the central area to the way images will be perceived in the periphery.

Spatial inhomogeneities are an important feature of the visual system's organization. Nonuniform processing starts with the spatially variable sampling rate of the photoreceptors, featuring a high density centrally and gradually decreasing density toward the retinal periphery. The nonuniform organization continues throughout the system up to the retinotopic mapping of the visual field onto the surface of the striate cortex[32]. This nonuniform structure, a visually unfavorable characteristic of the visual system (commonly considered biologically necessary), is assumed to be a response to limitations of the nonuniform imaging by the eye's optics or a method to reduce data rate in response to limited processing capabilities[40].

In contrast, we showed that the changes in contrast sensitivity across the retina may play an important role in maintaining size (distance) invariance[28]. The spatial frequency spectra of images frequently are defined in terms of cycles per picture-width rather than cycles per degree[6,11]. This is done under the assertion that "form perception is largely independent of distance" (ref. 6, p. 196). Such distance invariance has been reported for identification of bandpass filtered letters embedded in Gaussian noise[20], for recognition

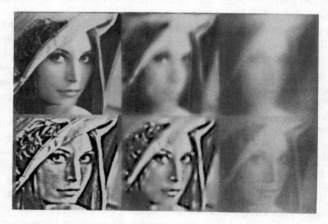

Figure 9. Simulations of the appearance of original images (top row) and enhanced face images (bottom row) for patients with central scotoma and cataract. Both patients were assumed to have the same contrast sensitivity function, and the images were assumed to span 4 deg of visual angle. The left column represents the original and enhanced images. The middle column simulates the appearance of both images to a patient with central scotoma (nonlinear processing). The right column illustrates the appearance of the same images to a patient with cataract (linear filtering). Note the improvement in visibility of detail for both simulated patients when the images are enhanced.

of bandpass filtered face images[13], and for identification of toy tanks' images[19]. Invariant perception also requires that important image features remain visible (do not drop below threshold) with changes in retinal spatial frequencies associated with the change in distance. This property of the visual system that causes its *detection* of image contrast to be nearly invariant to changes in size due to distance changes should be included in a proper simulation of vision. We have shown that the threshold distance invariance away from the fovea is as good as the invariance at the fovea[28]. For spatial frequencies straddling the peak of the CSF, the deviation from optimal invariance is small. The invariance model contains the foveal CSF in addition to the fundamental eccentricity constant (FEC), representing the drop in contrast sensitivity as a function of retinal eccentricity. Specifically, the FEC is the slope of the line representing contrast threshold as a function of eccentricity for a stimulus of 1 c/deg on a log-log graph. The CSF across the whole retina for all spatial frequencies can be described as a function of the foveal CSF and the FEC.

This enables the simulation of the appearance of wide angle images that are affected by the nonuniformity of the visual system. By using the same pyramidal image-contrast structure discussed above, together with the variation across the visual field, we can simulate the appearance of images with a nonuniform retina. As above, the image is sectioned into a series of bandpass filtered versions of 1-octave bandwidth. For each section, we calculated the corresponding local band-limited contrast for each point in the image. We then assigned a fixation locus, and for each point in the image the distance from this fixation point was determined. Based on that distance, in degrees, and the spatial frequency associated with the bandpass filtered version, each point can be tested against the appropriate threshold at that location to determine if it will be visible. A suprathreshold point is left unchanged while a subthreshold point is set to zero contrast. The appearance of the same image from two different distances is obtained by applying the same method of simulation while assigning a different angular span to the image depending on the observation distance. The simulations presented in Fig. 10 were obtained using the fit to the data of Cannon[2].

The simulated appearance of a scene to a normal observer from a distance where it spans 32 deg of visual angle is compared in Fig. 10 (top) to the appearance of the same scene spanning only 2 deg. In both cases, fixation is assumed to be at the center of the image, and there is little apparent change in image quality at different eccentricities. Furthermore, the two images appear similar despite the large difference in observation distances. The only noticeable effect is a slight blurring of the fine details of the "smaller" image. Such effects are associated with the suboptimality of the invariance and are included in our simulation. This constancy breaks down for an observer with a central visual loss of 5 deg radius as illustrated in Fig. 10 (bottom). Here we assumed that the observer placed the image of the scene on the retina adjacent to the scotomatous area, i.e. on the most centrally available functional retina[35]. At 32 deg, the wide field simulated image appears almost the same to the low vision observer as to the normal observer. However, when the scene spans only 2 deg of visual angle, the low vision observer suffers from a substantial loss of detail, and the invariant appearance of the image cannot be

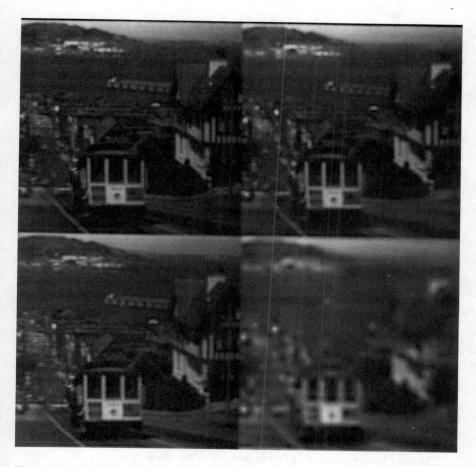

Figure 10. Changes in the appearance of a scene with a large change in observation distance are simulated for a normal observer (top) and for a patient with a 10 deg-diameter central scotoma (bottom). Images on the left represent the appearance of the scene to the observers when it spans 32 deg of visual angle. Images on the right represent the appearance of the same scene to the observers when it spans only 2 deg of visual angle. The normal observer is assumed to fixate at the center of the image in both cases. The patient is assumed to place the edge of the scotoma at the left edge of the image in both cases. The changes in appearance for the normal observer are small, limited to the very high spatial frequencies and compatible with the filtering of the image by the eye's optical media. The effect of change in distance is much more detrimental for the patient with a central scotoma. Note that at close range, the appearance of the scene to the patient is almost identical to its appearance to the normal observer. The effect in both cases is somewhat under represented in the simulation because the 512×512 pixels image at 32 deg contains information only up to 8 c/deg. The natural scene contains information at higher frequencies.

maintained. Thus, the same mechanism that serves to maintain the appearance of the image for normals across this 16-to-1 change in distance results in a deterioration of the appearance of the image for a patient with central scotoma.

4.2. Testing the Simulations of Nonuniform Retina

In testing the simulations of the appearance of wide images we look for the ability to distinguish the simulation from the unprocessed original using peripheral retina. The hypothesis in this case is that the two images become indistinguishable when the simulation closely represents the losses of image detail that occur with eccentricity. Changing the distance, however, should have little effect if our model of image invariance with change in distance[28] is of any value. In this case we also wish to determine which CSF stimuli are better estimaters of observers' perception and whether our estimate of the FEC is valid.

The testing stimuli were generated from two high resolution (1024×1024) images processed to simulate their appearance when fixated at the center and spanning 64 deg of visual angle[24]. Half of an original (unprocessed) image was displayed side by side with the simulation applied to the mirror image of the same image (Fig. 11) using two different CSF data sets. These data sets were obtained using 1-octave Gabor patches[28], and Cannon's[2] fixed aperture 2 deg extended gratings. We implemented these two types of simulations with the FEC values found for two tasks, 0.035 and 0.055 for contrast detection and discrimination of a vertical grating from a horizontal grating, respectively[28], and with two additional arbitrary levels on each side. The images were displayed on a large screen projection TV spanning 64 deg of visual angle. Image pairs were presented abruptly for 167 msec to prevent eye movements. Subjects were required to identify the processed (slightly blurred) half of the screen while maintaining fixation at the center of the screen. The central 6.4 deg of the field was masked with a gray circular patch of mean image luminance. Note that although these images contained no information above 8 c/deg the size of the central mask assures that for most of the image, the sensitivity of the observer's peripheral retina that had to be used was so poor that even with 100% contrast, higher frequencies could not be detected.

The most important result of this experiment is that the data actually fell along the active slope of the psychometric function (Fig. 12). Our prediction was that if the simulations were veridical, the threshold FEC (arbitrarily set to 75% correct response) should be close to either the 0.035 or the 0.055 values, where it is indeed found. This initial finding is encouraging. It illustrates that the simulations are not grossly incorrect. It would be easy, with simulations based on basic visual function measurements, to have images which are either completely distinguishable or completely indistinguishable.

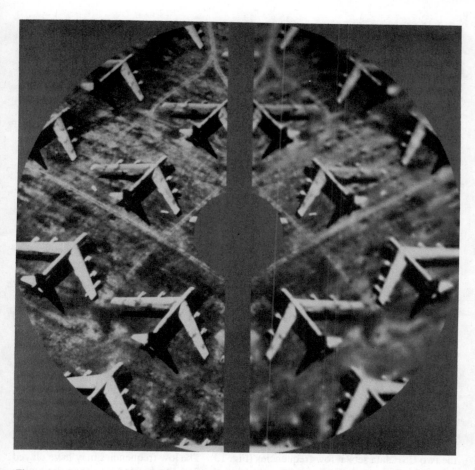

Figure 11. An example of the stimuli used in testing the simulation of wide images. The original unprocessed image on the left was compared with the simulation using the CSF obtained with Gabor patches of 1-octave bandwidth and an FEC of 0.1 on the right. This high value of the FEC results in clearly visible blurring at the edge of the image. The whole image spanned 64 deg at the observer's eye, and the central 6.4 deg were masked as shown. (This work was done in collaboration with G. Geri.)

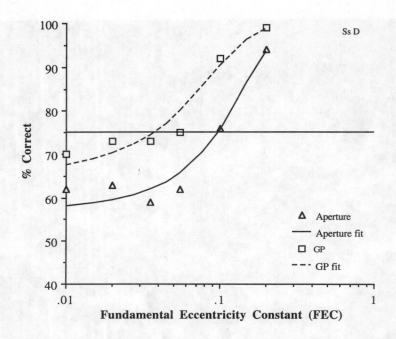

Figure 12. Results of testing the wide field simulations. Percent correct discrimination of the original from the simulation is plotted as a function of the FEC. Data are shown for two sets of simulations, one using 1-octave Gabor patch-CSF data (GP) and the other using Cannon's[2] data obtained with a fixed-aperture grating stimulus.

The Gabor patch based simulations resulted in FEC thresholds closer to our prediction than the fixed-aperture simulations. But this difference is not large despite fairly large differences in the corresponding CSFs. This might be the result of the similarity of the two CSF data sets at low frequencies (Fig. 13). The low frequencies may have played a more important role in the peripheral vision simulated and tested here than the higher frequencies where the CSFs, and therefore the simulations, differ.

A surprising result was that even for very low FEC values the detection of the simulation was much better than 50% (Fig. 12). Such a result is possible since even for an FEC of 0, the images are processed (using the effect of the foveal CSF), and therefore differ from the original. However, it is important to note that for the low values used, the simulations were processed so little that they were practically indistinguishable when examined carefully side by side on the screen with foveal vision for unlimited time. We believe that the high level of discrimination in the periphery is a result of the abrupt presentation[23]. However, extending the time of presentation to 500 msec did not change the results.

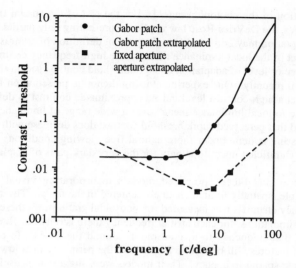

Figure 13. The foveal contrast threshold data sets used in testing the wide field simulations. Note the convergence of the two sets at low spatial frequencies.

Another consistent result was that for all our subjects, one of the images was easier to distinguish than the other. This difference should be explored further to determine the nature of the image content that led to this result. The issue of image dependence has been largely ignored. Watson[39] has recently shown the benefits that can be obtained from image dependent compression coding. The consideration of image dependent factors in simulation may also be of value in the analysis of image quality and image quality metrics. The simplest assumption is that the image dependent effect found is due to the relative spatial frequency content of different images. It is plausible that if an image has little high frequency information the original and the simulation will be harder to discriminate, since the effect of simulation will be smaller. The proper metrics for such spatial frequency content have not yet been determined.

5. Discussion

The basic assumption of this work is that local image contrast should be expressed as the dimensionless ratio of the local amplitude and the local average luminance in a way similar to that expressed in the definition of Michelson contrast or Weber fraction. The use of such a ratio implies that the human's sensitivity to the amplitude of change in luminance varies with the adaptation level associated with the local average luminance[31]. This is known to be the case for threshold contrast sensitivity at all spatial frequencies at high luminance levels. For low frequencies (less than 4 c/deg), the same relation is true for a large portion of the photopic range[14]. For the rest of the spatial frequencies and luminance ranges, the DeVries-Rose law applies, representing only partial adaptation.

Partial adaptation may be included in the present definition of contrast simply by reducing the effect of the local luminance mean on the high-frequency contrast to some degree. The degree or level of adaptation in suprathreshold contrast sensitivity has not been determined until recently. One experiment using dichoptic presentation found that contrast matching at a high-contrast level indeed approximated contrast as defined by the ratio of amplitude to local luminance mean[9] over a wide range of luminances. In a recent study, we found that perceived suprathreshold contrast does decrease with low luminance levels when testing is done under more natural free viewing conditions[29]. The effect, however, is of significant magnitude only for the very dark parts of displays viewed in a dark room.

García-Pérez[8] and Fleck[7] proposed models incorporating visual inhomogeneity based on multiple, spatially limited channels centered in the fovea. The spatial extent of various frequency channels was measured for sinusoidal gratings. In these models, which were used for simulations, for each spatial frequency there is only one threshold, limiting all features of that frequency to a fixed radius around the fovea. In our simulations, higher-contrast features will be visible farther into the periphery than lower-contrast features of the same spatial frequency. Their models were suggested as useful tools to analyze various visual perceptual phenomena such as the Gestalt frame of reference effect[8]. However, the role of the nonuniform visual system in aiding size-distance invariance was not considered.

This model[22] provides a new, more powerful tool to analyze the visibility of displays[3], generate equal visibility displays, or generate displays of pre-designed variable visibility. The model generalized the idea underlying Anstis'[1] equal visibility acuity chart. This generalization is achieved by adding the dimension of contrast and by providing a computationally efficient algorithm for its application to any image.

5.1. Future Work

Contrast measured by filtering, as suggested here, defines only incremental or decremental changes from the local background. This is analogous to the symmetric (cosine phase) responses of mechanisms or cells in the visual system. Another type of contrast may be defined as a transition from low to high luminance, or vice versa, in a band-limited signal[12]. The latter may be viewed as the response of the antisymmetric (sine phase) mechanisms. A complete description of contrast in a complex image should include both of these contrast representations in a way similar to the analysis of Stromeyer and Klein[33]. Incorporation of both symmetric and antisymmetric responses in a one-dimensional case using oriented filters is straightforward[17]. Complete two-dimensional application is difficult due to the lack of definition of Hilbert's transform for the two-dimensional case[21]. Without such a definition the contrast measure cannot be expanded to include the representation of antisymmetric mechanisms.

This work so far has addressed only the effects of contrast on perception at threshold. All of our work assumed contrast constancy to hold for suprathreshold contrast levels. The changes in suprathreshold contrast perception, and their effects on the perception of images, have to be examined and incorporated into an expanded model of contrast perception used in simulations. To that end, the proper metrics for the measurement of contrast of local features of various types in an image should be determined. We have already shown that a number of candidate metrics do not hold even for relatively simple patterns[12]. The effects of luminance on suprathreshold contrast perception were tested only for one spatial frequency. However, since the effect is spatial frequency dependent at threshold[37], the role of spatial frequency should be investigated at suprathreshold levels as well.

Acknowledgments

Supported in part by NIH grant EY05957 and by grants from the Ford Motor Company Fund and DigiVision, Inc. I thank R. Goldstein for valuable programming help, G. Young for help in data collection, and G. Geri for enabling the testing of the wide field simulations. Elisabeth Fine provided valuable editing help, and Miguel García-Pérez wrote an outstanding, detailed review that greatly improved the quality of this chapter.

References

1. S. N. Anstis, "A chart demonstrating variations in acuity with retinal position," *Vision Res.* **14** (1974) 589-592.
2. M. W. Cannon Jr., "Perceived contrast in the fovea and periphery," *J Opt. Soc. Am. [A]* **2** (1985) 1760-1768.
3. S. Daly, "The visual differences predictor: An algorithm for the assessment of image fidelity," *Proc. of the SPIE Vol. 1666 Human Vision, Visual Processing, and Digital Display III* (1992) 2-15.
4. M. Duval-Destin, "A spatio-temporal complete description of contrast," *Digest of Technical Papers Society for Information Display* (1991) 615-618.
5. E. Faye, "Functional classification of eye disease," in *Clinical Low Vision.* ed. E. E. Faye (Little Brown & Co., Boston, 1976), p. 218.
6. A. L. Fiorentini, L. Maffei, and G. Sandini, "The role of high spatial frequencies in face perception," *Perception* **12** (1983) 195-201.
7. H. J. Fleck, "Measurement and modeling of peripheral detection and discrimination thresholds," *Biol. Cybern.* **61** (1989) 437-446.
8. M. A. García-Pérez, "Visual inhomogeneity and reference frames," *Bulletin of Psychonomic Society* **27** (1989) 21-24.
9. M. A. Georgeson and G. D. Sullivan, "Contrast constancy: Deblurring in human vision by spatial frequency channels," *J Physiol.* **252** (1975) 627-656.

10. A. P. Ginsburg, "Is the illusory triangle physical or imaginary?," *Nature* **257** (1975) 219-220.

11. A. P. Ginsburg, "Visual information processing based on spatial filters constrained by biological data," *AMRL-TR-78-129 Vol. I and II* (Wright-Patterson Air Force Base, OH, 1978).

12. R. Goldstein, E. Peli, and G. Young, "Matching the contrast of luminance increments, decrements, and transitions," *ARVO Abstracts Invest. Ophthalmol. Vis. Sci.* **31(4, suppl)** (1991) 1271.

13. T. Hayes, M. C. Morrone, and D. C. Burr, "Recognition of positive and negative bandpass-filtered images," *Perception* **15** (1986) 595-602.

14. D. H. Kelly, "Visual contrast sensitivity," *Optica Acta* **24** (1977) 107-129.

15. B. L. Lundh, G. Derefeldt, S. Nyberg, and G. Lennerstrand, "Picture simulation of contrast sensitivity in organic and functional amblyopia," *Acta Ophthalmol. (Kbh)* **59** (1981) 774-783.

16. J. Larimer, "Designing tomorrow's displays," *NASA Tech Briefs* **17(4)** (1993) 14-16.

17. M. C. Morrone and D. C. Burr, "Feature detection in human vision: A phase-dependent energy model," *Proceedings of the Royal Society of London* **B235** (1988) 221-245.

18. B. Moulden, F. Kingdom, and L. F. Gatley, "The standard deviation of luminance as a metric for contrast in random-dot images," *Perception* **19** (1990) 79-101.

19. J. Norman and S. Ehrlich, "Spatial frequency filtering and target identification," *Vision Res.* **27** (1987) 87-96.

20. D. H. Parish and G. Sperling, "Object spatial frequencies, retinal spatial frequencies, noise and the efficiency of letter discrimination," *Vision Res.* **31** (1991) 1399-1415.

21. E. Peli, "Hilbert transform pairs mechanisms," *ARVO Abstracts Invest. Ophthalmol. Vis. Sci.* **30(4, suppl)** (1989) 110.

22. E. Peli, "Contrast in complex images," *J Opt. Soc. Am. [A]* **7** (1990) 2030-2040.

23. E. Peli, L. Arend, G. Young, and R. Goldstein, "Contrast sensitivity to patch stimuli: Effects of spatial bandwidth and temporal presentation," *Spatial Vis.* **7** (1993) 1-14.

24. E. Peli and G. Geri, "Putting simulations of peripheral vision to the test," *ARVO Abstracts Invest. Ophthalmol. Vis. Sci.* **34 (4, suppl)** (1993) 820.

25. E. Peli, R. B. Goldstein, G. M. Young, and L. E. Arend, "Contrast sensitivity functions for analysis and simulation of visual perception," *Noninvasive Assessment of the Visual System* **3** (1990) 126-129.

26. E. Peli, R. B. Goldstein, G. M. Young, C. L. Trempe, and S. M. Buzney, "Image enhancement for the visually impaired: Simulations and experimental results," *Invest. Ophthalmol. Vis. Sci.* **32** (1991) 2337-2350.

27. E. Peli and T. Peli, "Image enhancement for the visually impaired," *Opt. Eng.* **23** (1984) 47-51.

28. E. Peli, J. Yang, and R. Goldstein, "Image invariance with changes in size: The role of peripheral contrast thresholds," *J Opt. Soc. Am. [A]* **8** (1991) 1762-1774.

29. E. Peli, J. Yang, R. Goldstein, and A. Reeves, "Effect of luminance on suprathreshold contrast perception," *J .Opt. Soc. Am. [A]* **8** (1991) 1352-1359.

30. D. Pelli, *What is Low Vision?*, video tape presentation (Institute for Sensory Research, Syracuse University, Syracuse, NY, 1990).

31. J. G. Robson, "Linear and non-linear operations in the visual system," *ARVO Abstracts Invest. Ophthalmol. Vis. Sci.* **29(4, suppl)** (1988) 117.

32. E. L. Schwartz, "Spatial mapping in the primate sensory projection: Analytic structure and relevance to perception," *Biol. Cybern.* **25** (1977) 181-194.

33. C. F. Stromeyer III and S. Klein, "Evidence against narrow-band spatial frequency channels in human vision: The detectability of frequency modulated gratings," *Vision Res.* **15** (1975) 899-910.

34. L. N. Thibos and A. Bradley, "The limits of performance in central and peripheral vision," *Digest of Technical Papers Society for Information Display* **22** (1991) 301-303.

35. G. T. Timberlake, E. Peli, E. A. Essock, and R. A. Augliere, "Reading with macular scotoma. II: Retinal locus for scanning text," *Invest. Ophthalmol. Vis. Sci.* **28** (1987) 1268-1274.

36. C. W. Tyler, "Is the illusory triangle physical or imaginary?," *Perception* **6** (1977) 603-604.

37. F. L. Van Nes and M. A. Bouman, "Spatial modulation transfer in the human eye," *J. Opt. Soc. Am.* **57** (1967) 401-406.

38. A. B. Watson, "The cortex transform: Rapid computation of simulated neural images," *Computer Vision, Graphics, and Image Processing* **39** (1987) 311-327.

39. A. B. Watson, "DCTune: A technique for the visual optimization of DCT quantization matrices for individual images," *Society for Information Display '93 Digest* (1993) 946-949.

40. Y. Y. Zeevi, N. Peterfreund, and E. Shlomot, "Pyramidal image representation in nonuniform systems," *Proceedings of the SPIE* **1001** (1988) 563-571.

A MULTIPLE SPATIAL FILTER MODEL FOR SUPRATHRESHOLD CONTRAST PERCEPTION

MARK W. CANNON
Armstrong Laboratory AL/CFHP Bldg. 248
2255 H Street, Wright-Patterson AFB, OH 45433-7022, USA

Experiments to determine the apparent contrast of suprathreshold stimuli give a different picture of the gains and response pooling properties of tuned spatial filters than experiments designed to measure contrast thresholds. A model is derived that accounts for these differences and simulates both detection thresholds and suprathreshold contrast perception for stimuli composed of multiple sinewave components. The filters and contrast transducer functions are also used to explore possible models for human image sharpness estimates.

1. Introduction

One of the most pervasive theories in visual science today is that the perception of spatial form is mediated by operations performed on the outputs of multiple linear filters, each of which is tuned to a specific spatial frequency, orientation and spatial position. The outputs of these filters are thought to provide information about the local contrast, spatial frequency content and orientation in a scene that allows pattern processing algorithms in higher cognitive centers to identify objects against a complex background. Much of our knowledge about the properties of these filters has come from experiments designed to determine the contrast detection thresholds for sinewave gratings. In some of the earliest experiments, a contrast threshold function or its inverse, the contrast sensitivity function, was derived from sinewave grating threshold measurements[1]. The U shaped threshold function determined the lowest detectable contrast as a function of the spatial frequency of the grating and demonstrated that the contrast required to detect high or low spatial frequency gratings was higher than the contrast required to detect gratings of intermediate spatial frequency. The use of the inverse of the threshold function, the contrast sensitivity function, implied that the visual system was more sensitive to intermediate spatial frequencies than to high or low spatial frequencies. Subsequent experiments demonstrated that this threshold function was really an envelope describing the near peak sensitivities of many narrow band filters. The bandwidths of these filters in both the spatial frequency and orientation dimensions were first determined by measuring the threshold for a grating of one spatial frequency after adaptation by gratings of

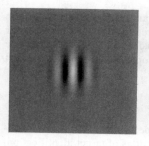 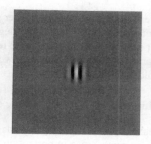 

Figure 1. Three vertically oriented spatial filters tuned to spatial frequencies one octave apart. The filter on the left is tuned to the lowest spatial frequency.

different spatial frequencies and orientations[2,3]. Other work in bandwidth determination involved measuring the threshold of a test grating presented on a masking background grating which had a different spatial frequency[4] and orientation[5] than the test or measuring the threshold for the sum of two different spatial frequency components[6] as the difference in spatial frequency between them was increased. Threshold determinations for sums of gratings and gratings of different spatial extent led to the concept of probability summation or response pooling across filters tuned to different spatial frequencies, orientations and spatial positions[7-9]. According to this theory, the outputs of all filters are contaminated by additive internal noise and a detection event occurs when at least one noisy filter produces a response greater than some criterion level. The probability that this detection event will be caused by a stimulus and not by internal noise, increases as the number of filters responding to the stimulus increases. Thus, stimuli of large spatial extent have a higher probability of being detected at a given contrast level than stimuli of small spatial extent.

Typical filter receptive fields derived from these experiments are illustrated in Fig. 1. The figure shows vertically oriented filters of three different sizes. Both psychophysical and neurophysiological data indicate that the visual system contains filters of many different sizes and orientations. The portion of an input image falling within the receptive field of the filter is spatially weighted by excitatory and inhibitory regions that are represented by light and dark areas in the figure. The output of the filter is the sum of those weighted inputs. Usually, the inhibition and excitation are balanced so the response of a single filter to a uniform illumination field is zero. If the input to a filter is a sinewave grating pattern, the filter exhibits both spatial frequency and orientation tuning. The filter responds maximally to gratings with a period equal to the spacing between the excitatory (or inhibitory) regions of the receptive field and oriented so that the grating bars are parallel to the long axis of excitatory and inhibitory regions.

These threshold experiments have led to a number of quantitative models that predict detection of complex spatial patterns[6,8]. A standard feature of these models is the adjustment of filter gain with spatial frequency so that model predictions of detection contrasts match the threshold contrast sensitivity function. The filter gain function has a maximum for filters tuned to spatial frequencies near 4 cycles per degree (c/deg) and decreases for filters tuned to higher or lower spatial frequencies. As the reader will see below, this type of a gain function is inappropriate for a model that is developed to account for contrast perception under suprathreshold conditions.

2. Contrast Perception in Human Vision

The question of suprathreshold contrast perception has been largely neglected by vision researchers, and this is unfortunate since important questions of target identification, image quality and image sharpness may depend more on our judgment of suprathreshold appearance than on threshold or discrimination performance. These judgments will depend on response pooling, spatial frequency tuning and orientation tuning under suprathreshold conditions. It is therefore important to understand these properties over the whole operating range of the human visual system.

2.1. Spatial Frequency Tuning of Contrast Perception

Contrast matching experiments by several researchers[10,11] demonstrated that the apparent contrast of high suprathreshold sinewave gratings do not show the increase at high and low spatial frequencies that is evident in the U shaped contrast threshold function. The following example will clarify the details of the experiment. Consider a grating of contrast c_1 and spatial frequency f_1 near the spatial frequency at which the contrast threshold function has a minimum. A typical contrast threshold function is labeled **Threshold** in Fig. 2. Choose this grating to be the standard in a contrast matching experiment. The object of the matching experiment is to adjust the contrast c_n of another grating at spatial frequency f_n so it has the same apparent contrast as the standard. If the matching is performed at a large number of spatial frequencies f_n, and if the contrasts c_n

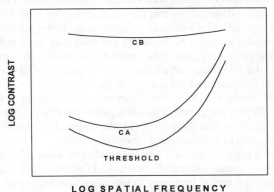

LOG SPATIAL FREQUENCY

Figure 2. A threshold curve and two typical equal perceived contrast contours (CA and CB) generated by contrast matching experiments.

that match c_1 are plotted as a function of f_n, a curve (usually smooth) that connects the values c_n is called an equal perceived contrast contour. All the points on the contour have the same perceived contrast. When the physical contrast of the test grating, c_1 is near threshold, the shape of the equal perceived contrast contour (CA) is similar to the contrast threshold function as shown in Fig. 2. It curves upward at spatial frequencies above and below f_1. The gain at those spatial frequencies is similar to the gain implied by the shape of the threshold contrast sensitivity function.

High and low spatial frequency gratings require more physical contrast than c_1 to achieve a match, in perceived contrast, with the grating at c_1, f_1. However, if c_1 is set to a contrast of about 0.5, the equal perceived contrast contour (CB) is flat over a large range of spatial frequencies, f_n. The flatness of curve CB implies that gratings at many spatial frequencies, f_n, have the same apparent contrast as the grating at c_1, f_1, when their physical contrast is equal to c_1. Apparently, filter gains change in a nonlinear manner as contrast increases and the visual system attempts to achieve a flat spatial frequency response for contrast perception under suprathreshold conditions.

2.2. Spatial Response Pooling for Contrast Perception

Consider the stimuli shown in Fig. 3. They are sinewave gratings of the same spatial frequency multiplied by Gaussian envelopes of different radii or half-widths. The number of cycles visible in each grating patch is determined by the half-width of the Gaussian envelope. This half-width is the distance in cycles of the underlying grating between the origin and the $1/e$ amplitude point of the envelope. The half-width is reduced by a factor of 4 as we move from the leftmost panel to the center panel and again by a factor of 4 as we move from the center to the right panel. We measured the thresholds of these patterns using a 2 interval forced choice technique and found that, as expected from the theory of probability summation, the thresholds increased as patch size decreased.

We also measured human perceived contrast responses to these stimuli using magnitude estimation and contrast matching techniques[12]. The data indicated that the differ-

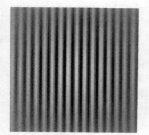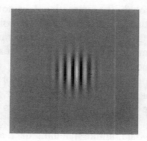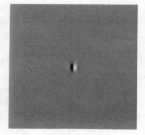

Figure 3. Three different sizes of stimulus patterns. The spatial half-widths or s values for the patterns from left to right are 8.0, 2.0 and 0.5. Thresholds decrease as size increases, but when contrast is greater than 0.1, the apparent contrasts of all three are equal when they have equal physical contrast.

ences attributed to probability summation at threshold gradually disappeared as contrast increased. At a spatial frequency of 4 c/deg all three patches exhibited equal perceived contrast for equal physical contrast when the physical contrast was greater than about 0.1. For those not familiar with the technique, the magnitude estimation experiments will now be considered in more detail.

During the course of a magnitude estimation experiment all three stimuli were presented at 12 different logarithmically spaced contrast levels. Stimuli and contrasts were randomized and each stimulus condition was presented three times. Presentation duration was 1 second followed by 6 seconds of uniformly illuminated screen. Average screen luminance under all conditions was 80 cd/m^2. Observers assigned a number, proportional to their perception of the contrast of the stimulus, to each presentation. No number scale was suggested. Observers used their own scale and data were normalized as follows.

Estimates at each contrast were averaged across sessions to produce a perceived contrast function for each subject. The geometric mean of perceived contrast for each function was computed as well as a geometric grand mean of perceived contrast for all functions. All individual observer means were then scaled to have a geometric mean equal to the grand geometric mean. The final mean perceived contrast function was the geometric mean of the scaled perceived contrast functions. Mean perceived contrast data from a group of 8 observers are illustrated in Fig. 4. The squares represent data for the largest patch size, circles are data for the smallest patch size. The vertical axis in the figure shows the mean perceived contrast estimate and the horizontal axis shows the physical contrast of the stimuli. The arrows pointing at the horizontal axis indicate the mean thresholds for the three stimuli determined with the same 8 observers. As expected from the theory of probability summation, the thresholds are separated along the contrast axis. Note, however, that the data gradually merge to the same perceived contrast at a physical contrast of about 0.1. The fact that the three curves are separate across a significant range of contrasts implies the existence of some type of response pooling different from that defined by probability summation. Probability summation addresses the probability of detection, in a system where stimulus response is mediated by many noisy, independent mechanisms. After detection occurs and contrast has reached a high enough value that the stimulus is always seen, probability summation does not apply. Any response pooling above this level is a pooling that is adding to the sensation of perceived contrast, not to the probability of detection. Over most of the contrast range in Fig. 4, where there are three separate curves, the stimulus is clearly visible. Thus, any differences in perceived contrast must be due to response pooling mediated by some type of actual physical connections among tuned mechanisms. In other words, the mechanisms are not independent. The separations among the lower regions of the three curves were also verified by contrast matching data, but interested readers will have to get those details elsewhere[13].

The magnitude estimation data, unlike matching data, allow one to make estimates of the form of the contrast transducer function. This is the functional relationship between the stimulus physical contrast and the contrast sensation perceived by the observer. Individual perceived contrast functions were very similar in form to the mean functions

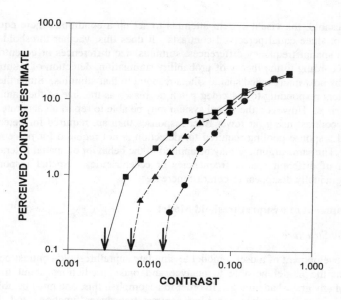

Figure 4. Mean perceived contrast functions for 8 observers.

shown in Fig. 4. They rose rather steeply from threshold and then merged with a slope of 0.5 at a contrast of about 0.1. Since these data are plotted in log-log coordinates, a slope of 0.5 means that, at high contrast, perceived contrast increased as a power function of physical contrast with an exponent of 0.5. Exponents in the literature range from 0.5 to 0.7.

2.3. Contrast Perception in Peripheral Vision

Experiments performed with peripherally viewed grating patches, in our lab, showed similar exponents and also demonstrated that perceived contrast in the periphery becomes independent of eccentricity at high physical contrasts[14]. The form of the data was similar to that shown in Fig. 4 except that the three curves would represent responses at three different eccentricities to gratings of the same spatial extent. Thresholds increase with eccentricity but perceived contrast functions, at all eccentricities where the stimulus is visible, merge at high contrasts.

2.4. General Features of Suprathreshold Contrast Perception

We have seen in the previous sections that the filter gains and response pooling properties for suprathreshold contrast perception cannot be inferred from filter gains and response pooling properties developed for threshold models. As stimulus contrasts rise above threshold, the visual system attempts to set up a condition where equal physical contrasts produce equal perceived contrasts. It does this whether threshold differences arise from spatial frequency differences, stimulus size differences or eccentricity differences. According to the theory of probability summation, detection of a stimulus is determined by how many tuned spatial filters respond to that stimulus. Since the number of spatial filters responding to a 4 c/deg patch decreases as the size of the patch decreases, threshold rises. However, the visual system may be able to report an accurate estimate of perceived contrast using far fewer filter responses than are required for detection, hence the spatial response pooling required for detection is not required for perception at high contrasts. The same argument may be applied to the behavior of spatial filters responding to stimuli of different spatial frequencies or eccentricities. Spatial response pooling seems to gradually disappear as contrast increases.

3. Development of a Suprathreshold Model

3.1. Model Structure

The development of a useful model to simulate suprathreshold contrast perception requires that the model be able to analyze and make predictions about the perceived contrast of any gray shade image. In order to accomplish this, one must be able to specify the spatial filter bandwidths, the filter contrast transducer functions and the rules by which filter outputs are combined. Psychophysical experiments designed to obtain the required parameters were necessarily limited to stimuli for which a well defined estimate of perceived contrast could be obtained. A very useful set of stimuli with these properties are sums of sinusoidal components spatially localized within Gaussian envelopes.

Development of the model was accomplished in two stages. The first stage was directed toward developing a model that would account for contrast perception of spatially localized grating stimuli at high physical contrast where perceived contrast appears to be independent of stimulus size[12]. This is the region shown in Fig. 4 where the three perceived contrast curves merge and increase as a power function of physical contrast with an exponent of 0.5. The second stage effort addressed the development of a contrast transducer function that would account for the lower portion of the same curves where the functions diverge to different thresholds[13]. The second stage effort also attempted to account for the perceived contrast of stimuli distributed across a wide range of spatial frequencies. The first stage effort will be discussed in this section. The second stage expanded model will be discussed in subsequent sections.

The perceived contrast for grating patch stimuli became independent of stimulus size at contrasts above 0.1 implied that spatial response pooling disappeared at high contrast levels. This assumption was reinforced by similar conclusions reached by other researchers on the basis of contrast discrimination and contrast matching data[10]. The equality of perceived contrast for the three different size grating patches also indicated that the receptive field size of the filters must not be much larger than the smallest grating patch shown in Fig. 3. Otherwise, this smallest stimulus would have produced a significantly smaller perceived contrast response than the other two.

The filters were modeled with Gabor functions, which have been used successfully by several researchers[6,15] to account for threshold phenomena. A Gabor filter is simply a sinewave grating multiplied by a Gaussian envelope. The half-width of the envelope is functionally related to the filter's spatial frequency bandwidth. The Gaussian envelope in this model is radially symmetric. Of course, other functions have been used to model spatial filters. These include difference of Gaussians[7], derivatives of Gaussians[16] and Cauchy functions[17]. Two primary reasons for choosing Gabors were their mathematical simplicity and lack of evidence indicating the clear superiority of one type over another when it comes to modeling a system composed of multiple filters.

Response pooling at high contrast was based upon the same Quick summation formula that has been used to describe response pooling effects at threshold. Response pooling was only permitted among mechanisms tuned to different spatial frequencies and orientations. Response pooling among mechanisms at different spatial positions was excluded since there appears to be no spatial summation at high contrast. The form of this response pooling equation is shown in Eq. (1).

$$R(x,y) = \left[\sum_f \sum_\theta F_{f,\theta}(x,y)^Q \right]^{1/Q}$$ (1)

$F(x,y)$ is the full wave rectified response of a filter tuned to a particular spatial frequency and orientation at location x, y. Q is an exponent that is usually 3.0 or 4.0 at threshold. $R(x,y)$ is the total pooled response of all the active filters centered at coordi-

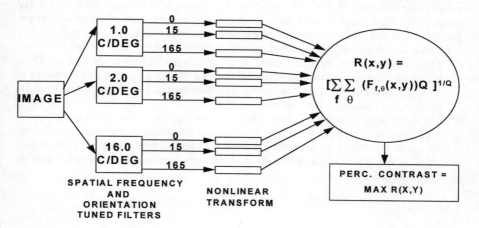

Figure 5. Model for contrast perception at physical contrasts greater than 0.1.

nates x, y. Note that if Q were 2 this equation would be the RMS value of the filter outputs.

A schematic diagram of the model is shown in Fig. 5. The diagram is similar to several spatial filter models in the literature in that it consists of parallel filters tuned to different spatial frequencies and orientations[6,8,11]. However, most of these models have filter parameters derived from threshold experiments. As the reader will see below, the filter parameters of this model were derived from contrast matching experiments where the standard grating was at a contrast of 0.3. The input to the model was a 256×256 pixel input image, representing a 4×4 degree spatial region. The filters were oriented Gabor sine filters with center frequencies ranging from 1 to 16 c/deg in 1/2 octave steps.

Filter spatial frequency is indicated by the numbers in the first column of boxes in Fig. 5. Each of the many parallel lines emerging from these boxes indicates the response of a filter with center frequency specified by the box, but with an orientation specified by the number on the line. Filter orientations ranged from 0 to 165 degrees in steps of 15 degrees. Each of these lines represents a full 256×256 pixel filtered image since all filters were assumed to be uniformly and densely distributed across the 4×4 input image. Each of these filtered images was full wave rectified and passed through a nonlinear power function transformation with an exponent of 0.5. These operations are indicated by the second column of boxes in the figure. The computation to pool image responses is shown in the circle. The computation for perceived contrast is shown in the box below the circle. The pooling computation can be envisioned as follows. Consider a stack of all the filtered and transduced images. Each layer in the stack represents an image produced by a spatial array of filters with the same spatial frequency and orientation tuning properties. Independent response pooling operations across all layers in the stack are conducted at each spatial position x, y. This computation produces a final pooled image, the same spatial size as all the others. However, the amplitude at each x, y in this final image is the nonlinear sum of responses from the same spatial position in all the filtered images. The final computation determines the maximum amplitude of the pooled image. It is this single value that corresponds to the model estimate of perceived contrast.

Two assumptions were made about the spatial filters involved in the model.

(1) The spatial shapes of the filters are all size scaled reproductions of each other. Thus, a 1 c/deg filter is has the same spatial shape as a 16 c/deg filter, but is expanded in size by a factor of 16. This size scaling was illustrated in Fig. 1. All filters have the same spatial half-width in cycles.

(2) The mean squared integrals of the filter amplitude profiles over space are all equal. This gives all filters equal gains and will allow the model to reproduce the flat response to sinewave gratings observed at high contrast. Interestingly, providing equal gains to the filters requires that their amplitudes increase in direct proportion to spatial frequency.

3.2. Determination of Filter Half-width and Response Pooling Equation

With these restrictions on the filters, there were only two model parameters to determine. These were the filter spatial half-width in cycles, s, and the value of Q in the response pooling equation. The first step in determining these parameters was the collection of data from three contrast matching experiments. The experiments involved matching a full screen sinewave grating test stimulus to a 0.3 contrast, spatially localized comparison stimulus. The three comparison stimuli were; (1) a 4 c/deg Gabor sine function with a half-width of 0.5 cycles, (2) a grating patch consisting of two orthogonal 4 c/deg gratings multiplied by a Gaussian envelope with a half-width of one cycle and (3) a pair of small spatially offset Gaussians, one positive and the other negative with respect to the average background luminance. Contrasts of the full screen grating necessary to match each of the three comparison stimuli were determined. Four observers took part in these experiments and the data were averaged across observers to provide a single estimate for each of the three matches. Each of the comparison stimuli at a contrast of 0.3 and three test gratings at contrasts required to match each of the comparison stimuli were used as inputs to the model. With the correct choice of Q and s, model responses to the comparison and its associated test stimulus, set at the experimentally determined matching contrast, should be equal. Model responses were recorded as filter s varied from 0.14 to 1.41 cycles and the Q of the response pooling equation varied from 2.0 to 4.0. The square of the differences between the model response to a full screen grating and its associated comparison stimuli were determined for all Q and s values tested. A mean square difference across the three experiments was computed for each set of Q and s. The values of Q and s that produced the smallest mean square difference between the model responses to the full screen grating and their associated comparison stimuli were 2.5 and 0.7 respectively. These values were fixed for the second stage of model development, which involved extending the model to low contrasts and threshold.

3.3. Rationale For Determination of the Contrast Transducer Function

In order to account for the transition between detection and perception, the model contrast transducer functions operating on the outputs of the linear filters must show the same characteristics as the perceived contrast functions in Fig. 4. The functions must be separated at low contrast, equal at high contrast and show a change of exponent at some intermediate contrast. Fortunately, a contrast transducer function with the proper characteristics has been proposed by other researchers on the basis of contrast discrimination experiments[18,19]. This contrast transducer function has the form shown in Eq. (2).

$$R = C^{\alpha+\beta} / \left(A^{\beta} + C^{\beta} \right) \qquad (2)$$

In Eq. (2), R is the output of the transducer, C is the contrast of the input stimulus, A is an adjustable parameter and the exponents α and β determine the exponents or slopes of the upper and lower parts of the function. If C is small with respect to A, the function in-

98

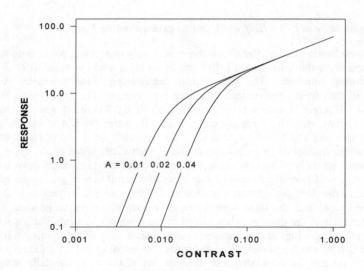

Figure 6. A candidate contrast transducer function.

creases as C to the $\alpha+\beta$ power. If C is large with respect to A, the function increases as C to the α power.

Equation 2 is plotted in Fig. 6 for three different values of A; 0.01, 0.02 and 0.04. The exponents are $\alpha = 0.5$ and $\beta = 3.0$. The three functions are separated for low values of C and overlap at high values of C. If we consider the response value of 0.1 to be some sort of criterion response level or threshold, the contrast necessary to exceed that threshold increases as A increases. Thus, the functions behave the way the contrast transducer function should behave if A were functionally related to stimulus spatial extent, spatial frequency or eccentricity. Eccentricity effects will be ignored in the present model for two reasons. (1) The model simulates spatial processing in a 4 degree by 4 degree region at the center of the visual field. (2) The stimuli used to calibrate and test the model fall off in contrast with eccentricity, so the perceived contrast estimate will be determined in the center of the image where image amplitude is largest. With this simplification, the problem has been reduced to determining a plausible computational scheme that can make A depend on the spatial frequency of the filter to which the transducer is connected and on the size of the stimulus. In subsequent sections of this chapter, the combination of linear filter and transducer function will be referred to as a non-linear filter mechanism.

Since thresholds increase above and below a spatial frequency range of about 3 to 4 c/deg for constant size gratings, filters tuned to spatial frequencies higher and lower than this minimum spatial frequency must have transducer functions with A values that are larger than those of filters tuned to 3 or 4 c/deg. Consequently, threshold behavior for sinewave gratings of the same spatial size can be accounted for by some sort of spatial frequency tuning function for A. This component of A increases as the spatial frequency difference between the stimulus and 4 c/deg increases. However, the other component of A is dependent on stimulus size. This component must decrease as stimulus size increases, and if the form of the contrast transducer function is to be preserved, the component must be independent of contrast. The equation finally chosen for the computation of parameter A is given below in Eq. (3).

$$A = K \cdot WT(f,\theta) \cdot \left(CR_{MAX} \, / \, Q_{POOL} \right) \tag{3}$$

Parameter K is a scaling constant and is the same for all spatial filters. The function $WT(f,q)$ is a weighting function that depends on the spatial frequency and orientation to which the filter is tuned. Filters tuned to 4 c/deg will have transducer functions with a smaller value of WT than filters tuned to 1 c/deg or to 16 c/deg. In the simulations to follow, it is assumed that all orientation responses are approximately equal so the dependence on orientation can be ignored, and the weighting functions can be referred to as $WT(f)$. The term Q_{POOL} accounts for the response pooling across space, orientation and spatial frequency that is known to exist near threshold. The mathematical expression for Q_{POOL} is shown in Eq. (4).

$$Q_{POOL} = \left[\sum_x \sum_y \sum_f \sum_\theta CR(x,y,f,\theta)^{3.0} \right]^{0.33} \tag{4}$$

The term CR represents the full wave rectified responses of individual filters tuned to specific spatial frequencies, orientations and spatial positions. The pooling equation performs the nonlinear sum over all filters. The term CR_{MAX}, in Eq. (3), is the maximal single filter response to the input. Even though Q_{POOL} is a nonlinear sum, its magnitude increases linearly with the amplitude of the CRs. Thus, the ratio CR_{MAX}/Q_{POOL} does not change as contrast increases, if the stimulus size is kept constant. Conversely, if stimulus contrast is kept constant, CR_{MAX} remains constant and the ratio CR_{MAX}/Q_{POOL} decreases as the size of the stimulus increases. This is exactly the type of behavior required for the contrast transducer functions.

3.4. Incorporation of the CTFS into the Model

A diagram of the full model is presented in Fig. 7. The filters shown in this figure are tuned to different spatial frequencies but only one orientation, q_j. Other orientations would be represented by parallel pathways similar to those of Fig. 7 arranged in layers above or below the page. All pathways originate from the same image block and terminate in the block containing the $PC(x,y)$ response pooling equation.

The filters are the same as those derived to fit the high contrast model shown in Fig. 5. In this model, however, the rectified filter outputs, CR, are fed into a global processing algorithm that computes CR_{MAX}/Q_{POOL} as well as into the parallel pathways that lead to the computation of perceived contrast. The output of the global processor multiplies the transducer function weights or gains, $WT(f)$, which are different for each filter central frequency. This multiplication computes parameter A of the contrast transducer function shown in Equation 3. The full contrast transducer equation for a particular x,y,f and q is shown at the bottom of Fig. 7. The outputs of the contrast transducer functions, the images $R(x,y)$, are the inputs to the suprathreshold response pooling operation, $PC(x,y)$. Note that $PC(x,y)$ is a second response pooling equation, independent of Q_{POOL}. The computation of perceived contrast is exactly the same as the process used in the high contrast model, illustrated in Fig. 5, even though the terms are labeled somewhat differently. The exponent Q is still 2.5.

3.5. Model Calibration

At this point the model had three free parameters; the scaling constant, K, the transducer response function exponent, β, and the spatial frequency weighting function $WT(f)$. Determination of values for K and β were accomplished with the weighting function $WT(f)$ set to a constant for all spatial frequencies. The form of $WT(f)$ was determined in subsequent simulations. The first simulations used a 4 c/deg, $s = 8.0$ cycles, Gabor patch

$$R_{x,y}\left(f_i,\theta_j\right) = \frac{\left[CR_{x,y}\left(f_i,\theta_j\right)\right]^{\alpha+\beta}}{\left[CR_{x,y}\left(f_i,\theta_j\right)\right]^{\beta} + K\left[WT\left(f_i\right)\bullet\dfrac{CR_{MAX}}{Q_{POOL}}\right]^{\beta}}$$

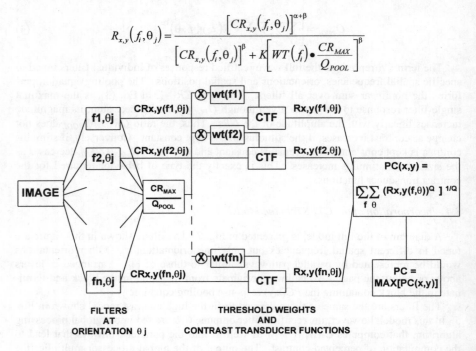

Figure 7. Model for contrast perception from threshold to high suprathreshold levels.

as input. This is the same stimulus that produced the leftmost perceived contrast function in Fig. 4. Parameters K and β were adjusted until a good fit of model responses to magnitude estimation data points and threshold was obtained. Threshold was treated fairly simply in the model. A criterion response level (CRL) of 0.1 was set as response threshold. Since any response below this would be invisible, CRL was subtracted from the perceived contrast computation. A noisy threshold could easily be obtained by adding noise to this level though this was not done in the current simulation. When the threshold adjusted perceived contrast computations (PC-CRL) are plotted on double logarithmic coordinates the curves become very steep at the contrast where PC approaches CRL. The contrast at which the threshold adjusted model perceived contrast curve crosses a perceived contrast level of 0.1 is assumed to be a good approximation of threshold. The best fit model curve for the $s = 8.0$ Gabor is shown as the leftmost curve in Fig. 8. It fits the data points rather well and crosses the perceived contrast = 0.1 level near the measured threshold (vertical arrow). The other two curves represent model responses to two smaller patches, ($s = 2.0$ and 0.5) generated with the same values of K and q and account fairly well for both threshold and perceived contrast.

The next task was to determine the form of the function $WT(f)$. Two interval forced choice threshold experiments were conducted with the same observers who generated the data shown in Fig. 8. The stimuli in these experiments were small sinewave patches with

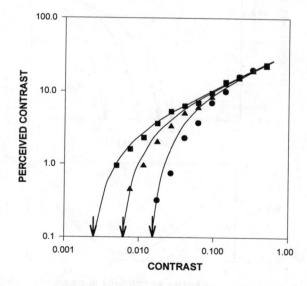

Figure 8. Model estimates of perceived contrast. The three curves are model responses to Gabor sine patches with $s = 8.0$, 2.0 and 0.5 indicated by the squares, triangles and circles respectively. The data points are average magnitude estimates from 8 observers. The vertical arrows are thresholds from the same 8 observers. Data were shown previously in Fig. 4.

Gaussian envelopes. The value of *s* for these patches was 0.5 cycles and spatial frequencies for the underlying gratings were 2, 4, 8 and 16 c/deg. These same stimuli were then used as inputs to the model. The values of *K* and β were fixed to the values that produced the responses shown in Fig. 8 and *WT(f)* was varied until model thresholds agreed with measured thresholds at all 4 spatial frequencies. The model perceived contrast functions for these stimuli are shown in the upper panel of Fig. 9. The resulting *WT(f)* curve is shown in the lower panel of Fig. 9. The *WT(f)* curve exhibits tuning similar to the contrast threshold function but does not rise as steeply as threshold with increasing spatial frequency. Measured thresholds, indicated by the vertical arrows in the upper panel of Fig. 9, range from 0.01 to 0.08. The *WT(f)* values only change by a factor of 3. Note also that the minimum of the *WT(f)* function is at 4 c/deg, while the lowest threshold for grating patches with *s* = 0.5 in the upper panel is at 2 c/deg. This demonstrates the fact that the model threshold is a function of stimulus size and the *WT(f)* function. Gratings that extend to the full 4×4 degree size have thresholds that show a minimum at 4 c/deg.

After the adjustment of the *WT(f)* function the model was re-tested with the *s* = 8.0,

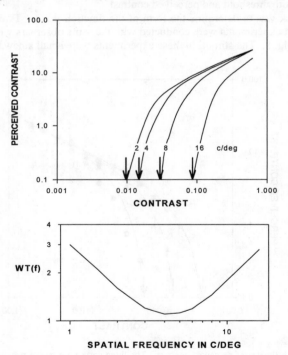

Figure 9. Parameter adjustment to define *WT(f)*. The upper panel shows measured thresholds (vertical arrows) and model responses for 4 small sinewave patches at spatial frequencies of 2, 4, 8 and 16 c/deg. The lower curve shows the *WT(f)* function required to achieve a match between model and measured thresholds.

2.0 and 05 cycle stimuli that produced the model perceived contrast functions shown in Fig. 8. Only negligible differences were seen so it was not deemed necessary to modify K and β from their previous values. This completed model parameter determination. All model parameters were fixed and further tests were run with stimuli not used in the calibration process.

3.6. Tests of Model Performance

The first test of model performance was a simulation of perceived contrast estimates for 16 c/deg grating patches with Gaussian envelope half-widths of 8, 2 and 0.5 cycles. Data were obtained for comparison purposes by obtaining thresholds and perceived contrast functions for these stimuli from the same observers who participated in the previous experiments. Magnitude estimation data were collected using the three 16 c/deg stimuli and a 4 c/deg $s = 8.0$ grating patch. The 4 c/deg patch was inserted into the experiment to assure that perceived contrast estimates for the 16 c/deg stimuli would be based on the same number scale as estimates for the 4 c/deg stimulus. Simulation results and psychophysical data points are illustrated in Fig. 10. The magnitude estimation data for 4 c/deg are a bit more noisy than the data shown in Fig. 8 but the model adequately accounts for both threshold and perceived contrast of the 16 c/deg stimuli.

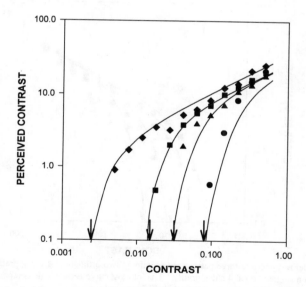

Figure 10. Perceived contrast data and model responses for three patch sizes at 16 c/deg and 1 patch size at 4 c/deg. The 4 c/deg patch is the leftmost curve. Data for $s = 8$, 2 and 0.5 are shown by the squares, triangles and circles, respectively. Agreement between data and model are good.

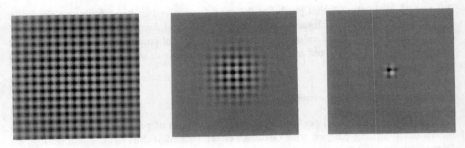

Figure 11. The sums of two orthogonal sinewave components multiplied by Gaussian envelopes with half-widths (from left to right) of 8, 2 and 0.5 cycles.

A second simulation tested the ability of the model to deal with sums of orthogonal gratings. Two orthogonal 4 c/deg gratings were added together and displayed to observers in a magnitude estimation experiment with the usual three Gaussian envelope half-widths, 8, 2 and 0.5 cycles. Thresholds were also measured. These stimuli are shown in Fig. 11.

An $s = 8$ cycle single component grating was also presented in the same experimental

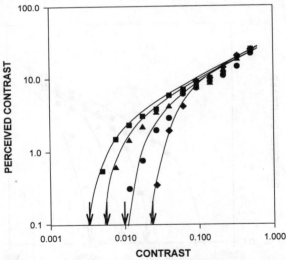

Figure 12. Model responses to three patch sizes containing two orthogonal 4 c/deg gratings and an $s = 8$ patch containing a single vertical 4 c/deg grating. The leftmost curve is the single component grating. The model predictions (smooth curves) account fairly well for the data.

session for two reasons. First, it was required to assure that observers were using the same number scale for both the orthogonal and the single component stimuli. Second, the new group of observers had a different mean threshold than the previous group for the $s = 8$ cycle single component grating. A perceived contrast function for the $s = 8$ grating provided a means to recalibrate the model to the new threshold for this stimulus. Parameter K was changed until the $s = 8$ simulation curve crossed the 0.1 perceived contrast axis at the newly measured threshold for that stimulus. With K set to this new value and all other parameters remaining fixed at their old values, model responses matched the data fairly well. The data and simulations are illustrated in Fig. 12. In other experiments, not illustrated here, the model was able to predict thresholds and perceived contrast functions for the sum of two orthogonal gratings of different spatial frequencies.

3.7. Comparison with other Models

It is appropriate at this time to discuss differences between the model presented here and many other parallel spatial filter models. Most other models filter the input with linear filters, operate on the filter outputs with a nonlinear contrast transducer function (CTF) and then perform response pooling on the outputs of the CTF stage. The filter gains usually vary across spatial frequency to match the contrast threshold function[6,8,11]. This type of model does not transition correctly into the suprathreshold contrast perception domain where spatial response pooling disappears and where equal perceived contrast contours across spatial frequencies are relatively flat. In order to produce flat equal perceived contrast contours with these models, the shape of the CTFs must vary as a function of spatial frequency. This variation has usually been done after the fact to fit the CTF to the data. The models have also not been able to account for the disappearance of spatial response pooling at high contrast. Several researchers have set up two separate models: one with spatial summation to deal with threshold conditions and one without spatial summation to deal with high suprathreshold conditions[11,19].

The model presented here has two distinct differences from earlier models. The first difference is that all filters have the same gain. The second difference is that modification of the form of the CTF is described in a well defined computation on the pooled responses of the filters. Equal filter gains, coupled with the fact that the upper branches of all perceived contrast functions are the same assures that the model will have nearly flat equal perceived contrast contours at high stimulus contrast levels. CTF dependence on spatial response pooling effects disappears at a contrast where the filter response, CR, substantially exceeds the R_{MAX} / Q_{POOL} term. Under these conditions the second response pooling operation [$PC(x,y)$ in Fig. 7] among the CTF outputs predominates. Thus, perceived contrast at high stimulus contrast levels is independent of stimulus size.

4. Application of the Model to a Study of Image Sharpness

4.1. Relevance of an Image Sharpness Metric

The concept of perceived image quality is becoming commercially more important with the likelihood of large investments in new video technology such as HDTV. The subject has been studied for many years giving rise to a large number of image quality metrics, few of which appear to be particularly successful in predicting human estimates of image quality[20-23]. Most of these metrics have attempted to remain image independent and predict human performance by including only the modulation transfer function (MTF) of the display device and some function of the human visual system such as the contrast threshold function and just noticeable differences (JNDs) for contrast. The lack of success of the earlier metrics can partially be explained by the fact that they have usually been derived by display engineers with little understanding of suprathreshold vision. The study reported here attempted to use the visual system model, derived above, to provide the filtering and contrast transduction processes on which an image quality metric can be based. The particular aspect of image quality addressed in this study is image sharpness perception for real world scenes degraded, by low pass filtering, to

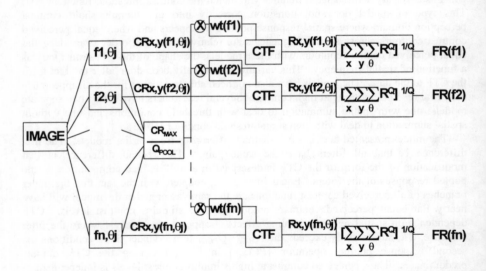

Figure 13. Model for analysis of image sharpness estimates. The model filters and transducer functions are the same as those in the perceived contrast model. In the present model, however, the computation of perceived contrast has been replaced by a response pooling operation across space and orientation of the images produced by each non-linear filter mechanism. This produces a single number at each spatial frequency. Two computational schemes for image sharpness, operating on these pooled outputs, were tested.

represent a range of display MTFs. The discussion to follow addresses only MTF based image degradation and cannot be used to address the subjective quality of noise degraded imagery.

4.2. Modeling Image Sharpness Estimates

All previous studies have agreed that image sharpness or image quality as a function of image blur was directly related to the spatial frequency content of the image. A reduction of high spatial frequency components in an image results in a lower estimate of image quality. Thus, the perceived contrast model was modified to emphasize the spatial frequency content of the filtered images. The modified model is shown in Fig. 13.

The rightmost column of processing blocks indicates that all images $R(x,y,f,q)$ are summed across space, (x,y), and orientation, q, with the nonlinear Quick response pooling equation. The outputs of these blocks, $FR(f)$ are a measure of the total activity produced by the image in the group of non linear filter mechanisms with pass band centered on spatial frequency f. In subsequent sections of this chapter, this grouping of non linear filter mechanisms with a common center frequency will be referred to as a **spatial frequency channel**. Note that the summation operation shown in Fig. 13 can be performed in parallel with the perceived contrast computation. Q values of 1 and 2 were tested as candidate exponents for the summations indicated in the rightmost blocks of Fig. 13. Since nearly identical image sharpness estimates were produced by the model in both cases, a value of 1 was used in the simulations reported below. This corresponds to simple linear summation. In order to expedite computations, this model used filters spaced every octave and orientations spaced every 30 deg, instead of the 1/2 octave and 15 deg spacing of the contrast perception model shown in Fig. 7. Several of the perceived contrast computations shown previously were repeated with the abbreviated model but no significant differences were observed. Thus, it was concluded that the reduced model was adequate for the image sharpness study. The purpose of the study to be described was to determine a computation on these filter mechanism outputs that would account for experimentally measured image sharpness estimates. Before we do any more with the modeling portion of the study, let us see what the experimental data looked like.

4.3. Image Sharpness Experiments

The images used in this study are shown in Fig. 14. These are 5 real world scenes scanned from photographs and digitized into 256×256 pixel arrays with 256 gray scale levels. The maximum "contrast" of each image was determined by computing the largest and smallest amplitudes and scaling them so that they had the same amplitudes on our display system as the peak and trough of a 0.5 contrast sinewave grating. The stimuli used to elicit image sharpness estimates were low pass filtered versions of the images shown in Fig. 14. Low pass filtering was accomplished in the Fourier domain using the filter function illustrated in Fig. 15.

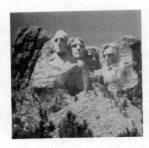
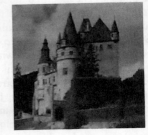
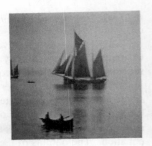
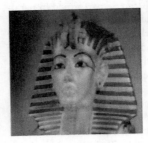
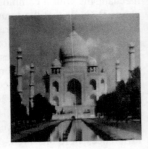

Figure 14. Real world scenes used in the image sharpness study.

Eight representations of each image were used in the experiments. Seven images were low pass filtered and the eighth image was unfiltered. Filter bandwidths (BW in Fig. 15) increased in half-octave steps from 2 c/deg to 16 c/deg. The MTF of the monitor was essentially flat out to 32 c/deg so the bandwidth available to the unfiltered picture was 32 c/deg. A set of filtered test images and their bandwidths are shown in Fig. 16.

Filtered images were normalized in contrast in the same way as the unfiltered image. This normalization scheme was also followed during the simulation runs, so both observers and the model "saw" the same images. Three different contrast levels were used in the experiment. They were the original contrast and contrasts equal to 0.5 and 0.25 times the original contrast. In a given session, each of the 8 observers saw 7 filtered images and one unfiltered image of the same scene at the three different contrast levels. Filter bandwidth and contrast level were randomized. Each image was repeated three times. Observers were told to ignore stimulus contrast as a factor and assign numbers they felt were proportional to the sharpness of each image as it appeared. Each image was presented in a different session, so we can't be sure that all images had the same rated sharpness for the unfiltered image. However, the shape of the perceived image sharpness functions from all observers were similar for all pictures. In order to compare data, responses to each picture were normalized so that the response for the 0.5 contrast unfiltered image was 1.0. Data for 8 observers, averaged across the 5 scenes are shown in Fig. 17. Image sharpness estimates increase with image bandwidth to around 8 c/deg and show no change above this value for the images used in this study. The fact that the three curves are very close indicate that observers were able to ignore contrast and that their estimates of sharpness were similar at all three contrast levels.

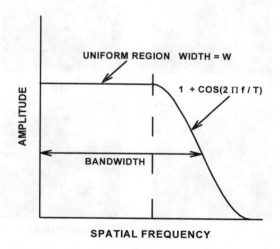

Figure 15. Low pass filter function used for filtering pictures. The width of the 1+cos region increased in direct proportion to the bandwidth. This gave the roll-off portion a constant shape in log coordinates.

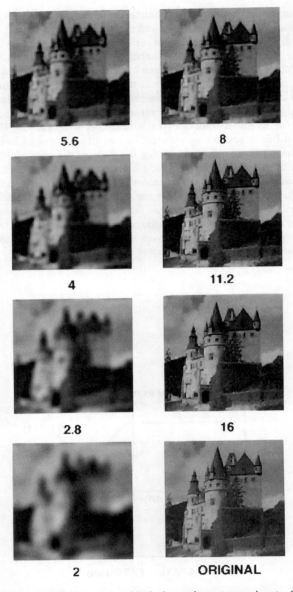

Figure 16. A set of low pass filtered images used in the image sharpness experiments. The number below each image is the bandwidth in cycles per degree of the low pass filter used to process that image.

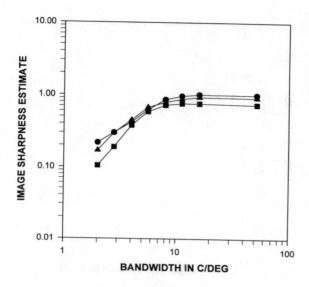

Figure 17. Average image sharpness estimates as a function of image bandwidth in c/deg. Squares, tri-angles and circles represent image "contrasts" of 0.125, 0.25 and 0.5 respectively. Although an ordering effect due to image contrast can be seen, the effect is small.

4.4. Models for Image Sharpness Perception

The purpose of the simulation was to find a reasonable computation on the outputs of the model shown in Fig. 13, that would account for the image sharpness data shown in Fig. 17. An approach that consisted of summing all the channel responses, which would be similar to the image quality concept of modulation transfer function area or MTFA, would not work since this computation would be highly dependent on stimulus contrast. It appears that image sharpness depends on the responses of high spatial frequency channels since it is primarily these channels that show reduced amplitude with the filtering performed on the real world scenes. Thus, a promising approach to account for image sharpness estimates was to divide the response of the two highest spatial frequency channels by the sum of the responses of all channels. This scheme would provide contrast normalization and emphasize the importance of high spatial frequency responses. A typical model response to one of the images at a contrast of 0.5 is shown in Fig. 18.

The amplitude of the curve at the data points for 1, 2, 4, 8 and 16 c/deg are model channel responses. In order to simulate human responses, the model response to the unfiltered high contrast version of each picture was normalized to 1.0. Model responses to lower contrast presentations of the same picture were multiplied by the normalization factor required to normalize the high contrast image. Normalized model estimates of im-

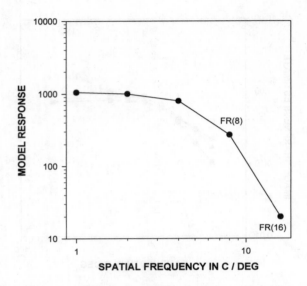

Figure 18. Model responses to a typical picture at a contrast of 0.5. The data points represent the responses of tuned mechanisms that are summed, with the Quick summation rule, across space and orientation. Image sharpness was based on the sum of the responses to the 8 and 16 c/deg channels, *FR*(8) and *FR*(16), divided by the sum of all channel responses.

age sharpness averaged across the 5 images are illustrated in Fig. 19.

The three curves in this figure show responses for the three different contrast levels. The point where the slope of the curves becomes horizontal is reproduced quite well by the model. The break point is about 8 c/deg. However, the separation among the three curves is much greater for low bandwidth images than the data shown in Fig. 17. This rapid drop-off is caused by the fact that the slopes of the perceived contrast functions become steeper at low contrast. Since this is built into the portion of the model derived from the perceived contrast data it must remain the same in this study. Thus, this does not seem to be an appropriate coding scheme for image sharpness. Another processing scheme that would not be as sensitive to the low contrast slope was investigated.

When the channel outputs from the model in Fig. 13 are plotted as a function of the spatial frequency to which the channel is tuned, the response function is always low pass in character for real world scenes. This follows from the fact that the spatial frequency spectrum of the unfiltered scene decreases as the reciprocal of the spatial frequency. The plot in Fig. 18 can be envisioned as a spatial pattern of channel responses where the channels are arranged along some spatial dimension, which in this case labels the logarithm of the spatial frequency to which the channel is tuned. The pattern always decreases from left to right and will shift to the left as image bandwidth decreases. Now, assume the existence of a pattern analysis network, "looking" at this output pattern. Further, assume

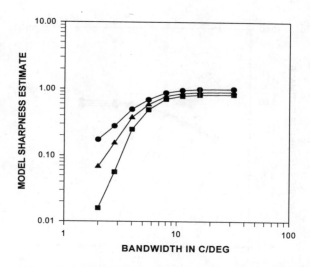

Figure 19. Mean model responses to filtered images averaged across images. Circles, triangles and squares represent picture contrasts of 0.5, 0.25 and 0.125 respectively. While the function breakpoints are similar to those of Fig. 17, the separation at the bottom of the curves is too large.

that this network can identify the horizontal axis coordinate where the function passes through an amplitude equal to half the amplitude at the left side of the pattern. This coordinate would define a measure of image sharpness since it would shift to smaller spatial frequency values as the image bandwidth decreased. It was also hoped that this half amplitude point would be more independent of stimulus contrast than the previous measure for image sharpness. This network could be simulated by simply determining the spatial frequency of the half amplitude points for model response plots similar to those shown in Fig. 18.

Since the spatial frequency channels in the model were spaced an octave apart, while a real system might have mechanisms distributed densely along the spatial frequency axis, interpolation was required to determine the spatial frequency of the half amplitude point from response plots of the type shown in Fig. 18. The results for this hypothetical network operating on the responses of the channel model are illustrated in Fig. 20.

The vertical axis is the position of the half amplitude point along the spatial frequency axis. Each curve represents the mean spatial frequency averaged across the 5 pictures. The mean spatial frequency for the unfiltered, contrast = 0.5, pictures was normalized to 1. All other responses were scaled by the scaling factor that normalized the 0.5 contrast unfiltered pictures. The positions of the half amplitude points agree rather well with the experimental image sharpness data shown in Fig. 17. The three curves lie close to each other indicating near independence of contrast and the saturation point occurs at about a bandwidth of 8 c/deg. In particular, the low contrast differences among the image sharpness estimates has disappeared. These results indicate that the half amplitude tracking

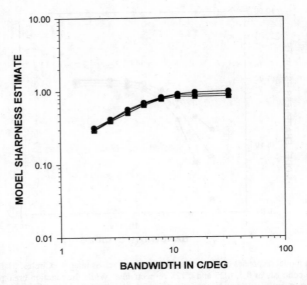

Figure 20. Model estimate of image sharpness from the position along the spatial axis of the half amplitude point of the channel responses. The three curves again indicate three picture contrasts but the curves nearly overlap demonstrating that this measure is relatively independent of contrast.

scheme coupled with the nonlinear filter model does an adequate job of accounting for human image sharpness estimates on real world scenes. It will require future experiments with other specially designed stimuli, with spectra that do not decrease as $1/f$, to explore the limitations of this analysis scheme for image sharpness.

5. Summary

One of the primary goals of this chapter has been to make the reader aware of the fact that data collected in threshold experiments may not be useful in predicting image appearance or perceived contrast responses at suprathreshold levels. A case in point is the tendency of many non-vision scientists to interpret the threshold contrast sensitivity function as a gain function for the spatial frequency tuned mechanisms in the visual system. We have seen that successful simulation of the suprathreshold response of the system requires filter mechanisms that have constant gain across spatial frequency. This may be surprising for scientists who have not considered suprathreshold phenomena, but cannot be ignored by any modeler who attempts to represent human perception of the appearance of real objects under suprathreshold conditions. The model also revealed that suprathreshold responses can be accounted for by a common contrast transducer function at all spatial frequencies if the form of the function depends on the spatial properties of the filter outputs. Thus, one is not required to fit different contrast transducer functions to mechanisms that are tuned to different spatial frequencies. The data presented earlier and the model derived from the data indicate a general operating principle for human visual system performance: the visual system strives toward constant gain across spatial frequencies at high contrasts to overcome spatial frequency spectrum distortions introduced at threshold. This trend to constant gain applies whether the threshold distortions are caused by spatial frequency, spatial size or eccentricity in the visual field.

An interesting question introduced by this work is the role of probability summation at threshold. Both magnitude estimation and contrast matching experiments performed in support of the modeling work have made it clear that the difference in thresholds for stimuli of different sizes is translated into a difference in perceived contrast for moderately suprathreshold contrasts. This difference in perceived contrast disappears gradually as contrast is increased further. Probability summation assumes that detection occurs when at least one of a group of noisy mechanisms produces a response that is above some criterion level or threshold. The number of mechanisms capable of producing this response increases as the size of the stimulus increases. Thus, the lower threshold for the larger stimulus is attributed entirely to the probability that a single mechanism will exceed threshold. Obviously, this explanation cannot account for perceived contrast effects just above threshold. The perceived contrasts of the stimuli in this contrast range increase with stimulus size. This effect must be due to some type of hardwired response pooling among the mechanisms responding to the stimuli. In this interpretation, the larger perceived contrast for the larger stimulus is due simply to the increase in the number of responding mechanisms contributing to the pool.

Response pooling calculations at threshold are usually considered to be a convenient approximation to the "true" process of probability summation. However, a real hardwired response pooling operation provides an alternate explanation for size dependent threshold differences. If it is the strength of the pooled responses that determine threshold, the pooled response of a large stimulus would exceed threshold at a lower contrast than the pooled response of a small stimulus. The response pooling equation in the Q_{POOL} term of the model makes no differentiation between subthreshold and suprathreshold response pooling. This allows a smooth transition from detection to perception. In this sense, the model attributes size dependent differences in response at both subthreshold and suprathreshold levels to a hardwired response pooling operation. It is possible that threshold detection is a combination of both probability summation and real response pooling, but for ease of computation, thresholds in the model are accounted for by response pooling alone.

The model responds correctly to a variety of elemental stimuli, such as multiple component sinewave grating patches. Thus, it offers a front end for exploring higher order computations such as the image sharpness algorithm derived above. A particularly interesting application of the model would be as a front end for a pattern classification system. The filters tuned to different spatial frequencies, spatial positions and orientations offer a rich parameter space for any pattern classification scheme. Daugman[24] has recently demonstrated the power of this richness in an extremely reliable algorithm that uses Gabor filter responses to the spatial patterns in the human iris as a basis for personal identification.

References

1. O. H. Schade, *J. Opt Soc. Am.* **46** (1956) 721-739.
2. C. Blakemore and F. W. Campbell, *J. Physiol.* **203** (1969) 237-260.
3. A. Pantle and R. Sekuler, *Vision Research* **9 (1969)** 397-406.
4. H. R. Wilson, D. K. McFarlane, and G. C. Phillips, *Vision Research* **23** (1983) 873-882.
5. C. Blakemore and J. Nachmias, *J.Physiol.* **213** (1971) 157-174.
6. A. B. Watson, *Vision Research* **22** (1982) 17-25.
7. R. F. Quick, *Kybernetik* **16** (1974) 65-67.
8. H. R. Wilson and J. R. Bergen, *Vision Research* **19** (1979) 19-32.
9. J. R. Bergen, H. R. Wilson, and J. D. Cowan, *J. Opt. Soc. Am.* **69** (1979) 1580-1587.
10. M. A. Georgeson and G. D. Sullivan, *J. Physiol.* **252** (1975) 627-656.
11. W. H. Swanson, H. R. Wilson, and S. C. Giese, *Vision Research* **24** (1984) 63-75.
12. M. W. Cannon and S. C. Fullenkamp, *Vision Research* **28** (1988) 695-709.
13. M. W. Cannon and S. C. Fullenkamp, *Vision Research* **31** (1991) 983-998.
14. M. W. Cannon, *J. Opt. Soc. Am. A* **2** (1985) 1760-1768.
15. J. G. Daugman, *J. Opt. Soc. Am. A* **2** (1985) 1160-1169.
16. R. A. Young, *Spatial Vision* **2** (1987) 273-293.
17. S. A. Klein and D. M. Levi, *J. Opt. Soc. Am. A* **2** (1985) 1170-1190.
18. H. R. Wilson, *Biol. Cybernet.* **38** (1980) 171-178.
19. G. E. Legge and J. M. Foley, *J. Opt Soc. Am.* **70** (1980) 1458-1471.
20. R. J. Beaton, *Proceedings of the Human Factors Society, 27th Annual Meeting* (1983) 41-45.
21. H. L. Task, Tech Report AMRL-TR-79-9 (Armstrong Laboratory Wright-Patterson Air Force Base, Ohio, 1979).
22. H. L. Snyder, Tech Report HFL-80-1 (Virginia Polytechnic Institute and State University, Blacksburg, VA, 1980).
23. C. R. Carlson and R. W. Cohen, Report ONR-CR-213-120-120-4F (Office of Naval Research, Arlington, VA, 1978).
24. J. G. Daugman, *IEEE Trans. Patt. Anal. Mach. Intell.* **15** (1993) 1148-1161.

DISCRIMINATION INFORMATION IN NATURAL RADIANCE SPECTRA

WILSON S. GEISLER
Center for Vision and Image Sciences
Mezes 330
University of Texas
Austin, TX 78712

Vision is based upon detecting and identifying differences in the radiance spectra arriving at the eye or camera from different directions. Radiance spectra can differ in total radiance (intensity), in shape (color), or both. Ideal-observer theory was used to measure the relative amounts of intensity and chromatic information available to discriminate pairs of natural radiance spectra created by illuminating natural surfaces (Krinov, 1947) with a natural daylight source (D65). Two ideal observers were evaluated -- one operating at the input to the eye or camera, and one at the level of the photopigments in the human cone photoreceptors. The relative amount of intensity and chromatic information in each discrimination pair was quantified by the effective increase in contrast due to the chromatic information. The analyses showed that chromatic information increases the effective contrast by an average of 30% to 70% at the input to the eye, but only by 5% to 10% at the level of the photopigments. It appears that much of the chromatic information in natural radiance spectra is lost between the cornea and photopigments, and that the chromatic information available at the level of the photopigments, for the purpose of discriminating between regions or detecting region boundaries, is usually small relative to intensity information.

1. Introduction

In the natural environment, indirect light sources, such as the sun and sky, irradiate the surfaces of objects. Each surface absorbs some fraction of the light incident upon it and reflects the remaining fraction.[1] This reflected light is a highly useful source of information because different surface materials have different reflectance spectra, and because the amount of light reflected from a surface varies systematically with the orientation of the surface relative to the light source.[2] The light reaching the observer from a surface is

---

[1] Some fraction of the light may also be absorbed and then re-emitted at longer wavelengths (fluorescence). For most natural materials, this is a minor component of the total light radiating from a surface.

[2] The light reflected toward the observer may also depend upon the orientation of the surface relative to the line-of-sight, and the location of the light source with respect to the observer.

described by a radiance spectrum (intensity as a function of wavelength). It is traditional to divide a radiance spectrum into two parts: the total radiance (the area under the radiance spectrum), and shape of the radiance spectrum (the wavelength distribution). Loosely speaking, the total radiance corresponds to the intensity or gray-level, and the shape of the radiance spectrum corresponds to the color or chromatic content.

The human visual system has evolved to make use of both intensity and color information. However, the two components may not be of equal value for performing visual tasks. For some tasks (e.g., edge detection), intensity information may be critical and chromatic information unimportant, and for other tasks (e.g., materials identification) the reverse may be the case. The fact that all species with vision have the ability to encode intensity differences, whereas many do not have the ability to encode color differences, suggests that color information may be less useful than intensity information for many basic visual tasks.

To evaluate these issues, I have attempted to use ideal-observer theory to quantify the relative amounts of intensity and chromatic information in natural radiance spectra, that is, radiance spectra produced by combining natural reflectance spectra with natural irradiance spectra. The interest in analyzing natural radiance spectra derives from the presumption that they are important in everyday visual performance, and were important in the evolution of the human visual system.

Ideal-observer theory is a well-accepted tool for analyzing the performance limitations imposed by the information contained in sensory stimuli. It has been extensively applied in the study of both intensity discrimination (e.g., Rose, 1948; Barlow, 1958; Green & Swets, 1974; Geisler, 1989; Pelli, 1990) and chromatic discrimination (e.g., Vos & Walraven, 1972; Buchsbaum & Goldstein, 1979; Massof & Starr, 1980; Geisler, 1989). Indeed, the ideal-observer calculations described here are for a standard discrimination task in which the observer is required to detect whether or not a difference exits between two regions of an image. However, because the analysis involves computing the *relative* amounts of intensity and color information, the conclusions will generalize to a range of other tasks (for further discussion see Jordan et al., 1990).

2. Methods and Results

2.1. Discrimination Task

The discrimination task is illustrated in Figure 1. On a given observation trial, one of two possible patterns is presented. Stimulus A consists of two regions with identical radiance spectra, $P_1(\lambda)$, and stimulus B consists of two regions with different radiance spectra, $P_1(\lambda)$ and $P_2(\lambda)$. Without loss of generality, we can suppose that the two stimuli are presented with equal probability. The observer's task is to identify whether each observation trial contains stimulus A or stimulus B. The observer's goal is to maximize accuracy (total percent correct). In the present analysis, the particular size, duration, and shape of the two regions are irrelevant because the calculations concern the relative amounts of intensity and chromatic information available to perform the task. Indeed, each of the two regions may consist of any number and any configuration of subregions (as long as all subregions have the same radiance spectrum). Thus, the conclusions that can be drawn from the present analysis are fairly general.

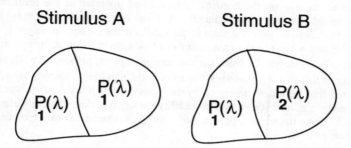

Figure 1. Illustration of the discrimination task. On each observation trial the observer is presented with either stimulus A (two regions with the same radiance spectrum) or stimulus B (two regions with different radiance spectra). The task is to identify which stimulus was presented.

2.2. The Radiance Spectra

The natural radiance spectra that I analyzed were derived from the 337 reflectance spectra reported by Krinov (1947). Krinov's sample includes trees, grass, river banks, fields of flowers, dirt roads, bricks, snow, lake water, and so on. To obtain a representative sample of outdoor natural radiance spectra, the Krinov reflectance spectra were multiplied by a standard (D65) daylight irradiance spectrum (Wyszecki & Stiles, 1982). All the radiance spectra were then converted from energy units $[P(\lambda)]$ to quantum units $[n(\lambda)]$,

$$n_1(\lambda) = P_1(\lambda)\lambda \tag{1}$$

$$n_2(\lambda) = P_2(\lambda)\lambda. \tag{2}$$

(The specific quantum and energy units are irrelevant because the analysis only considers the relative amounts of intensity and chromatic information.) The analysis reported here did not consider the effects of surface orientation.

2.3. Description of the Ideal Observer at the Cornea

Discrimination of one radiance spectrum from another may be based upon either the difference in the total radiance (intensity), the difference in the wavelength distribution (color), or both. To determine how much information for discriminating between the pairs of radiance spectra is contained in the intensity differences and how much in the chromatic differences, the performance of an ideal observer that used only the intensity differences was compared with the performance of an ideal observer that used both the intensity and chromatic differences.[3] Two separate ideal observers were considered. The first operated at the input to the eye (at the cornea). The second operated at the level of photon absorptions in the receptor photopigments. At these two levels in the stream of visual processing, the dominant source of noise is quantal fluctuations (photon noise).

Let $n_1(\lambda_i)$ and $n_2(\lambda_i)$ be the mean number of photons arriving at the eye, in a given time period, at wavelength λ_i, from the two image regions, respectively. It is a well-known physical fact that the random fluctuation in the number of photons arriving at the eye (in a fixed time period) is described by the Poisson probability density, which can be approximated by a normal (Gaussian) probability density function with the variance equal to the mean.[4] Using the normal approximation, the performance accuracy (percent correct) of the ideal observer is

$$PC = \Phi\left(\frac{d'_I}{2}\right) \tag{3}$$

where $\Phi(\cdot)$ is the standard normal integral function, and d'_I is the "signal-to-noise ratio" (the difference in the mean intensities divided by the square root of the average variance):

$$d'_I = \frac{\left|\sum_{i=1}^{n} n_2(\lambda_i) - \sum_{i=1}^{n} n_1(\lambda_i)\right|}{\sqrt{0.5\left(\sum_{i=1}^{n} n_2(\lambda_i) + \sum_{i=1}^{n} n_1(\lambda_i)\right)}} \tag{4}$$

When both chromatic and intensity information are used, ideal performance is given by the following formula:

$$PC = \Phi\left(\frac{d'_{I+C}}{2}\right) \tag{5}$$

where

---

[3] An ideal observer is a theoretical device that performs a task at the maximum level possible given the available information; thus its performance serves as a precise measure of the available information.

[4] The normal density provides a good approximation to the Poisson density only when the mean number of photons is large; however, when the normal approximation is being used to compute discrimination performance, it is accurate even at very low means (Geisler, 1984; Geisler et al., 1991).

$$d'_{I+C} = \frac{\sum_{i=1}^{n}[n_2(\lambda_i) - n_1(\lambda_i)]\ln[n_2(\lambda_i)/n_1(\lambda_i)]}{\sqrt{0.5\sum_{i=1}^{n}[n_2(\lambda_i) + n_1(\lambda_i)]\ln^2[n_2(\lambda_i)/n_1(\lambda_i)]}} \tag{6}$$

Equations (4) and (6) are standard and follow directly from the formulas derived in Geisler (1984) and Helstrom (1964). The summations in Eqs. (4) and (6) were taken over the range of 400 nm to 650 nm in 10 nm steps (because that is how the Krinov data are reported). However, given the smoothness of the spectra, it is unlikely that the results reported here would have been different with a finer sampling.

There are a number of essentially equivalent ways that one could report the computed ideal-observer performances. One would be to report the values of PC or d' for intensity information alone and for intensity-plus-chromatic information (note that PC and d' are monotonically related to each other). However, it is difficult to relate specific values of d' to the subjective appearances of images, and the PC values are compressed into a small range at high levels of d'. Therefore, I report instead a measure that compares the contrast between regions with the "equivalent contrast" between the regions due to the combined intensity and chromatic information. In this measure, contrast (C) is defined in the usual fashion (the so-called Michelson contrast),

$$C = \frac{I_{max} - I_{min}}{I_{max} + I_{min}} = \frac{\left|\sum_{i=1}^{n}n_2(\lambda_i) - \sum_{i=1}^{n}n_1(\lambda_i)\right|}{\sum_{i=1}^{n}n_1(\lambda_i) + \sum_{i=1}^{n}n_2(\lambda_i).} \tag{7}$$

Combining Eqs. (4) and (7) gives the relationship between d'_I, contrast, and mean intensity:

$$d'_I = 2\sqrt{\overline{N}}C \tag{8}$$

where the mean intensity, $\overline{N}$, is given by,

$$\overline{N} = 0.5\left(\sum_{i=1}^{n}n_1(\lambda_i) + \sum_{i=1}^{n}n_2(\lambda_i)\right). \tag{9}$$

To derive the equivalent contrast measure, note that any given contrast between the two surface regions (at constant mean intensity) is associated with a particular value of d'_I. When chromatic information is included, the signal-to-noise ratio, d'_{I+C}, must either remain the same or increase. In other words, d'_{I+C} must be greater than or equal to d'_I. The *equivalent contrast*, C_e, is defined to be the contrast that would produce d'_{I+C} (while holding the mean intensity, $\overline{N}$, fixed). Thus, C_e is obtained by finding d'_{I+C} with Eq. (6), substituting d'_{I+C} for d'_I in Eq. (8), and then solving for contrast:

$$C_e = \frac{d'_{I+C}}{2\sqrt{\overline{N}}}. \tag{10}$$

The figures that follow plot the proportional increase in contrast due to chromatic information, C_e / C. This measure has the virtue of being independent of the size, shape and duration of the regions being discriminated. Combining Eqs. (8) and (10) shows that the ratio of the contrasts is equal to the ratio of the d's,

$$\frac{C_e}{C} = \frac{d'_{I+C}}{d'_I}. \tag{11}$$

2.4. Performance of the Ideal Observer at the Cornea

Now, consider the chromatic and intensity information available in the natural radiance spectra synthesized from the Krinov reflectance spectra. The first analysis was to compute both the contrasts and the equivalent contrasts for all 56,616 possible pairs of spectra. Figure 2 displays a two-dimensional histogram of the results. The horizontal axis on the right gives the Michelson contrast between pairs of spectra. The horizontal axis on the left gives the percentage increase in contrast due to the chromatic information (i.e., $100 \times C_e / C$). Finally, the vertical axis is the frequency of pairs falling in a bin, normalized to a peak value of 1.0. As can be seen, the contrasts between natural radiance spectra cluster around 30-50%. Also, as might be expected, the percentage increase in contrast due to color is greatest when the contrasts (C) are low (this is seen in the increased spread of the distribution at low contrasts). Overall, there is a fairly substantial increase in effective contrast due to chromatic information -- chromatic information effectively increased the contrast by an average of 32% (0.12 log units).

It might be argued that the above analysis is biased against chromatic information in that the Krinov spectra contain a number of rather extreme cases, such as snow and asphalt, which would produce very large intensity differences and small chromatic differences. Thus, a second analysis included only those spectra whose intensities fell in the middle two quartiles (i.e., high and low intensity radiance spectra were excluded). The results are shown in Figure 3. The average contrast improvement was 70% (0.23 log units). This is a substantial increase in effective contrast.

The fact that the contrast (or equivalently, the signal-to-noise ratio) increased an average of 32% and 70% in the above two analyses implies that chromatic information can be of value in discriminating between regions in natural images. Thus, the results suggest that there may be some value to using chromatic information in, for example, boundary and region detection algorithms.

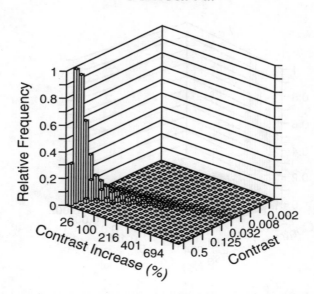

Figure 2. Frequency histogram of percent contrast increase due to chromatic information for 56,616 pairings of 337 natural radiance spectra. The right horizontal axis plots the Michelson contrast between pairs of spectra. The left horizontal axis plots the percent increase in contrast due to chromatic information, as measured by an ideal observer operating at the level of the input to the eye or camera. "Contrast Increase" can also be interpreted as the percent increase in d'.

2.5. Description of the Ideal Observer at the Human Photoreceptors

The performance of the ideal observer at the cornea showed that there is considerable chromatic information available in natural radiance spectra. However, the human visual system has only three types of cone photoreceptors with rather broad spectral sensitivities. With so few types of receptor, the human cone system may only extract a fraction of the useful chromatic information from natural radiance spectra. Thus, an important question is how much of the chromatic information available at the cornea remains available at the level of the photoreceptors.

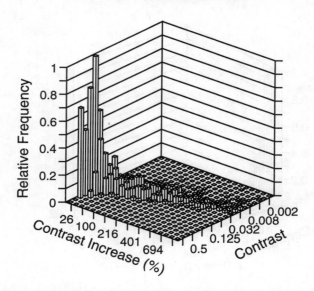

Figure 3. Frequency histogram of percent contrast increase due to chromatic information for 14,028 pairings of 168 natural radiance spectra. These spectra represent the middle two quartiles of intensity from the original 337 spectra (see Figure 2).

Subjectively, when the Krinov spectra are rendered on a color monitor, they vary quite a bit in both apparent brightness and color, suggesting that both chromatic and intensity information might be useful for discriminating between them. However, subjective impressions can be misleading; for example, neural circuits could amplify small spectral differences into large subjective differences. To determine how much of the chromatic information useful for discriminating between natural spectra is available in the cones, the Krinov spectra were analyzed with an ideal observer operating at the level of photon absorptions in the photopigments (as opposed to at the cornea).

The mean rate of photon absorptions in the individual photoreceptors were computed using the following equations,

$$r = \kappa \sum_{i=1}^{n} n(\lambda_i) t(\lambda_i) a_r(\lambda_i) \tag{12}$$

$$g = \kappa \sum_{i=1}^{n} n(\lambda_i) t(\lambda_i) a_g(\lambda_i) \tag{13}$$

$$b = \kappa \sum_{i=1}^{n} n(\lambda_i) t(\lambda_i) a_b(\lambda_i) \tag{14}$$

where $n(\lambda)$ is a radiance spectrum (in quantum units), $t(\lambda)$ is the transmittance function of the ocular media, κ is the receptor aperture (the light collection area), and $a_r(\lambda)$, $a_g(\lambda)$, and $a_b(\lambda)$ are the absorption spectra of the red (long wavelength), green (middle wavelength), and blue (short wavelength) sensitive photopigments.

The formula for ideal-observer performance (at the photopigments), when only the intensity information is used, is given by

$$d'_I = \frac{\sqrt{m}}{\sqrt{0.5}} \frac{\left| p_r(r_2 - r_1) + p_g(g_2 - g_1) + p_b(b_2 - b_1) \right|}{\sqrt{p_r(r_2 + r_1) + p_g(g_2 + g_1) + p_b(b_2 + b_1)}} \tag{15}$$

where (r_1, g_1, b_1) and (r_2, g_2, b_2) are the mean quantal absorptions in the red, green and blue cones for the two spectra being discriminated, m is the total number of cones under the retinal image of the test patch, and (p_r, p_g, p_b) are the proportions of red, green and blue cones. When both chromatic and intensity information are used, performance is given by the following formula:

$$d'_{I+C} = \frac{\sqrt{2m} \left[p_r(r_2 - r_1)\ln\left(\frac{r_2}{r_1}\right) + p_g(g_2 - g_1)\ln\left(\frac{g_2}{g_1}\right) + p_b(b_2 - b_1)\ln\left(\frac{b_2}{b_1}\right) \right]}{\sqrt{p_r(r_2 + r_1)\ln^2\left(\frac{r_2}{r_1}\right) + p_g(g_2 + g_1)\ln^2\left(\frac{g_2}{g_1}\right) + p_b(b_2 + b_1)\ln^2\left(\frac{b_2}{b_1}\right).}} \tag{16}$$

Equations (15) and (16) are directly analogous to Eqs. (4) and (6).

To apply these equations I assumed (a) cone absorption spectra based upon the Smith and Pokorny (1975) fundamentals, (b) the ocular transmittance function given in Wyszecki and Stiles (1982), and (c) that there are twice as many red cones as green cones and three times as many green cones as blue cones. No assumptions for m and κ were necessary because they cancel when computing the ratio of the d's (i.e., C_e / C). (For more details, see Geisler, 1989; Jordan et al., 1990.)

2.6 Performance of the Ideal Observer at the Human Photoreceptors

Now, consider the chromatic and intensity information available at the photoreceptors for discriminating between natural radiance spectra. As before, the first analysis was to compute both the contrasts and the equivalent contrasts for all 56,616 possible pairs of spectra. Figure 4 displays a two-dimensional histogram of the results. At the

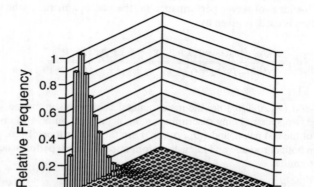

Figure 4. Frequency histogram of percent contrast increase due to chromatic information for 56,616 pairings of 337 natural radiance spectra. The right horizontal axis plots the Michelson contrast between pairs of spectra computed at the level of photon absorptions in the photoreceptors. The left horizontal axis plots the percent increase in contrast due to chromatic information as measured by an ideal observer operating at the level of receptor photopigments. "Contrast Increase" can also be interpreted as the percent increase in d'.

photoreceptors, the average percent increase in contrast due to chromatic information was only 5% (0.02 log units), and only 7% of the pairs showed an improvement greater than

0.05 log units. This suggests that at the level of the photopigments, the chromatic information for discriminating between pairs of natural spectra is usually very small (relative to intensity information). However, it might be argued again that this analysis is unfair because the Krinov spectra include some rather extreme variations in intensity. Thus, a second analysis included only those spectra whose intensities (at the photopigments) were in the middle two quartiles. The results are shown in Figure 5. The average contrast improvement was 11% (0.047 log units). This is still a small improvement.

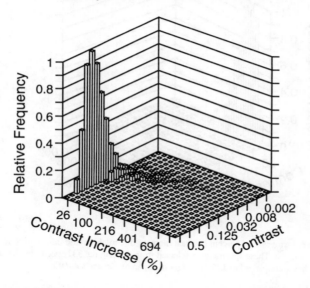

Figure 5. Frequency histogram of percent contrast increase due to chromatic information for 14,028 pairings of 168 natural radiance spectra. These spectra represent the middle two quartiles of intensity from the original 337 spectra (see Figure 4).

The Krinov spectra might be biased against the chromatic information in another way: they might contain too many samples with the same or similar spectral shapes, compared to the actual numbers that occur in nature. In other words, the Krinov spectra may include too many samples of the same or similar color. To explore this possibility, I tried, in a third analysis, to bias the sample in favor of the chromatic information by selecting a small subset of spectra that appeared (subjectively) to be maximally spread out in hue and saturation. The results of the analysis for this subset are shown in Figure 6. Again, the chromatic information seems to be very small. The average contrast improvement was 10% (0.04 log units).

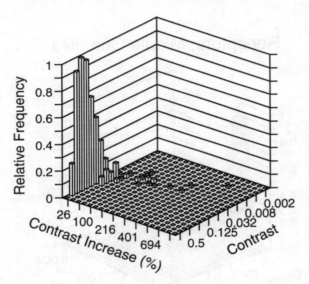

Figure 6. Frequency histogram of percent contrast increase due to chromatic information for 45 pairings of 10 natural radiance spectra. These spectra were selected from the original 337 spectra by the author, based on color appearance; they were picked to differ strongly in apparent hue and saturation.

3. Discussion

The summary statistics for all the analyses (both at the cornea and at the photopigments) are shown in Table 1. The percentage increases in contrast at the photopigments are very small, but at the cornea they are large enough to be valuable. Thus, it appears that considerable chromatic information for discriminating between regions in natural images is lost due to preneural factors. (Undoubtedly this is due in part to the large spectral overlap of the red and green cones.)

There are several criticisms that might be leveled against the information analyses described here. First, it could be argued that discriminations between radiance spectra in the real world involve high degrees of position uncertainty in space and time; whereas the present ideal observers were "signal-known-exactly," and hence they "knew" the exact positions in space and time. However, position uncertainty is likely to have little effect because the values of d' for intensity alone (d'_I) and intensity-plus-color (d'_{I+C}) will be affected similarly by uncertainty effects, and hence their ratio, which equals C_e / C, will remain nearly the same.

Table 1. Summary of ideal-observer calculations.

**Average Contrast Increase
Due to Chromatic Information**

	All Spectra	Mid Intensities	Selected
Cornea	32% (0.12)	70% (0.23)	49% (0.17)
Photopigments	5% (0.023)	11% (0.047)	10% (0.0414)

**Percentage of Pairs
Where Contrast Increase Exceeds 0.05 Log Units**

	All Spectra	Mid Intensities	Selected
Cornea	35%	57%	53%
Photopigments	7.5%	15.4%	13.7%

A second criticism might be based upon the fact that pairs of Krinov reflectance spectra produce rather large intensity and chromatic differences, which under many viewing conditions would be well above detection threshold. It might be argued that a more useful stimulus set would consist of pairs of natural reflectances nearer human detection threshold. One response to this criticism is that detection thresholds depend not only on the magnitude of the intensity and color differences, but on the area, duration, and mean luminance of the stimuli; thus there are many conditions where pairs of Krinov spectra *will* produce near threshold differences. For example, consider the visibility of adjacent image regions when navigating through the environment. As a pair of regions is approached, the visual angles expand and the information for discriminating between the regions increases until the observer is able to make the discrimination (i.e., detect the boundary between the regions). At the cornea, the information for discriminating between the regions is (on average) substantially greater if chromatic information is considered; hence, accurate discrimination would be possible at substantially greater distances. On other hand, at the level of the photopigments the chromatic information would be of much less value in expanding the distance over which the regions could be discriminated.

Another response to this criticism is based on the likely possibility that many of the more subtle differences in reflectance which occur in the environment might be modeled by pairs of regions which are each a weighted sum of two or more Krinov reflectance spectra (e.g., two types of grass growing together in a field and viewed from a distance). I have not yet analyzed such combination spectra in detail, but some preliminary analyses suggest that the major conclusions of the present paper will continue to hold. For example, simulations show that if a less discriminable pair of reflectance spectra is created by adding the same reflectance spectrum to a pair of Krinov reflectance spectra, there is little effect on the proportion increase in contrast due to chromatic information (C_e / C), even though the contrast between the regions is reduced.

A third criticism might be that many of the Krinov reflectance spectra are for natural terrain surfaces viewed at large distances, and hence they may not be representative of the natural reflectance spectra encountered at smaller distances. José Ramón Jiménez Cuesta (of the University of Grenada, Spain) and I are carrying out an ideal-observer analysis of the reflectance spectra of (a) various fruits and their leaves, and (b) a large collection of man-made materials. Preliminary results indicate that the average increase in effective contrast due to chromatic information is somewhat larger for these stimuli than for the Krinov spectra, but that the increase is still rather small (0.053 and 0.062 log units at the photopigments for the fruits and leaves, and man-made materials, respectively).

Finally, it could be argued that a precise analysis of the chromatic information for discriminating between regions in natural images should take into account the relative frequencies at which the different spectra appear side-by-side in nature, as well as the survival value of particular discriminations. Such considerations seem unlikely to help the case for color, because color made a weak contribution even when I attempted to bias the analysis in its favor. Thus, one is led to conclude (at least on the basis of the Krinov data) that in the real world, the chromatic information available at the level of the photopigments, for the purpose of discriminating between regions or detecting boundaries, is small relative to intensity information.

On the other hand, it is important to recognize that the chromatic information in natural radiance spectra may be much greater in some visual tasks. For example, if the task were not to discriminate two regions, but to identify the material composition of surfaces, then it is likely that the chromatic information would be greater than the intensity information, even at the level of the photoreceptors.[5] For example, intensity information may be sufficient for detecting the boundaries between the surface of a fruit and the leaves behind or in front of it, but may well be insufficient if the task is to identify the type of fruit and

---

[5] Recall that the information available to perform a task is quantified by the performance of the specific ideal observer for that task. Therefore, when the task changes, the relative amounts of intensity and chromatic information can change.

whether it is ripe (and hence edible). For such an identification task, the chromatic information may be substantially greater than the intensity information.

Acknowledgments

This research was supported in part by NIH grant EY02688 and AFOSR grant F49620-93-1-0307. I thank Larry Maloney for providing the Krinov data files.

References

1. H. B. Barlow, "Temporal and spatial summation in human vision at different background intensities," *Journal of Physiology, London* **141** (1958) 337-350.
2. G. Buchsbaum and J. L. Goldstein, "Optimum probabilistic processing in colour perception I: Colour discrimination," *Proc. R. Soc. Lond.* **205** (1979) 229-247.
3. W. S. Geisler, Physical limits of acuity and hyperacuity. *Journal of the Optical Society of America A* **1** (1984) 775-782.
4. W. S. Geisler, "Sequential ideal-observer analysis of visual discriminations," *Psychological Review* **96** (1989) 267-314.
5. W. S. Geisler, D. G. Albrecht, R. J. Salvi, and S. S. Saunders, "Discrimination performance of single neurons: Rate and temporal-pattern information," *Journal of Neurophysiology* **66** (1991) 334-361.
6. D. M. Green and J. A. Swets, *"Signal Detection Theory and Psychophysics,"* (New York: Krieger, 1974).
7. C. W. Helstrom, "The detection and resolution of optical signals," *IEEE Transactions on Information Theory* **IT-10** (1964) 275-287.
8. J. R. Jordan, W. S. Geisler, and A. C. Bovik, "Color as a source of information in the stereo correspondence process," *Vision Research* **30** (1990) 1955-1970.
9. E. Krinov, *"Spectral Reflectance Properties of Natural Formations,"* Technical translation TT-439 (National Research Council of Canada, Ottawa, 1947).
10. R. W. Massof and S. J. Starr, "Vector magnitude operation in color vision models: Derivations from signal detection theory," *Journal of the Optical Society of America* **70** (1980) 870-872.
11. D. G. Pelli, "The quantum efficiency of vision," In *Vision: Coding and Efficiency* ed. C. Blakemore (Cambridge University Press, Cambridge, 1990) pp. 3-24.
12. A. Rose, "The sensitivity performance of the human eye on an absolute scale," *Journal of the Optical Society of America* **38** (1948) 196-208.
13. V. C. Smith and J. Pokorny, "Spectral sensitivity of color-blind observers and the cone photopigments," *Vision Research* **12** (1975) 2059-2071.
14. J. J. Vos and P. L. Walraven, "An analytical description of the line element in the zone-fluctuation model of color vision: 1. Basic concepts," *Vision Research* **12** (1972) 1327-1344.
15. G. Wyszecki and W. S. Stiles, *"Color Science,"* (New York: Wiley, 1982).

Models Applications
and
Evaluation

THE ORACLE APPROACH TO TARGET ACQUISITION AND SEARCH MODELLING

KEVIN J. COOKE,
PHILIP A. STANLEY and JEREMY L. HINTON
British Aerospace Sowerby Research Centre, Bristol BS12 7QW,UK.

The ORACLE model has been developed to represent as many features as possible of human visual processing in a simplified mathematical form, and can be applied to practical problems such as those involved with the prediction of visual task performance when using optical and electro-optical aids. As knowledge about specific processes of human vision grows, attempts are made to update the appropriate parts of the model. This chapter describes some of the component parts of the model as they are currently represented. It describes the treatment of detection and recognition of image components as a function of scene parameters such as background luminance. The initial calculation is of the 50% detection threshold for a particular target. However the model exploits aspects of observer variance to generate a performance prediction for a particular task and contrast relative to the detection threshold contrast for that target. The statistical variance for a population of observers is assumed to be a constant ratio relative to the threshold (50% probability of detection) value and enables probabilities of acquisition to be calculated for any target position in the visual field(the visual lobe). Acquisition probabilities for successive fixations within a field of view can be determined from consideration of the common area of the visual lobe and the search field, but adequate modelling of search is only achieved by acknowledging the time course of observer variation, and the use of 'soft shell' visual lobes.

1. Introduction

In inviting a presentation describing the ORACLE visual performance model given at a meeting of the Armstrong Laboratory Advisory Group (ALAG) in 1991, Art Menendez asked for an overview of the underlying concepts of a model that was currently flexible enough to address a variety of practical problems. This chapter describes the ORACLE model basic concepts and how they have been revised over the years with the growth of visual performance information. Art also requested that we address 'the critical issues', and wanted to investigate how we could combine the deeper theoretical approaches with the requirement for simpler practical models. To have some validity simplified models should result from assumptions and trade-offs made from underlying detailed theories. The validity can be established by comparing the results with test data. This paper does not attempt to answer the question 'Does the model work?', by the accuracy with which it should be able to predict experimental data; rather it concentrates on describing how aspects of human vision can be modelled. Component parts of the model have been experimentally tested at each stage of its development both by laboratory and field studies, and in many cases the prediction of psychophysical data is satisfactory. It has not, however, been possible to test all the interactions as fully as we would desire due to an apparent absence of fundamental data, some instances of which are highlighted in this chapter. In this regard it would be beneficial to vision modellers to have a common database against which to test their models.

Individuals or groups with specialist knowledge of an area could then be responsible for maintaining parts of such a database so that development could take place in a coordinated way.

The principal objective in creating the ORACLE vision model has been to establish in a single mathematical model the ability to predict the performance statistics for human visual response under a wide range of viewing conditions. Performance is evaluated in terms of threshold sizes, contrasts, and probabilities for search, detection, recognition and identification. The visual system's response to image characteristics (e.g. motion, colour etc) is evaluated in terms of effects on these processes. The model necessarily neglects many associated phenomena some examples being velocity perception and colour appearance.

Research has provided data from a variety of sources which give a well established set of mean contrast threshold values for simple shapes in plain backgrounds. In practical situations targets are seldom simple and backgrounds are usually structured. The aim in developing a model is to be able to extrapolate from simple conditions towards novel and complex conditions. To do this it is not enough to represent ideal thresholds with an empirical model because this becomes very limiting when attempting to deal with complex stimuli. It was therefore decided to direct the model development towards a representation of the known physiology and anatomy of the visual system. On this basis, if the stimulus is adequately characterised then a model of visual response should be capable of representing visual performance independently of the display devices used or the task that the observer is required to perform. This chapter describes the development of a threshold model which in the first instance was an attempt to represent the contrast threshold response of the visual system as a function of target size and different scene luminances.

Fundamentally ORACLE is a human visual performance model but since electro-optical technology now also permits energy at many wavelengths of the electromagnetic spectrum to be presented in a visible format, the issues associated with this transformation need to be considered. Such processes can generally be represented by an understanding of the physics of the sensor system in generating the visible image. Knowing the parameters to which the human visual system is sensitive should make it possible to model current and future systems by representing the transfer functions from detector through to the display.

1.1. Theoretical Basis of the Model

As with all optical imaging systems, light entering the eye is spread before reaching the detectors. The image reaching the retina is subjected to optical spreading both by the optics of the eye and by diffusion through neural tissue which overlays the retinal receptor layer. Such an optical modification, which results in the blurring of the image, is an imperfection but in human vision the blurring is used as an advantage. Even when approaching diffraction limited conditions, the image spread resulting from the dioptrics of the eye is quite large with respect to the distance between receptors, and this is useful for distributing the information so that it can be sampled by the receptor matrix without the possibility of spatial aliasing, at least at the fovea.

The retina contains four types of receptors comprising three different types of cones and the rods. The distribution of retinal cone cells has been mapped by Østerberg[1] and Curcio et al.[2] from which emerges a consistent picture of coarser sampling with increasing angle from the fovea. The process of converting photons into neural signals is subject to the limitations of this non-uniform receptor sampling, and also to the effective temporal rates at which these signals are processed in the retina. The first stages of processing of the retinal image occur in the neural layers close to the receptors. These implement some aspects of adaptation, and transform the nature of the stimulus which is subsequently transmitted to the cortex. Then three main layers of processing produce signals which are functions of the differences between the output of adjacent receptors. These signals are subject to noise, and their strength relative to noise determines whether an observer will detect a target.

Observer threshold levels are not constant, being subject to periodic variations over time varying between a few minutes and several weeks. In addition the threshold level at any one instant of time will depend on the criterion adopted. A variety of experimental techniques have been used to measure observer thresholds and depending on technique the resulting thresholds may differ considerably. The more an observer is constrained in his choice of response (forced choice) the lower his threshold is likely to be. Effectively, in a forced choice situation the observer's criterion will equate to much smaller signal-to-noise levels than when the observer is free to choose.

The historical development of the model rested on the assumption that it is the edges of a target rather than the total energy contained within its area which are significant. The visual threshold detection process can therefore be described by quantifying the signal strength in terms of the maximum illuminance gradient as sampled by adjacent receptors at the retina. This signal strength measure, in conjunction with the number of receptors which contribute, provides the potential for predicting detection performance. Therefore target signatures are specified in terms of their perimeters and contrasts.

1.2. The Basic ORACLE Model

Early processes in the visual system transmit difference signals from adjacent receptors. If the target object is an optical point source then the signals reaching the cortex are derived from the differences between a central receptor responding to a peak illuminance input and a surrounding ring of adjacent receptors. For a larger uniform luminance target object the maximum illuminance gradients will occur across many receptor pairs around its perimeter. Target acquisition requires that at some point in the visual system the total signal must exceed a limiting value determined by the noise level and the observer's operating criterion. It is necessary to consider how the signals generated by individual receptors combine to provide a total signal for a given target object.

The ideal model would be a representation of the anatomical network of connections and the associated mechanisms of signal transduction and summation. Given the limited understanding of the visual system when the threshold model was first developed[3] this was not considered to be a practical proposition. A simplified approach was adopted to represent the average signal strength of the receptors together with a simplified summation function. More recent understanding of visual mechanisms does not appear to contradict this approach, which has been found to be adequate for the representation of simple target acquisition, and from which approaches for handling more complex situations have been developed.

The flow of the processes represented in the calculation of threshold performance in basic ORACLE is outlined below. Some terms and functions are introduced here, but will remain to be defined later on in the text.

- The mean scene luminance is used to calculate a measure of the adaptation level of the visual system $K_1 g_3(E_r)$.
- The mean scene luminance is used together with the size of the field of view area to calculate the pupil diameter.
- From the pupil diameter, the modulation transfer function and equivalent point spread function are calculated.
- The point spread function in conjunction with target size and the input luminance contrast, C, provides a measure of the illuminance gradient on the retina producing the value of $K_2 C$.
- In the case of recognition the previous calculation is based on only a fraction of the target dimension as a means of representing the resolvable detail.
- The function of the number of receptor pairs $g_2(n)$ around the perimeter of the target object image is calculated based on a receptor spacing of 0.145 milliradians.
- For very small targets the function of number of receptors is limited to the ring of receptors around the half height circumference of the optical point spread function.
- The threshold equation (1) combines these functions to provide a ratio of the available signal to the required threshold signal. This ratio can then be converted into probability.

The basic form of the ORACLE equation is:

$$K_2 C = \frac{K_1 g_3(E_r)}{g_2(n)} + d_c \qquad (1)$$

where K_2 is the average illuminance gradient between two adjacent receptors at the region of maximum slope of the illuminance profile, C is the luminance contrast between the target and its immediate background, $K_1 g_3(E_r)$ is a measure of adaptation level, $g_2(n)$ is a function of the number of receptor pairs on the perimeter of the target object image, and d_c is a constant representing the minimum signal that can be discriminated. These descriptions will be expanded in the following paragraphs. Contrast used in this chapter is psychometric contrast (C) and is

$$C = \frac{(L_t - L_b)}{L_b} = \frac{L_t}{L_b} - 1 \qquad (2)$$

where L_t is the luminance of the target, and L_b is that of the background.

1.3. The Retinal Image

The retinal image of a target object with a perfect quality edge provides the maximum retinal illuminance gradient that can be achieved between adjacent foveal receptors. The sharpness of the image on the retina is determined from optical spread functions representative of the observer's eye under the prevailing viewing conditions. The optical spread functions measured by Campbell and Gubisch[4] were shown to be dependent on the pupil diameter. Their

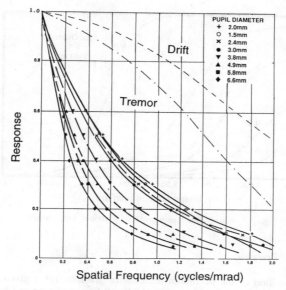

Figure 1. MTF of the eye: optical and motion components.

measurements excluded effects from tremor and drift of the eye, but these are included in the ORACLE representation as part of the total pre-receptor spread function. The optical spread function is the illuminance profile across the retina resulting from a point source. It can be converted to its frequency domain counterpart, the modulation transfer function (MTF), by taking the Fourier transform of the illuminance distribution (Figure 1). The retinal illuminance gradient can be determined from the spread function. Since it is common practice to measure the quality of optical and electro-optical systems by measuring MTFs, it is useful to be able to convert such measures into spread functions for predicting visual performance. It is possible for a given size of pupil, and knowing the shape of the optical spread function, to calculate the maximum illuminance gradient for an image at the retina.

Figure 2 shows retinal illuminance profiles for a variety of target sizes. The difference of retinal illuminance across adjacent receptors in the region of maximum gradient can be determined from such profiles. The curves in Figure 2 are derived from the eye spread function for a 3.0 mm pupil diameter and foveal viewing. For target disc diameters greater than about 9 minutes of arc the gradient is constant and the same as that shown for the 9 minute of arc disc. This limiting gradient for large targets gives a difference of 0.163 between adjacent receptors, where receptor spacing is assumed to be 0.5 mins of arc. The maximum gradient for discs smaller than 9 minutes of arc reduces, as it does with any degradation due to a poorer eye optical spread function or a poorer quality displayed target. In ORACLE K_2 adopts the value of 0.163 the result for best image quality.

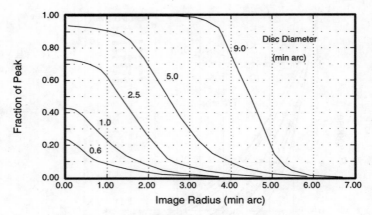

Figure 2. Retinal illuminance profiles for various width targets.

1.4. The Number of Receptors

Knowing the position of the maximum illuminance gradient, for a given target size it is possible to determine the number of receptors which will be sampling it and hence the number of receptors used in the detection process will reach a minimum and constant value for very small target objects and this will be governed by the width of the optical spread function. This width is generally the width of the function at half of the peak illuminance. For objects which are very small with respect to the point spread function (effectively point sources with diameters of less than 0.6 minutes of arc) the target signal is reduced in proportion to the peak of the illuminance profile at the retina, which itself is reduced in proportion to the area of the target. Thus, in the limit, contrast threshold must become inversely proportional to the stimulus area due to optical considerations alone. It is known[5] that when viewing a simple circular stimulus of very small angular subtense at the eye the contrast required to see it is indeed inversely related to the area. These trends are embodied in Ricco's law which states that the product of the threshold contrast and the area of the target is a constant. The proportionality of the function K_2 to target area effectively implements Ricco's Law[6] in the ORACLE equation for small targets. This is essentially a result of the optical properties of the eye.

At the other extreme of stimulus size, very large targets with a diameter in excess of 0.5 degrees of visual angle cannot be completely imaged on the fovea centralis. Outside this region the density of retinal receptors, and hence resolution, decreases rapidly. Consideration of this falling density of receptors must be included in any modelling of very large object threshold contrast performance.

The precise number of receptors (n) contributing to a cortical response will depend on the receptor arrangement and density. From the work of Pirenne[7] we have assumed a cone receptor spacing of 0.5 minutes of arc in the central fovea. According to Campbell[8] there are predominantly two different cone types in the fovea combining to provide foveal colour response. In earlier versions of ORACLE the assumption was made that the arrangement was a hexagonal close packed matrix, with difference processing being maximal between like cones and this led to a calculated spacing between like cones of 0.7 minutes of arc (0.2 mrad). We no longer hold this view and currently assume a 0.5 minute of arc inter-receptor spacing for foveal response to luminance, with difference processing not being sensitive to cone type.

The effective perimeter size of small targets is also influenced because the eye is never in a completely stationary state, the image being subject to motion across small angular distances due to tremor and drift.[9] The number of retinal receptors calculated as sampling the illuminance profile over the average glimpse or fixation time (a third of a second) makes allowance for the blurring effects of tremor and drift. These involuntary eye movements cause the image to move across the retina, increasing the effective length of the contour of maximum illuminance gradient and the number of receptors (n) sampling it. The increased size is calculated by assuming the drift to be linear motion over 1.5 minutes of arc and the tremor to have an amplitude of typically 1-3 minutes of arc. Saccadic eye movement does not need to be considered as vision is assumed to be suppressed during the saccade.

A method for representing approximately the rate of reduction of signal across receptors as the target size reduces is to operate on the illuminance gradient value K_2 to reduce the effective retinal signal with decreasing target size:

$$f(K_2) = \frac{0.163\ X}{(X^4+1)^{0.25}} \tag{3}$$

where X is the target dimension multiplied by a constant representing system image sharpness.

For relatively large image sizes the length of the contour of maximum gradient remains roughly the same as the length of the geometrical image contour. If the contour is closed, then the internal number of receptors will be less than the external, but on average the number of receptor pairs per unit length of perimeter can be assumed to remain the same regardless of which portion of the perimeter we are considering. Therefore it was decided to base the function of n on the actual perimeter length (Eq. 4), but with due allowance for smaller targets never reducing below a limiting ring of receptors, as determined by the spread function described earlier.

$$n = \frac{Perimeter}{Inter-cone\ \ distance} \tag{4}$$

As the model developed, it was necessary to establish what function of the number of receptors, when combined with the local signal strength, best matches experimental contrast thresholds. The simplest model for matching contrast thresholds for multiple glimpse viewing, (Eq. 5), required an inverse square law for the signal contribution from each receptor pair:

$$g_2(n) = n^{-2} \tag{5}$$

Model predictions were compared with Blackwell[10] classic data for the case of 10 foot lambert luminance (34.3 cd m^{-2}) and effectively infinite viewing time. The target signatures were characterised by using the values of contrast in conjunction with the target size converted to a count of the number of receptor pairs around the perimeter to give a value for n. Then using the $g_2(n)$ function (Eq. 5) the values were entered into Eq. (1). This produced values for $K_1 = 0.48$ and $d_c = 0.00036$ which are respectively the slope of the function and the intercept with the y axis.

A similar exercise was conducted for the Taylor[11] data, again restricted to foveal viewing, but employing a shorter presentation time than was the case in the Blackwell studies. The viewing time in Taylor's experiment restricted the observer to a single glimpse, and an $n^{-1.5}$ relationship provided the best fit between data and model. This apparent reduction in receptor contribution was considered to be due to a proportion of detectors responding below the noise level in a single glimpse, and therefore not contributing to the short-duration threshold performance.

The basic model was also tested to see if it could be used to match experimental threshold values for rectangular targets using short presentation times. Results for Lamar et al's[12] subset of square targets were examined in detail. Model predictions for these data were also optimum for $n^{-1.5}$. In conclusion, for brief presentations (i.e. up to ⅓ of a second), the function of n underlying detection performance is $n^{-1.5}$, whereas for longer presentations the function becomes n^{-2}.

1.5. Modelling the Two-Dimensional Small Size Contrast Function

With rectangular targets it is necessary to use a two-dimensional modelling approach. Although an object may have a uniform luminance, the image may give rise to illuminance gradients which differ for the two dimensions, particularly if one dimension is considerably smaller than the other. The two-dimensional form of modelling operates primarily on the function $f(K_2)$. This causes the input contrast to be reduced according to the peak of the point spread function when the target perimeter is very small. The two dimensional version of the model allows the decrease in contrast in one dimension to be separated from the other dimension, such that a long thin rectangular bar will produce a reduced contrast across the width but not along the length. This is represented in the following function:

$$f(K_2) = 0.163 \left(\frac{(XY)}{(1+X^{n_\theta})^{\frac{1}{n_\theta}} (1+Y^{n_\theta})^{\frac{1}{n_\theta}}} \right) \tag{6}$$

where X is h, the target height, multiplied by an image sharpness function. Y is w, the target width, multiplied by an image sharpness function, and n_θ dependent on eccentricity.

1.6. Contrast Polarity

Blackwell[10] concluded that there was no significant difference within the limits of his experiments between positive and negative luminance contrasts as far as achieving threshold was concerned. However, close inspection of his 1946 data suggested that there may have been a difference for very small sizes and hence high contrasts. An experimental comparison was reported by Church and Hawkins[13] using a fixed negative contrast of -0.75. They found it necessary to increase the positive contrast to levels of between 1.2 and 2.0 to achieve threshold for an identical size target under the same controlled ambient viewing conditions. The reason for this difference is unclear but the effect is acknowledged in the model in the form of an empirical compressive non-linearity.

1.7. The Expanded ORACLE Model

The basic model so far described has been expanded to include functions representing adaptation, noise and peripheral vision and is :

$$f(K_2)C = \left[\left(\frac{K_1 g_1(\theta)}{g_2(n)} + 0.1 d_c\right) g_3(E_r) + d_c\right] \frac{N}{N_e}(1 + a_p \sigma) \tag{7}$$

where $f(K_2)$ is a function of the image signal strength of the target which decreases when the image becomes very small, or the presentation time is reduced. C is the available target contrast. K_1 is a constant taking the value 0.48. $g_1(\theta)$ is a function of the changing receptor density with retinal eccentricity. $g_2(n)$ is a function of the number of retinal receptor signals combining to produce a threshold response. d_c is a decision criterion level below which on average an observer will not signal detection. $g_3(E_r)$ is a function of the retinal illuminance level to which the eye has adapted. N/N_e is a ratio of the total display and eye noise to the eye noise alone, a_p represents the ratio of available target signal to threshold signal in terms of the numbers of standard deviations from the mean, σ is the standard deviation and therefore the combination $(1 + a_p \sigma)$ is convertible to probability. Expansion of this form of the model has enabled parallel spatial processing of visual information to be included for bar patterns thresholds to be modelled.

2. Bar Pattern Response

Bar pattern thresholds are modelled by using a scheme wherein receptive fields of different sizes are represented, and each receptive field surround forms the centre of the receptive field at the next spatial scale, as this enables information to be encoded efficiently. Overington[14] adopted a pyramid of 4 spatial levels along similar lines to that described by Baker and Sullivan.[15] The model was devised to consider aperiodic targets but has been further developed to consider spatial frequency response. However, the modelling of periodic patterns is reduced to the consideration of one bar of the grating for simplicity. The attenuation of input signal was redefined as an attenuation of the input modulation by the combined MTF of the display system plus the dioptrics of the eye. Overington[16] developed a model of the response to sinusoidal bar patterns, and then treated square waves by decomposing them into their component fundamental sinusoidal frequencies and associated harmonics. Fourier theory shows that a square wave can be considered as the sum of a number of sine-wave components whose frequencies are odd multiples of the fundamental frequency. Thus a square wave which is a function of x having unit amplitude (peak to peak=2) and period X can be considered as the sum of the infinite series

Thus the amplitude of the fundamental (first harmonic) component of a square wave grating of contrast m is $4m/\pi$, while the amplitudes of the third, fifth and higher harmonics are respectively $4m/3\pi$, $4m/5\pi$ and so on. The effective contrast for the fundamental sinusoidal

$$\frac{4}{\pi}\left[\sin\frac{2\pi x}{X}+\frac{1}{3}\sin\frac{6\pi x}{X}+\frac{1}{5}\sin\frac{10\pi x}{X}+......\right] \tag{8}$$

component of a square wave is 1.27 times the square wave contrast. A cautionary note is that the definition of contrast when considering periodic and aperiodic stimuli is different and in general the modulation contrast (C_m) appropriate to bar pattern response, is half the psychometric contrast $(\delta L/L)$ since $C_m=\delta L/2L$.

The input contrast for the target is adjusted as above for the considered frequencies but must also be attenuated according to the system transmission properties as defined by the total system MTF and specifically by the system transmission at the frequency under consideration.

The local maximum luminance gradient between adjacent receptors when sampling a sine wave is approximated by:

$$\sin(\omega\frac{\delta x}{2}) \tag{9}$$

where δx is the retinal receptor spacing, ω is $2\pi f$, and f is the spatial frequency of the bar pattern (c/mrad) at the retina.

For periodic patterns, the function $f(K_2)C$ in normal ORACLE was therefore replaced with:

$$2F_1(C)T(f)\sin(\frac{\pi\delta x}{w}) \tag{10}$$

where $F_1(C)$ is the effective contrast (amplitude) of the frequency considered for the bar pattern, w is the bar width $(1/f)$, and $T(f)$ is the (display + eye) MTF.

The resulting ORACLE equation for mean threshold for bar targets of the type used in MRTD modelling, and to which the Johnson criteria relate, was therefore:

$$F_1(C)T(f)\,2\sin(\pi f\delta x) = \left[\left(\frac{K_1g_1(\theta)}{g_2(n)}+0.1d_c\right)g_3(E_r)+d_c\right]\frac{N}{N_e}(1+a_p\sigma) \tag{11}$$

2.1. Multiple Channel Modelling with ORACLE

In effect ORACLE was originally a single channel model. We refer to this smallest spatial channel as the midget system, following the use of the term in the description of the neuroanatomy of the retina. The channel is represented with a receptor spacing required to provide the maximum observed acuity, and is consistent with the smallest spatial channel proposed by Marr et al.[17] There is much debate about the exact properties and relative sensitivities of visual channels and the interpretation of the relevant psychophysical data. As a consequence in early development of a multiple channel model, a series of spatial channels were assumed in which the inhibitory surround diameter is used to provide the centre of the next largest spatial receptive field which results in efficient signal processing and minimal noise. A set of four parallel channels has been adopted sufficient to model typical contrast sensitivity functions and include the performance for lower spatial frequencies. These channels have centre diameters of 1, 3, 9 and 27 cone widths, that is, 0.145, 0.435, 1.305, 3.915 mrad (Figure 3).

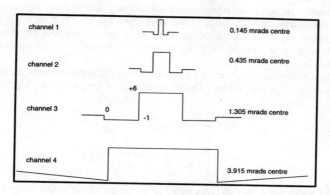

Figure 3. Spatial response of the proposed visual channels.

We assume that they operate in a similar way to the midget system based on a single cone centre as described earlier, but with a progressive scaling of the receptive field size. The effect of this receptive field size scaling is to increase the maximum illuminance gradient across the receptive field, to decrease the effective MTF of the channel and to decrease the number of receptive fields that are sampling the target edge signal.

For the smallest channel the maximum gradient for an edge was determined by convolving the 3.0 mm pupil diameter eye point spread function with an extended edge. We have calculated the maximum illuminance gradient for the larger receptor diameters and the following values are suggested for the revised model, 0.16, 0.38, 0.73, 1.0. These replace K_2 in the equation for the respective channels. The bar pattern luminance gradient is derived for the sine bar by use of Eq. (9) where the value for δx, the inter-receptor spacing, is increased for the larger receptive field sizes until the full luminance gradient is sampled.

The left hand side of Eq. (11), which calculates average signal strength, can now be represented for a series of receptive field sizes. The right hand side includes the function of number of receptors and can be revised by scaling the number of detectors per unit length of target edge proportionally to the diameters of the receptive field sizes for the different size channels. The same power law of the number of receptive fields which was developed for the single cone-centred channel to provide an adequate relationship to threshold data is included for each of the multiple channels.

The adaptation state of these channels may well be independent but we have insufficient data to determine the functions which would apply to the proposed channels and have therefore implemented a model on the assumption that gain control mechanisms are operating with effectively the same properties for all channels. This enables us to use the same retinal illuminance functions to represent response to differing levels of ambient illumination. Finally ORACLE is calibrated against laboratory forced choice data, and rather than representing the internal noise and assumed summation laws across detectors in detail there is an empirically derived signal limit below which the visual system is modelled not to respond (d_c). The value for d_c was calibrated for a single receptive field size but with a four channel model this signal limit must operate in all channels. Again we are not aware of data that permit specific definition of values for the independent channels so we have modelled the limit with a receptive field weighting included. In so doing the actual value of d_c for the smallest (formerly the only) channel has been revised from 0.00036 up to 0.0008 to allow for the contribution of the additional channels.

In the presence of display noise we need also to consider the implications of the changing size of receptive field on noise integration. The retina-referred display noise N_d is given as:

$$N_d = \frac{\delta L}{\left(\dfrac{A_e^2 + A_d^2}{A_d^2}\right)^{0.25} \left(\dfrac{t_e^2 + t_d^2}{t_d^2}\right)^{0.25} L_B} \tag{12}$$

where L_B is the background display luminance. A_e and t_e are the effective integration area and time respectively for the eye, and A_d and t_d are the effective integration area and time of the display. The integration area A_e becomes dependent on the receptive field size: see Section 2.4.

The total retina-referred noise N is then given as:

$$N = (N_d^2 + N_e^2)^{0.5} \tag{13}$$

where N_e, the equivalent input noise of the visual, system takes a value dependent on the adaptation state of the observer (see Section 3.). The ratio of the display noise relative to the eye noise is used as a scalar of contrast requirement to reach threshold for each channel.

The output of each channel is a ratio of the input contrast to channel threshold contrast in terms of standard deviations. These can then be summed in quadrature and the total converted to an acquisition probability.

In the case of the rectangular stimulus which is evaluated as equivalent sine waves, because of the limited number of receptive field sizes used to model performance at one retinal location, more than one harmonic may provide a signal to the same channel. This is because the bandwidths of the channels deriving from our receptive field assumptions are broader than those proposed by other researchers. As a consequence only the strongest harmonic signal to each channel is considered in 'grating' applications of the model. This only becomes significant for low frequency bar patterns.

The foveal bar pattern response model has not been formally developed to deal with response to patterns whose bars extend into extra-foveal regions. The effect can be seen in Figure 4 which shows extended sine, square and foveal sine grating thresholds re-plotted from Howell and Hess[18]. A bar length of 2 degrees was assumed in extracting the foveal data.

It is presumed that for these extended stimuli additional probability will be summated from the surrounding coarse receptive fields. It has only been found possible to apply this model to very

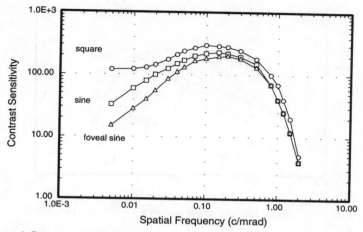

Figure 4. Contrast sensitivity for square, sine and foveal extent sine patterns taken from Howell and Hess[18].

low spatial frequency extended bar patterns by considering many harmonics and many different sized receptive fields. In so doing it is necessary to consider the extent of the stimulus that would be sampled by each receptive field. At present the practical significance of such stimuli does not justify the increase in model complexity.

The spatial frequency response of the four channels is shown in Figure 5. The combined probabilistic output of these channels compares well with the foveal sine contrast sensitivity data of Howell and Hess[18] which are also re-plotted in the same figure.

2.2. Square-Wave Response

The response to square bar patterns can be modelled either by converting the signal from the bar into its fourier transform as a set of sinusoidal equivalents or by directly dealing with the edge strength of the bar. The differences between a rectangular grating and an isolated bar receive different emphasis in the two descriptions. The retinal contrast of the middle bars of a grating, when convolved with the optical spread function of the eye, can be reduced by the overlapping of the spread function from two adjacent bars. This has to be calculated in the model and the sampling function in Eq. (9) provides the effective contrast reduction that is experienced between adjacent bars.

The length of the test pattern and the number of bars influence detection thresholds. Imaging system measurements such as Minimum Resolvable Temperature Differences (MRTD) conventionally operate with 7:1 aspect ratio length to width 4 bar patterns, whereas many psychophysical experiments have been conducted with both a very large number of bars (spatial frequency dependent) and of large angular subtense at the retina. Once again some of the earliest relevant observations can be found in Howell and Hess[18] since that time a number of studies have employed frequency scaled grating area in the interest of maintaining constant cortical magnification.

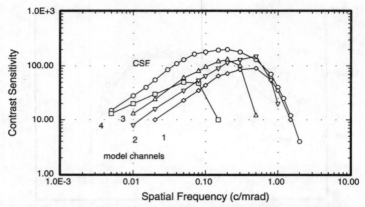

Figure 5. ORACLE model response for 4 parallel channels and foveal extent sinusoidal CSF from Howell and Hess.[18]

2.3. Multiple Channel ORACLE - Summary

The 4 channels proposed earlier can be modelled with the same basic equation:

$$F_1(C_w) T(f) 2\sin(\pi f \delta x) = \left[\left(\frac{K_1 g_1(\theta)}{g_2(n)} + 0.1d_c \right) g_3(E_r) + d_c \right] \frac{N}{N_e} (1 + a_p \sigma) \qquad (14)$$

where the terms are similar to those used in Eq. (11), but expanding C_w and d_c,

$$d_c = 0.00080 \sqrt{\frac{R}{0.145}} \qquad (15)$$

$$C_w = C_R \sin\left(\frac{\omega \delta x}{2} \right) \qquad (16)$$

where R is the radius of the receptive field, C_w is the effective contrast available to adjacent receptive field units, C_R is the contrast available to the observer at the display, δx is the retinal receptor spacing, ω is $2\pi f$, f being the spatial frequency of the bar pattern (cycles per milliradian) at the retina. $F_1(C_w)$ is the effective contrast (amplitude) of the frequency considered for the bar pattern. $T(f)$ is the (display + eye) MTF.

The only necessary amendment to the noise term N/N_e is to calculate an effective spatial integration area (A_e) for each of the four receptive fields: see Eq.(12 and 13).

$$A_e = \pi \left(\frac{R}{2} \right)^2 \tag{17}$$

3. Adaptation

By various means the human visual system manages to operate successfully over the very large range of luminances encountered in natural scenes despite the 'handicap' of neural mechanisms of limited dynamic range. The process by which the system adjusts to prevailing light level is known as adaptation. Some aspects of this process, such as pupil size variation, are relatively well understood. Retinal components are more complex and our understanding, particularly of neurophysiological mechanisms, is still incomplete. Nevertheless there seems to be a degree of consensus, at least when psychophysical evidence is considered, that several mechanisms are involved. These probably include both subtractive and multiplicative adaptation at more than one site.[19] A variety of such processes have been proposed[20] including receptor response compression, compensatory range control by pigment depletion or other internal photoreceptor mechanism, post-receptoral gain control and high-pass filtering perhaps resulting from lateral inhibition. Many of these can be primarily considered as 'anti-saturation' mechanisms.[21] However, under some conditions, their action may produce a second desirable effect. This is the 'preservation' of contrast relationships in the visual signals, as described by Weber's Law, permitting the system to sense scene reflectance.

The process of adaptation is perhaps most clearly illustrated by threshold versus intensity (t.v.i.) functions wherein, for a given set of experimental conditions (size, duration), the threshold target intensity increment is plotted against the intensity of the adapting background. Figure 6 shows the typical form of such functions. Under many conditions at higher intensities, the slope of this function approaches unity, satisfying Weber's law. There is general agreement that this cannot easily be explained without invoking some form of gain control mechanism. The published models aim to predict such t.v.i. data. They appear to fall into two categories. Some authors[20,22] employ a combination of response compression, subtractive and multiplicative mechanisms to reproduce the function. For cone vision this approach requires four stages and a number of constants must be defined by iteration. Others workers have emphasised the contribution of noise processes,[23] perhaps relying on a single gain control mechanism in the Weber region.[21] It is likely that a complete model would require integration of all these ideas but it is clear that the result would be a relatively large number of constants to which values could not easily be assigned on the basis of current data. In this circumstance it seems prudent to adopt the noise-based approach which is most easily compatible with existing ORACLE concepts.

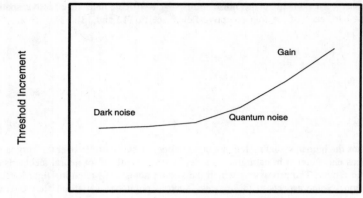

Figure 6. Representation of a three stage adaptation function.

3.1. ORACLE Luminance Functions

The ORACLE treatment of luminance effects has been made more explicit by the implementation of a three regime cone adaptation function. At low luminance dark light is the controlling factor, at intermediate values performance is quantum limited and at high levels thresholds tend away from a square root dependence on retinal illuminance towards the proportionality of Weber's law due to the action of a single adaptation mechanism. It does not seem necessary to incorporate cone saturation since, with steady backgrounds, cones appear to operate up to the damage limit. In the first instance a function based on the approach of Shapley and Enroth-Cugell[21] has been used for simplicity.

The adaptation function acts as a new noise term in Eq.(7), both the noise ratio and function of retinal illuminance being removed. This ensures, amongst other things, the correct treatment of external (device) noise as luminance varies. The combined operation of gain and noise in a single term seems intuitive and has the advantage that the term can, in principle, be independently verified by measurement of equivalent input noise.[24] In detail it is suggested that the function describing sensitivity should be the quadrature sum of three terms:

$$N_e = \left(N_d^2 + N_q^2 + \left(N_n/G\right)^2\right)^{0.5}$$ (18)

where N_e is the root mean square (RMS) equivalent input noise of the visual system, N_d is the 'dark noise' of the visual system (ie. the spontaneous firing occurring prior to the adaptation (gain) mechanism, often quoted as an equivalent illuminance but here considered to be an equivalent receptive field quantum catch). N_q is the quantum catch arising from the background i.e. the quantum noise term, N_n is the RMS neural noise arising from any source central to the adaptation mechanism (expressed arbitrarily in the same units as N_d), which varies inversely with G, the gain of the system.

Following Shapley and Enroth-Cugell[21] we adopt the gain function observed in retinal ganglion cells:

$$G = \left(1 + \frac{F}{F_c}\right)^{-n} \qquad (19)$$

where F is the effective luminous flux in the receptive field in question, F_c is the critical flux required to reduce gain to 2^{-n}, believed to be 10 to 100 times greater than 'dark light', n is an exponent, often measured to be 0.9, but taking ideal value (1.0) for present purposes, resulting in a gain of 0.5 when the flux is equal to F_c.

It is the third term in the quadrature sum which gives rise to Weber or near-Weber behaviour at higher luminance levels.

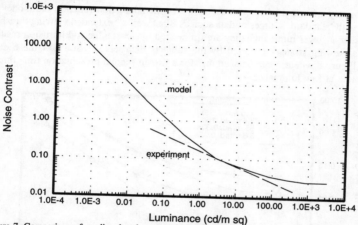

Figure 7. Comparison of predicted and measured equivalent input noise as a function of adapting luminance.

The detail of the calculation of total noise[25] which draws on the work of Geisler, Banks and colleagues[26,27] is omitted here for brevity but Figure 7 illustrates how *rms* noise contrast varies with input luminance for the following assumptions:

- Foveal viewing
- Diameter of receptive field centre—0.5 min arc
- Transduction efficiency—34%
- Effective integration time—60 ms
- Dark light—10 Trolands
- Gain constant—100 Trolands
- RMS neural noise central to the gain mechanism—7.5 equivalent quanta.

For comparison, Figure 7 also shows the straight line fit to the measurements of equivalent input noise presented by Burgess and Colborne[28] which can be plausibly predicted (over the intermediate range) by the combined action of quantum noise and pupil variation.[29] It is clear that the addition of dark noise and neural noise to the calculation appears to cause these curves to diverge significantly. As intended, the predicted curve asymptotes to constant (Weber) contrast at high luminance and shows inverse proportionality to low luminance. Unfortunately we cannot compare data with theory over such a large luminance range since equivalent input noise does not appear to have been measured under cone isolation conditions or at luminances above about 300 cd m^{-2}. There is a pressing need for such measurements and as will be seen similar data are needed for peripheral vision.

3.2. Limitations of Comparison Data

Unfortunately when equipped with the revised cone adaptation function the model cannot be compared with 'standard' sources of data such as Blackwell's[10] extended viewing thresholds since it is clear that at lower luminance they are influenced by substantial rod intrusion resulting from an off-axis viewing strategy reported by the subjects themselves. Some of these data are re-plotted in Figure 8 where it can be seen that for a fifteen second presentation time thresholds do not asymptote at low luminance.

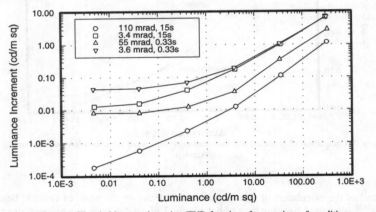

Figure 8. Threshold versus intensity (TVI) functions for a variety of conditions.

The basic threshold data used for calibration of luminance effects under single glimpse conditions are those of Blackwell and McCready[30] (also shown in Fig. 8) with which the model will naturally show reasonable agreement. These data are for foveal presentation only whereas, at present, the model incorporating the new adaptation function shows a strong (and perhaps excessive) dependence on eccentricity. To fully validate the model we require cone isolation threshold data for a variety of luminances and eccentricities. There are few relevant studies. One experiment, reported by Taylor,[31] is restricted to a very small (0.91 mrad perimeter), very brief (10 ms) target leaving large sections of the threshold surface un-validated. Targets as small as this are obviously very susceptible to the effects of the optical quality of the eye. This introduces considerable uncertainty into any off-axis performance comparison.

3.3. The Rod Contribution

It is possible to base a description of adaptation in rod vision[†] [,32] on mechanisms directly analogous to those used in the cone model but employing different constants. The relevant constants which were derived, in part, by iterative comparison with the rod isolation data of Barlow[23] are listed below for completeness only:

- Transduction efficiency—25%
- Effective integration time—100 ms
- Dark light—0.022 Scotopic Trolands
- Gain constant—1.2 Scotopic Trolands
- RMS neural noise central to the gain mechanism—10 equivalent quanta.

With such a large number of free parameters there is little point in pursuing data comparisons beyond the point of establishing the principle. Since it has not been possible to validate the revision of the cone element of the model for peripheral vision no attempt has been made to examine combined output since this would rely heavily on performance at off-axis locations where the rod contribution is still more significant.

In conclusion we find that further modelling awaits the collection of fundamental data on the foveal and peripheral detection of aperiodic stimuli under rod and cone isolation conditions. Such information, if combined with measurements of equivalent input noise under the same conditions would resolve some of the uncertainty found in even this simplified description of adaptation.

4. Pupil Diameter Dependence on Field Luminance and Size

Pupil diameter has a significant impact on both the illuminance and sharpness of the retinal image. Data relating pupil size and retinal illuminance were collated by DeGroot and Gebhard[33] and from these it has proved possible to establish a simple mathematical relationship. The data presented show a rather large variance and the authors suggest that this may be due, in part, to differences in stimulus area employed (but unfortunately not reported) by different workers. The implicit assumption here is that the mechanism of pupil control is based on luminous flux rather than luminance. If true, this places a significant limitation on the utility of the equation particularly where displays and sighting systems of limited field-of-view are concerned.

In order to resolve this question Stanley and Davies[34] conducted experiments to determine the steady state pupil diameter resulting from foveal fixation of fields-of-view of various luminances and diameters. If these results are plotted against corneal flux density (i.e. the product of

---

[†] The rod performance model itself is not described in this chapter.

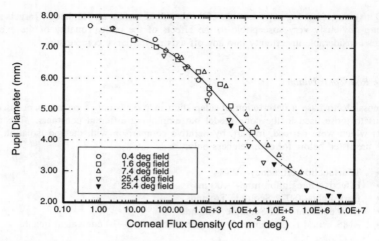

Figure 9. A single relationship combines the area and luminance control of the pupil.

luminance and subtended area) they appear to approach a single function (Figure 9). It seems reasonable to conclude that, over the range of conditions studied, the pupil control mechanism acts like a simple area integrator. These data also suggest that the observed relationship between pupil diameter and viewing distance[35] may be an uncontrolled effect of subtense.

The data can be described to a first approximation by the equation:

$$p = 7.75 - 5.75 \left(\frac{(F/846)^{0.41}}{(F/846)^{0.41} + 2} \right) \tag{20}$$

where p is the pupil diameter in mm and F is the corneal flux density in cd m^{-2} deg^2.

5. Peripheral Visual Performance

5.1. Peripheral Performance Modelling

Several major data sets have described the change of threshold performance with eccentricity. Taylor[11,28] found a rise in contrast thresholds relative to the fovea for peripheral viewing at high luminance, with a corresponding decrease out to a few degrees at very low light levels. This is in keeping with the expected contributions of rod and cone performance. The luminance contrast thresholds given in Figure 10 are a summary of the results of Taylor's[11] studies.

The trends for rod and cone density with retinal eccentricity are shown in Figure 11. Cone density falls rapidly over the first 10 degrees and then reduces at a slower rate over the remainder of the visual field. A simple and approximate function to model this changing density of cones per unit area is obtained by normalising the density to the fovea (i.e relative foveal density =

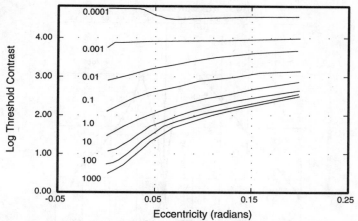

Figure 10. Taylor's experimental threshold contrasts with eccentricity at luminances given in cd/m².

1.0), then the density change with eccentricity is adequately represented for the first 20 degrees by the reciprocal of 1 plus the eccentricity in degrees.

$$g_1(\theta) \propto \frac{1}{\theta+1} \tag{21}$$

where $g_1(\theta)$ is the cone density relative to the fovea, and θ is the angle of eccentricity in degrees.

The function is representative of the changing density over the central area of the retina and correlates reasonably well with the measured contrast threshold data for small targets measured over the same central region.

The approach to peripheral visual performance has been to consider the visual processes to be essentially the same at any one retinal location other than for the change in image quality, receptor size and density. Work on grating sensitivity by Rovamo[36] and acuity by Cowey and Rolls[37] has attempted to demonstrate the equivalence of vision at different retinal locations. Rovamo measured contrast sensitivity functions for retinal positions from the fovea to 30 degrees into the periphery. His data show that peripheral sensitivity progressively reduces. It was found that, by adjusting the grating sizes and spatial frequencies for the individual peripheral locations, the resulting observer response functions could all be neatly overlaid. Functions that would provide the correct scaling of contrast sensitivity with angle relate to the concept of cortical magnification factor (CMF). CMF is defined as the linear extent of visual striate cortex to which each degree of the retina projects. Rolls and Cowey[37] attempted to relate CMF to ganglion cell density but found difficulty in determining the projection for the central receptors to the ganglions as they are displaced by the foveal pit. Drasdo[38] applied a correction factor and arrived at a relationship between the percentage of ganglion cells and peripheral angle not significantly different from that given by Eq. (21).

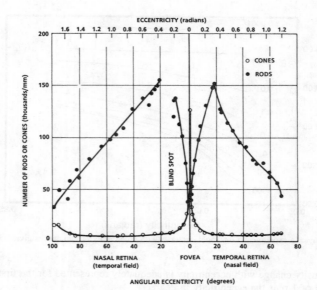

Figure 11. Rod and cone density with eccentricity.

The small and large target threshold trends with eccentricity are treated separately in the model. If a target is viewed foveally and it is smaller than the foveal blur circle then the illuminance gradient is reduced on the retina between adjacent foveal receptors. This is modelled by treating the target size as a constant equivalent to the circumference of the blur circle, and reducing the retinal signal proportional to the target area relative to the area of the blur circle.

With peripheral viewing we need to consider the nature of the blur and the decreasing receptor density, and hence the increased distance between adjacent receptors. The increase in inter-receptor distance will mean that the illuminance gradient of an edge is sampled more coarsely but provides a larger difference signal.

In ORACLE, avoiding the complexities of off-axis aliasing, we assume the effective blur circle radius increases in the same proportion as the receptor linear density reduces. For a small target which is unresolved foveally, the maximum illuminance gradient reduces proportional to the area of the local blur circle (i.e. by a factor of $\theta+1$), whilst the linear sampling interval increases by a factor of $(\theta+1)^{0.5}$. The result is that the sampled illuminance gradient changes by a factor $(\theta+1)^{0.5}/(\theta+1)$ or $(\theta+1)^{-0.5}$, whilst the number of samples contributing to detection decreases by the linear factor $((\theta+1)^{0.5})$ producing an overall rate of threshold contrast increase of $\theta+1$.

For larger (resolved) stimuli edge illuminance gradient reduces in proportion to the blur circle radius which is matched by the linear receptor sampling producing no change in sampled illuminance gradient. The number of contributing samples declines as $(\theta+1)^{0.5}$ and contrast threshold increases at a corresponding rate.

In the case of very large targets such as the 2 degree diameter disc used by Taylor the rate of change of threshold with eccentricity appears to be less than $(\theta+1)^{0.5}$. There may be many reasons for this finding but it is difficult to interpret since such a stimulus is of equivalent size to the whole fovea and the sampling of its entire perimeter cannot approach the highest foveal cone density.

The effects of blur in peripheral vision have been incorporated into the visual efficiency function, which is a relationship between the actual image sharpness and the best achievable foveal image sharpness. The peripheral blur is calculated from the MTF for the eye by scaling the foveal MTF by the linear sampling interval as represented above by $(\theta+1)^{0.5}$. The visual efficiency $\eta_v(\theta)$ for peripheral vision is therefore:

$$\eta_v(\theta) = \frac{\int\limits_0^\infty \exp-\left((\theta+1)^{0.5}f/f_c\right)^n \delta f}{\int\limits_0^\infty \exp\left(-f/f_c\right)^n \delta f} \tag{22}$$

where f is the spatial frequency in cycles per milliradian, f_c and n are derived from the pupil size and are used in an exponential power function to generate eye MTF's and θ is the peripheral angle away from the fovea in degrees.

The model incorporates peripheral image quality interactions for small target sizes by including $\eta_v(\theta)$ in the calculation of the retinal illuminance gradient. This operates in the model on the signal strength function $f(K_2)$ and on the function of the number of receptors for the height and width components $g_n(1)$ and $g_n(2)$.

$$f(K_2) = 0.163\left[\frac{\left(\frac{g_n(1)(XY)}{(1+X^{n_\theta})^{1/n_\theta}}\right)+\left(\frac{g_n(2)(XY)}{(1+Y^{n_\theta})^{1/n_\theta}}\right)}{g_n(1)+g_n(2)}\right] \tag{23}$$

where X is $2.66h\eta_v(\theta)$. Similarly Y is $2.66w\,\eta_v(\theta)$ and n_θ is a value dependent on eccentricity.

5.2. Horizontal and Vertical Measurements

It was confirmed by Millodot et al[39] that the circular asymmetries in the retina result in different acuity performance for the vertical and horizontal meridians of the visual field. The vertical decline in acuity with eccentricity tends to be greater than the horizontal. Hinton,[40] as part of a study of the effects of afterimages on target detection, investigated differences in probabilities for the detection of a disc target measured in the vertical or horizontal meridian. The resultant performance curves of probability against eccentricity are referred to as visual lobes. The experiment employed a 10 minute of arc diameter disc target against a plain background of 15 cd m^{-2} and a positive luminance contrast of 0.140. Five observers were used in the study and eccentricities out to 5 degrees were explored. Targets were exposed for 300 milliseconds. The results are shown in Figure 12 and demonstrate the superior performance along the horizontal meridian. The model has not in general been configured to accommodate these asymmetries as they require extensive additional computation only justified in specific applications.

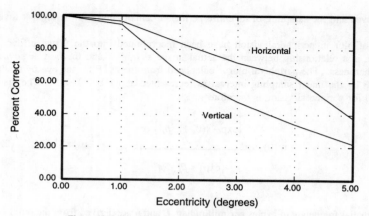

Figure 12. Lobe differences between the horizontal and vertical meridian.

5.3. Peripheral Recognition Performance and Application to Search

Use of peripheral vision is not restricted to detection tasks, higher level discrimination being carried out at least to the extent required to guide fixations. The effect is as if task-related visual lobes operate in parallel. Thus large lobes may be defined for the detection of a particular stimulus, small lobes for its identification, with a continuum of intermediate angles over which intermediate tasks can be performed. To model search in a cluttered or structured scene accurately, a representation of the various levels of information processing is required, to produce fixation patterns based on the strength of the signal and the information content. Such a model would be difficult to develop and would be very scene dependent. The alternative option, which has at present been adopted, is to determine the average visual lobe that usefully represents the task that we are attempting to model.

To calibrate the model for search in a structured scene, an attempt was made to measure the visual lobe for discriminating targets from non-targets where targets were described as vehicles of 'military significance'.[41] The experimental method ensured that many of the targets presented appeared in the periphery of the observer's vision, and therefore a visual lobe was constructed which was directly applicable to the detection of tanks in complex real-world scenes.

The target and background scenes were taken from a 300:1 scale physical terrain model, painted and recorded in a manner so as to simulate thermal imagery. A total of 560 targets were included in 1000 scenes. Each scene was exposed to the observers for 0.333 seconds and the observers were required to indicate the location of the target. The targets appeared in one of 16 locations which were chosen to coincide with eccentricities of 0, 3, 6, or 9 degrees when the observer was fixating the centre of the screen.

Data from this experiment provide the average visual lobe that was used to calibrate the model for observers searching for the target vehicles in structured terrain. A further use of the data is in direct calibration of the model fractional perimeter value which is further discussed in the next section. For every observation, ORACLE predictions for corresponding conditions such as details of the target signature, were compared with the subject's response and a maximum likelihood statistic was used to determine the best fitting fractional perimeter value.

6. Recognition Modelling

Few experiments have adequately explored the effects of contrast on recognition to provide information for modelling purposes. The approach adopted by Van Meeteren[42] and in ORACLE is to relate recognition to the detection of features or detail within the target signature. However, one main difference in performance between detection and recognition is that the detection process obeys Ricco's Law such that contrast threshold is proportional to the area of the target. This enables detection of very small objects to be achieved by compensating increase in contrast. The same does not appear to be true for recognition. The recognition task becomes size limited and further increases in contrast do not provide enhanced recognition performance. As van Meeteren suggested that the detection of just one critical feature is not sufficient for recognition. A number of features must be detected to distinguish between target types. Therefore two adjacent features of critical size must not merge. The ability to recognise must therefore limit as soon as the blur circle is twice the size of the critical feature. For detection the visual response is calculated as a dependence on the slope of the maximum contrast gradient across adjacent receptors and the number of receptive field units that are sampling that gradient. The optical spread function due to the optics and neural layers of the eye always spread the finest point of light so that it falls on limiting number of receptors. In the model, for detection of small targets the number of receptors limits and the contrast is attenuated to model Ricco's law.

Recognition is modelled as the detection of a fraction of the actual target perimeter. The fractional perimeter value scales the target size down to a fractional size dependent on task level. This corresponds with detection of smaller feature elements. It is additionally necessary to introduce a size limit below which no increase in contrast could restore recognition performance. The options are either to operate on contrast, size or a combination of both.

Data casting some light on this question are to be found in the Snellen letter legibility results obtained by Ginsburg,[43] shown in Figure 13. The importance of this work lies in the measurement of both detection and recognition of letters and recorded threshold contrasts for a wide range of sizes.

Snellen letter sizes are classified by the distance at which the stroke width would subtend 1 minute of arc at the eye. Normal acuity being 6/6 and a target 10 times larger would be 6/60. Ginsburg's results are evaluated here in terms of the nature of the retinal signal after convolving the target stroke width with the eye's line spread function. The appropriate spread function was determined from the background luminance of 60 cd m^{-2}. Table 1 provides summary results of convolving the line spread function with the cross-sectional stroke width of the letters. The results are summarised for each target size in terms of the maximum achieved luminance as a percentage of the total possible. The table compares the ratios of recognition to detection contrast thresholds with the luminance reduction ratio.

To model object detection we have so far used the retinal illuminance gradient and target size information. Comparison of columns 4 and 5 in Table 1 indicates that in the move to recognition, the reduction of the illuminance peak may also be a useful predictor. From this it is concluded that, in addition to modelling the recognition process as the detection of fractional

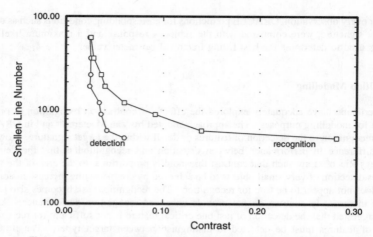

Figure 13. Ginsburg's experimental size thresholds for various contrast Snellen letters.

size of the detail, we must acknowledge that in the limit the effective contrast of that feature is attenuated and the contrast attenuation is proportional to the change in peak (or trough) illuminance.

Table 1. Experimental contrast threshold data for detection and recognition of letters from Ginsburg. The threshold ratios are compared to loss of peak luminance after letter stroke width convolution with eye point spread function.

Snellen letter acuity	Detection threshold contrast	Recognition threshold contrast	Ratio of recognition to detection	Ratio of peak to actual illuminance
6/60	0.024	0.025	1.04	1.05
6/36	0.025	0.028	1.12	1.09
6/24	0.025	0.036	1.44	1.17
6/18	0.024	0.040	1.66	1.37
6/12	0.034	0.060	1.76	1.72
6/9	0.036	0.092	2.55	2.63
6/6	0.042	0.140	3.33	3.84

The actual ORACLE implementation of the size limit to recognition is not described in detail here but is based on the attenuation of effective contrast between two independent target elements optically collapsing into a single object.

7. Suprathreshold Modelling

For many practical situations, it is important to be able to predict the conspicuity of objects that are well above detection threshold. Johnson[44] investigated the ability of ORACLE to predict the conspicuity of supra-threshold stimuli. In brief, subjects compared the conspicuity of stimulus targets of various shapes and colours presented against various coloured backgrounds. The target stimuli were ranked in order of their relative conspicuity, and the ranking was compared to the target conspicuity predicted by the model. The model was used to calculate the available signal in terms of the number of standard deviations above threshold.

It is worth digressing to clarify the treatment of threshold statistics. We assume a constant relationship between the standard deviation and the mean (i.e. threshold contrast value) which enables probability to be calculated for any condition. An analysis of large scale data sources[10] shows that this ratio is never less than 0.1 and reaches a maximum of 0.4. Although data generated from a small number of observers and limited trials tends to produce a standard deviation relative to the mean of 0.25, the ORACLE model uses 0.4, aiming to reflect the maximum spread of performance of a population.

The comparison revealed that the logarithm of the number of standard deviations provided a linear correlation with conspicuity (Figure 14). This value is equal to zero for threshold stimuli, becomes negative for sub-threshold stimuli, and becomes positive for suprathreshold stimuli.

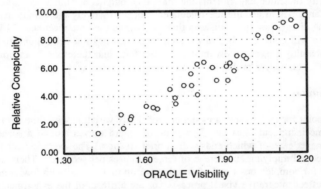

Figure 14. Measured relative conspicuity vs. ORACLE visibility for luminance contrast

8. Static Search

The modelling described so far has been predominantly concerned with the acquisition of a target object at a known position. This section considers the acquisition of targets at an unknown location in a fixed field-of-view. Static field search performance can involve a variety of tasks such as finding stationary targets or moving targets, or approaching or receding targets. Target growth in the approaching case will be due to target motion or observer motion or both moving together. For fast approaching targets the rate of change of acquisition probability with time is controlled mainly by the rate of target growth in size. However it is also important to consider the change of contrast, especially where atmospheric effects or sensor resolution are pertinent.

During a search process an observer moves his eyes to fixate on different locations in the scene (a glimpse). The aim is to continually bring objects of interest in a scene onto the fovea, which is the highest resolution area of the retina. These objects of interest are presumably preselected using the coarser sampling of peripheral vision. The average number of fixations made in many viewing situations are three per second and the process of relocating and fixation we refer to as a glimpse.

Search is not a simple process but is simplified for modelling purposes by assuming independence between glimpses. This allows us to deal with the situation where there is overlap in the areas of the scene processed in successive glimpses. The justification for doing this is supported by the exponential nature of many cumulative probability distributions against time for search tasks, which would otherwise be linear for sequential processing.

An additional problem is encountered because the strategy of an observer in a search task changes as the search progresses within a trial. In structured scenes containing new background information, there is evidence that early glimpses are devoted to orientating the observer such that he can formulate a logical search strategy. Then search consists of a sequence of visual fixations eventually stopping at the target, resulting finally in the foveal process of classification.

In the majority of search experiments the main data outputs are times to acquire the target, from which mean times to acquire are calculated,[45] or alternatively the cumulative probability with time. If the distribution of acquisition times is normal then the mean and 50% cumulative probability times will coincide. For raw search times this has not been found to be the case. Cumulative probability curves follow an exponential form and therefore mean times can often be twice the 50% cumulative probability time.

8.1. Glimpse Duration

The starting point for establishing a model of probability variation with time is to decide what the practical time increment must be. Eye point of regard moves around a scene by regular saccadic movements each of which ends with a brief fixation. The average inter-fixation time is a third of a second implying an average of three glimpses per second.[46] There are reports of longer fixations for complex tasks and of durations of up to a second with low contrast stimuli, whether these reflect integrative visual processes or are artifacts of the experimental definition of a glimpse remains to be seen. Meanwhile it seems prudent to retain the simplified modelling assumption of a constant average 0.33 second glimpse time throughout the search task.

8.2. Visual Lobes in Search

The retina is described as having a decreasing density of receptors with increasing retinal eccentricity. For photopic vision this demands an increased contrast and/or target size to maintain a constant level of target visibility with eccentricity. The probability of acquiring a given target therefore decreases the further that target is from the fovea, and hence the need to glimpse around a scene. A small target is likely only to be resolved a short way into the periphery, whereas a large target may be acquired at the limits of the visual field. The single measure of eccentricity angle where one observer is able to make his decision between acquiring and not acquiring the target is known as the hard shell visual lobe. The distribution of these decision angles constitutes the soft-shell visual lobe.[6] The soft shell lobe is the essential building brick on which search modelling for the performance of a population of observers is built. (Figure 15).

In measuring acquisition times in a search task it is important to accurately establish performance associated with the first few glimpses since at this time probability is most sensitive to the size and shape of the underlying lobe.

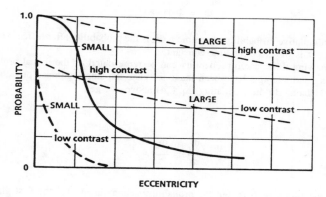

Figure 15. Some examples of visual lobes.

8.3. Field Factors

Many models have used field factors to model change in performance from laboratory to field conditions, e.g. Akerman and Kinzley.[47] The Rand model developed by Bailey[48] uses a factor of 5.5 to multiply laboratory thresholds to predict field performance. This value is an average of the thresholds taken from Taylor[11] and Blackwell and McCready.[30] The majority of field factors give poor results when applied to a different task. In ORACLE we have included a factor that represents the difference between decision levels for a laboratory forced-choice task and a free-choice situation in which the observer is allowed to respond at will. This is represented in the model by (c') or confidence level.[49] The concept is essentially one of an increase in required signal-to-noise ratio from some baseline to match field or free choice performance. We apply a S/N ratio difference across the whole range of target sizes. In search experiments the calibration of this signal-to-noise ratio is achieved by matching the initial rise of the cumulative probability curve. Some allowance is needed to ensure that reaction time is removed from the measures. In parallel the value has been calibrated by measuring contrast threshold for targets using both forced and free choice tasks. The resultant value used for free choice threshold modelling is 2.8, which coincides well with the values measured by Kelly and Savoie[50] in a similar context.

8.4. Search Accumulators with Time

A common approach to simplified search modelling has been to fit simple exponential functions to experimental search times. Then for any assumed visual lobe (for either a single observer or a population) there are two factors used to describe the accumulation of probability with time. These are the time constant of the representative exponential rise of probability and the maximum probability after a long period of search. This is represented by:

$$\Phi_t = \Phi_\infty \left[1 - e^{-\frac{t}{\tau}} \right] \tag{24}$$

where Φ_t is the cumulative probability after time t, Φ_∞ is the probability after (effectively) infinite viewing time, and τ is the effective time constant.

The infinite viewing time search probability can be represented by the foveal probability for long time viewing and attempts have been made to relate the single glimpse probability to the effective time constant. By differentiating Eq. (24) above, we get;

$$d\frac{\Phi_t}{dt} = \frac{\Phi_\infty}{\tau} e^{-\frac{t}{\tau}} \tag{25}$$

which at zero time becomes Φ_∞/τ, but the probability accumulated over the first glimpse P_g is conventionally the single glimpse probability P_g. Therefore,

$$P_g = \frac{\Phi_\infty}{\tau} 0.33 \quad or \quad \tau = \frac{\Phi_\infty}{3P_g} \tag{26}$$

This is a basic form of search probability accumulation but this simplification was never found to be totally adequate and the following more complex approach is used with the ORACLE threshold equation.

An observer confidence scaling factor was applied to represent the free choice situation and the resulting visual lobe provides the single glimpse probability from which the search accumulation is developed. It is necessary to determine the single glimpse probability for a given lobe size within a given field-of-view. The hard shell approximation takes the lobe angle associated with 50% probability, or 50% of peak probability, and overlays this across the search field-of-view and hence calculates the probability for one single glimpse.

The hard shell search model is as follows:

$$\phi_t = P_f(1-(1-P_g)^n) \quad where \quad P_g = \left(\frac{\theta}{\theta_f} - \frac{\theta^2}{4\theta^2_f} \right) \tag{27}$$

where θ is the visual angle at 50% of peak, θ_f is the field-of-view angle (degrees), P_f is the foveal probability, P_g is the single glimpse probability, n is the number of glimpses, and ρ_t is the probability at time t.

The probability of acquisition is a calculation of the common area between a circular symmetric visual lobe and the area of the display field-of-view. In any random glimpse distribution there is an area of the visual lobe which does not remain within the field. The worst case is when the observer is fixating at the edge of the field-of-view if we assume that all fixations fall within the field-of-view. The above equation includes the effects of wasted visual performance outside the search area, following the work of Davies.[51]

If this approach is applied using a hard-shell approximation to a population soft-shell visual lobe, then it does not adequately allow for the variety of visual lobes that have been measured. Typically for large targets, lobes tend to be flatter than for small targets. For such flat lobes the single hard-shell approximation has proved to be a very bad performance predictor.

The ORACLE approach is to divide the lobe into subsets of the population. The probability axis of the soft-shell lobe may be interpreted as the variability of performance for individuals over a long period of time, or the proportion of the population operating at that level at a specific time. Performance probabilities for the subsets of the population are individually accumulated using the hard shell accumulator for each subset of the population, and then averaged after each glimpse. This probability accumulator results in a slower rate of probability increase compared to probability accumulators based on hard shell lobes, or alternatively from using the integrated area under the visual lobe.

The assumption in this approach is that at the start of the search task individual observer's performances are significantly different. From the work of Ronchi,[52] it is apparent that a lot of within-observer variance occurs within a short period of time, and therefore the use of a constant hard-shell lobe representing a subset of the population is inadequate. Including a rate of spread of observer performance for sub-samples of the population as the task proceeds provides both slower rates of probability accumulation and also limits to the maximum achieved probability. The rate of change of an observer's lobe radius is not a well defined quantity and the best estimates that we can make are based on experimentally derived cumulative probability curves of search.

It seems unlikely that observer performance will drift rapidly from one extreme to another. The rate of change of performance should ideally represent the many internal circadian rhythms that are known to occur, some operating over seconds, hours or days. The Ronchi data suggest that much of the variance occurs in tens of seconds and therefore the longer duration rhythms contribute little. On the same basis change will not be erratic enough to show violent jumps in fractions of a second. We have modelled the rate of change as being equivalent to the toe of a sigmoid for very short durations, being more rapid over several seconds, and then slowly tailing away for long times, following essentially an S-shaped curve. The curve is modelled using three simple mathematical functions covering the whole S curve in a progressive manner.

If $n_g < 5$ then

$$y = 1.2 \left(0.3 \frac{n_g}{5.14} \right) \tag{28}$$

If $5 < n_g < 19$ then

$$y = 1.2 \left(0.3 \log_e \frac{n_g}{5.14} + 0.3 \right) \tag{29}$$

If $n_g > 19$ then

$$y = 1.2 \left(1.0 - 0.3 \frac{19.44}{n_g} \right) \tag{30}$$

$$\phi_p = 1.0 - 2^{-[x \pm y]^{2.8}} \tag{31}$$

where y takes a value between 0.0 and 1.2 representing the degree of change, x is the starting value for a population sub set, n_g is the number of glimpses, and ϕ_p is the lobe probability.

The visual lobe is considered to represent proportions of the population who at a given time would detect the target at a given lobe radius. These are divided into sub groupings and we use these expressions to expand the upper and lower limits of the lobe sub populations. In choosing the subdivisions of the population, one approach would be to subdivide the lobe into equal probability increments, but this was not thought to be the best solution in that it gives equal weighting to the extremes of the distribution and to the centre. Ideally the interval should be associated with the statistical normal distribution. We therefore chose to subdivide into equal increments of population standard deviation, resulting in nine subdivisions.

Probability in a glimpse is calculated by taking the integral of the area contained under the lobe between the maximum and minimum probability value and relating this to the field-of-view size to give an average detection probability for the subsection of the population in the glimpse. The nine subsets are calculated independently and then averaged to give total population performance.

The next task is to regulate the rate of observer threshold spread such that individual subsets of the population are changing their performance in a logical manner and in accordance with the measured temporal variation. Assuming that all subsets of the population eventually encompass all behaviour levels over infinite time then each subset, initially represented by a small sub section of the visual lobe, will eventually be represented by the total visual lobe. This assumes that the search task is of long enough duration.

Independent glimpses are then accumulated for the subsections of the population, each weighted by the population increment, but with the maximum and minimum value of each sub-population progressively expanding with each glimpse. By this method each sub-population grouping is effectively tending towards the mean of the total population with time.

The above functions were tested against experimental data sets to arrive at an optimal rate of performance change.

8.5. Search in Structured Scenes

When all the objects in an image are well above threshold conditions, experiments where eye movements are recorded show that fixations occur more frequently on objects which have target-like characteristics.[53] This we suggest to be a recognition process and it forms the basis for modelling the process of search in structured scenes. The lobe required for modelling search in a structured scene is selected on the basis of the level of discrimination that will guide observers' fixation patterns. The closer the clutter approximates to the target then the harder is the discrimination task, and the representative lobe shifts progressively away from a pure detection task through recognition to identification.

The nature of the search task in a specific scene is dependant on strategy and secondary sources of information, the effort in modelling at an equivalent level of detail is far greater than the reward for many practical situations. What we are able to do is to select the average lobe that will produce experimentally measured cumulative search probabilities when using the search accumulation model which has been validated for plain field search. In theory therefore an observer may operate with lobes which range from pure energy detection lobes for wide eccentricities progressively down to fine detail discrimination in foveal vision. The calibration exercise enables the average useful visual lobe for a search task to be determined for the types of scenes and targets that will be represented in the model.

Task related fractional perimeter distributions are used for search. These effectively provide a measure of the size of the detail that needs to be resolved in order to achieve a certain level of discrimination. The variance of the observer response is included in the basic threshold model and the variance of the target/non target distribution is contained in the statistics of the fractional perimeter values used to represent a specific task with a range of different stimuli.

The search modelling can now extend this variance to encompass the target detection task where the scene contains variable levels of confusable clutter. As the clutter approximates to the target then the average fractional perimeter value required is representative of the identification task. If the scene contains few clutter objects the fractional perimeter value required is similar to that appropriate for a pure detection task.

9. Current Status of the Model

We have software implementations of the model operating on PC and compatible computer systems which are menu operated to provide ease of running for optical sights, thermal imagers and naked eye viewing. Development of software is continuing with the intention of coding further areas of the modelling to match user requirements, some of the potential areas for software development include components of colour performance and response to target motion.

ORACLE has been developed for colour threshold performance by using the cone response sensitivities as a function of wavelength. The luminance contrast is derived from the sum of the long (R) and medium (G) wavelength cone mechanisms and the colour difference from the difference of the R and G cones. In both cases the signal is relative to the average of the R and G cones. The colour channel is modelled with a lower spatial frequency response than the luminance channel. This spatial level enables thresholds to be predicted for isoluminant and short wavelength stimuli. This model still needs to be tested for detection thresholds for small stimuli. Most well calibrated colour thresholds quoted in the literature relate to 2 degree or 10 degree stimuli.

The ORACLE aperiodic model considers the effects of target motion at 2 spatial levels enabling modelling of the effects of target motion on contrast thresholds. The model is not yet able to predict the effects of awareness of motion on target recognition. Characteristics of vehicle movement provide extra cues to recognition, especially in a search task. Effort is being directed to include this effect.

The model described in this chapter deals with human observer performance. Linked to this we have system models for thermal imagers, image intensifiers and optical sights. The approach has been to model the variables that affect human visual performance in a detailed way so that the human performance model can be combined directly with any display model which characterises the signal in terms that the human vision model can handle. With a thermal imager the apparent temperature of a target after passage through the atmosphere is sensed by a detector and the radiant energy transferred to visible spectrum wavelengths at a display. The variables that need to be quantified to model the displayed thermal image are, the image quality as a system MTF, the target size and contrast allowing for detector sampling and magnification, and treatment of the sensor and system noise so that these are represented as an equivalent white noise with an associated RMS luminance fluctuation at the display. It is then possible to model thermal imagers in detail and predict the practical effect of changing system parameters such as gain and offset.

Similarly incorporation of the results of detailed studies which have established internal noise of the visual system at a variety of ambient light levels, permits an assessment of acceptable level of display system noise.

One other problem often encountered in thermal image modelling is to deal adequately with a structured target signature which may be dominated by a set of hot spots. To address this problem we have carried out experiments in which detection thresholds were measured for a set of rectangular targets. Thresholds were also measured for composite stimuli, made up of various combinations of the rectangular targets. The results have been used to set up a model which will predict detection of multi-contrast targets. This model has been able to predict when elements of a target signature contribute to the overall detectability of a target and also when components cease to aid detectability.

The ORACLE model has been under continuous development for many years and is still subject to review and update dependent on the demands of our customers and the increasing information emerging from research into human visual processes.

References

1. G. A. Østerberg, Topography of the layers of rods and cones. *Acta Opthalmol. Supplement*, **6** (1935) 1-103.
2. C. A. Curcio, K. R. Sloan, R. E. Kalina & A. E. Hendrickson, Human photoreceptor topography. *J Comp Neurol.* **292** (1990) 497-523.

3. I. Overington & E. P. Lavin, A model of threshold detection performance for the central fovea. *Optica Acta* **18** (1971) 341-357.

4. F. W. Campbell & R. W. Gubisch, Optical quality of the human eye. *J. Physiol.* **186** (1966) 558-578.

5. A. Ricco, Relazzione fra il minimo angelo visuale e l'intensitaluminosa. *Annali Ottalmologia* **6** (1877) 373-479.

6. I. Overington, *Vision and Acquisition.* Pentech Press (1976) .

7. M. H. Pirenne, *Vision and the eye.* Chapman and Hall Ltd (1967).

8. F. W. Campbell & J. G. Robson, Application of Fourier analysis to the visibility of gratings. *J Physiol.* **197** (1968) 551-566.

9. R. W. Ditchburn & J. A. Foley-Fisher, Assembled data on eye movements. *Optica Acta.* **14** (1967) 113.

10. H. R. Blackwell, Contrast thresholds of the human eye. *J Opt Soc Amer.* **36** (1946) 624.

11. J. H. Taylor, Contrast thresholds as a function of retinal position and target size for the light adapted eye. *Proceedings of the NAS-NRL Vision Committee.* (1962).

12. E. S. Lamar, S. Hecht, S. Schlaer & C. D. Hendley, Size, shape and contrast in the detection of targets by daylight vision 1. Data and analytical description. *J Opt Soc Amer.* **7** (1947) 531-543.

13. N. T. Church & K. Hawkins, Contrast sign dependence. Min. Tech. Contract No KV/B/813/CB64B, Study Note No 2 Sept (1969).

14. I. Overington, Towards a complete model of photopic visual threshold performance. *Opt Eng.* **21** (1982) 2-13.

15. K. D. Baker & G. D. Sullivan, Multiple bandpass filters in image processing. *IEE Proc.* (1980) 127.

16 I. Overington, Practical Application of Contrast Sensitivity for the determination of the Performance of Visual Aids plus Observer. *BAe Report* ST13071 (1975).

17. D. Marr, T. Poggio, E. Hildreth, Smallest Channel in early human vision. *J Opt Soc Am.* **70** (1980) 868-870.

18. E. R. Howell & R. F. Hess, The functional area for summation to threshold for sinusoidal gratings. *Vision Research.* **18** (1978) 369-374.

19. J. Walraven, C. Enroth-Cugell, D. C. Hood, D. I. A. MacLeod & J. L. Schnapf, The control of visual sensitivity. in: *Visual Perception: The Neurophysiological Foundations* (L. Spillmann & J.S.Werner, Eds.). Academic Press, London (1990).

20. J. Walraven & J. M. Valeton, Visual adaptation and response saturation. In: *Limits in Perception* (A.J. van Doorn, W.A. van de Grind & J.J. Koenderink, Eds.). VNU Science Press, Utrecht (1984).

21. R. Shapley & C. Enroth-Cugell, Visual adaptation and retinal gain controls. In: *Progress in Retinal Research* (N. Osborne and G. Chader, Eds.), **3** (1984) 263-346. Pergamon Press, Oxford.

22. D. C. Hood & M. A. Finkelstein, Sensitivity to light. In: *Handbook of Perception and Human Performance* (K.R. Boff, L. Kaufman and J. Thomas, Eds.). Wiley, New York (1986).

23. H. B. Barlow, Increment thresholds at low intensities considered as signal/noise discriminations. *J Physiol.* **136** (1957) 469-488.

24. D. G. Pelli, Effects of visual noise. PhD thesis. University of Cambridge (1981).

25. P. A. Stanley, Modelling visual adaptation. *B.Ae Sowerby Research Centre Human Factors Technical Memorandum* HF30 (1991).

26. W. S. Geisler, The physical limits of acuity and hyperacuity. *J Opt Soc Am. [A]* **1** (1984) 775-782.

27. M. S. Banks, A. B. Sekuler, & S. J. Anderson, Peripheral spatial vision: Limits imposed by optics, photoreceptors and receptor pooling. *J Opt Soc Am. [A]* **8**, (1991) 1775-1787.

28. A. E. Burgess,& B. Colborne, Visual signal detection. IV. Observer inconsistency. *J Opt Soc Am. [A]* **5** (1988) 617-627.

29. P. A. Stanley, The source of 'internal' noise in the visual system. *B.Ae Sowerby Research Centre, Human Factors Technical Memorandum* HF28 (1990).

30. H. R. Blackwell & D. W. McCready, Foveal detection thresholds for various durations of target presentations. *Minutes and Proceedings of NAS-NRC Vision Committee*, AGSIL/53/4405 (1952) 249.

31. J. H. Taylor, Factors underlying visual search performance. *Presented at NATO Symposium on Image Evaluation, Munich, Germany. Scripps Institute of Oceanography* Ref.69-22 (1969).

32. J. L. Hinton, Low light extension to the ORACLE model of human visual performance. *B.Ae. Report* JS11586 (1990).

33. S. H. DeGroot & J. W. Gebhard, Pupil size as determined by adapting luminance. *J Opt Soc Am* **42**, (1952) 492-495.

34. P. A. Stanley & A. K. Davies, The effect of field of view size on steady state pupil diameter. Submitted to *Ophthal Physiol Opt* (1995).

35. C. J. Bartleson, Pupil diameters and retinal illuminances in interocular brightness matching. *J Opt Soc Am* **58**, (1968) 583-855.

36. J. Rovamo, Cortical Magnification factor predicts the photopic contrast sensitivity of peripheral vision. *Nature* **271**, (1978) 54-56.

37. E. T. Rolls & A. Cowey, Topography of the retina and striate cortex and its relationship to visual acuity in rhesus and squirrel monkeys. *Exp Brain Res.* **10**, (1970) 298-310.

38. N. Drasdo, The neural representation of visual space. *Nature,* **266**, (1977) 554-556.

39. M. Millidot & A. Lamont, Peripheral acuity in the vertical plane. *Vision Res.* **14**, (1974) 1497.

40. J. L. Hinton, The use of afterimages in the simulation of scotoma effects on visual performance. *British Aerospace Sowerby Research Centre Report* JS10307 (1985).

41. J. B. Bell, Visual lobes for complex scenes. *BAeD Report* BT13006 (1982).

42. A. van Meeteren, Characterisation of task performance with viewing instruments. *J Opt Soc Am. [A]* **17**, (1990) 2016-2023.

43. A. P. Ginsburg, Visual information processing based on spatial filters constrained by biological data. *PhD Thesis, University of Cambridge* (1978).

44. D. F. Johnson, Suprathreshold conspicuity of coloured stimuli in high ambient lighting. *BAe Report* JS11511 (1990).

45. E. S. Krendel & J. Wodinsky,Search in an unstructured visual field. *J Opt Soc Am.* **50**, (1960) 562-568.

46. R. M. Boynton, Summary and Discussion. In A. Morris and E P. Horne, Eds: *Visual Search Techniques* (Washington: National Academy of Sciences - National Research Council.) (1960) pp 231-250.

171

47. A. Akerman & R. E. Kinzley, Predicting aircraft detectability. *Human Factors,* **21,** (1979) 277-291.
48. H. H. Bailey, Target detection through visual recognition: a quantitative model. : *The Rand Corporation Report* No RM-6158-PR. Santa Monica, California. (1970).
49. K. J. Cooke, Modelling of Visual Search Performance. BAe Report No. BT14588 (1983).
50. D. H. Kelly & R. E. Savoie, A study of sine-wave contrast sensitivity by two psychophysical methods. *Perc. and Psych.* **14,** (1973) 313-318.
51. E. B. Davies, Visual search theory with particular reference to air-to-ground vision. *R.A.E. Technical Report* No. TR68055 (1968).
52. L .Ronchi, An annotated bibliography on variability and periodicities of visual responsiveness, Fondazione 'Giorgio Ronchi', XVII, Firenze (1972).
53. L. G. Williams, A study of visual search using eye movement recordings. *Honeywell Inc* Document 12009-IR1, (1967).

CHARACTERIZATION OF TASK PERFORMANCE WITH VIEWING INSTRUMENTS

AART VAN MEETEREN
TNO Human Factors Research Institute
P.O. Box 23, 3769 ZG
Soesterberg, The Netherlands

The chapters in this book are based, to a large extent, on presentations made at the Armstrong Laboratory Advisory Group Conference "Applied Spatial Models for Target Detection and Recognition" organized by Dr. Arthur Menendez in May 1991. The proceedings of the conference were recorded and transcribed. This chapter is, with minor changes, the transcript of Dr. van Meeteren's presentation at the conference. Presenting his work in this format is intended to preserve for the reader the free spirit and uninhibited exchange of ideas that was fostered by Dr. Menendez at this meeting. This spirit of scientific camaraderie was the reason and cause for the publication of this book.

Dr. Menendez: It is my pleasure to introduce Dr. Aart van Meeteren, who is presently the director of the TNO Institute for Perception in the Netherlands, an organization which has many well-known visual psychophysicists, and has a long history of applied research both for the Dutch and the NATO military.

Dr. van Meeteren: Thanks. Ladies and gentlemen, I am very grateful for the invitation to participate in this laboratory advisory group meeting, and it is a pleasure to describe recognition experiments which we did with thermal viewing devices and image intensifiers—in general, viewing devices to be used in the field—and to also explain the prediction model that we have derived from those experiments to you.

The central question—it occurred to me when I was talking with military users of those viewing devices—always was of the sort: At what distance can I recognize, see, detect the enemy?

So the range of the viewing devices—the distance at which we can perform certain visual observation tasks really seems to be a very practical performance measure.

It is also attractive from a theoretical point of view if you realize that the targets are scaled to distance, and if we think about images built up sample-wise, the distance is also scaled to the number of samples taken from the target.

And it is really a small step then to think that perhaps in the recognition of the targets, this number of independent samples that can be taken from the target may be an important criterion.

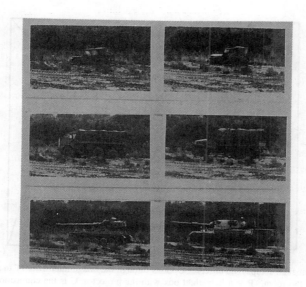

Figure 1. Target set.

This approach has about the same rationale as the introduction of visual acuity in order to predict the distance at which we can read letters of different sizes. So from this point of view, it is my objective to propose a similar sort of visual acuity measure, not for letter recognition but for the performance of complicated observation tasks in the field.

More specifically, I will try to show to you that recognition of a set of military targets may be characterized just by the detection of a simple contrasting disk upon a uniform background. And for that reason, I think I will call the model which I will describe to you the equivalent disk model.

Now, if you start with object recognition experiments, the first thing to do is to define the target set. This is the target set we have used (Fig. 1). There are six different military vehicles, individually different. They are also grouped in three different classes: two jeeps, two trucks, and two tanks.

It is important to emphasize, we think, that a recognition task, a recognition experiment, needs to start with the definition of a target set. There is no such thing as recognizing one particular individual tank. The recognition of that tank would always depend on what other targets there are in the target set.

If I am talking now about recognition, it is always referring to this target set. Note the particular features by which the individual targets can be distinguished from one another. These are always those shiny parts, small patches of light contrasting with a background, patches of different forms and sizes and in different relative position to each other. These are the features by which we can distinguish the targets.

So the detection of those patches of light must be an important factor in target recogni-

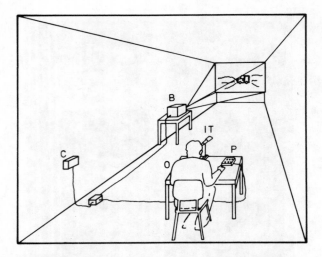

Figure 2. Experimental setup. The observer O looks through the image intensifier IT to a scene projected at the far end of the room. B is a light-tight box with the projector, C is the connection with computer control, and P is the response panel.

tion, and maybe it is the most dominant factor. Maybe if we have detected those patches of light, we may be very close to recognition of the target.

For that reason, we really thought very early in our experimental experiences that maybe object recognition might be characterized by the detection of a test object like this one, a simple circular disk upon a uniform background.

Before I come back to explaining the model, I will first describe the object recognition experiments which we have done.

The next slide (Fig. 2) shows the experimental set-up. This is an elongated, tunnel-shaped room in the basement of our building, and it was totally pitch dark. If you had entered during the experiment, it would be pitch dark in this room.

There is a subject looking through an image intensifier system at a scenery with a very low luminance level, projected by a slide projector which is covered in a light-tight box. The very low luminance of the scenery was controlled with the aid of neutral density filters.

The whole experiment is under computer control. There are sessions in which 76 slides of those sceneries with targets in the center were presented to the observer. And he paced the presentations himself. There was a response panel here, and he had to answer a simple question: What targets do you recognize?

And there was one key for each of the possible targets. Now, if he was in doubt about the choice between two targets, he was asked to press both buttons, and then the score was distributed over the two responses, so one point was distributed—but even if he was in doubt between four targets, he would push four keys.

And the experiments were performed session-wise. In each session, 76 presentations of this kind: one target in the center, so there was no search involved—it is important to underline that—and this sort of background.

Dr. Kosnik: How long was the target left on for?

Dr. van Meeteren: As long as the observer found necessary. He was pacing the experiment by giving his response. After he had given the response, the next presentation followed.

Dr. Thibos: And the subject was very familiar with these photographs to begin with?

Dr. van Meeteren: Yes. It belongs to the definition of the recognition experiments that he knows the targets *a priori* very well; he knows the response keys. So he is always working within that setting.

And I think that really is not artificial. I mean, if you go out in the field, people always will also be expecting a certain number of targets that they think of or are relevant in their particular situation.

Now, among those 76 slide presentations, there are three groups simulating three different distances. So in one session we obtain data referring to three different distances.

Test object	Responses						
	Munga	Nekaf	DAF	GMC	AMX	Leop.	Empty scene
Munga	0.32	0.32	0.02	0.04	0.01	0.02	0.27
Nekaf	0.40	0.37	0.01	0.03	0.03	0.01	0.15
DAF	0.02	0.02	0.61	0.19	0.07	0.04	0.05
GMC	0.02	0.02	0.22	0.57	0.08	0.06	0.03
AMX	0.00	0.00	0.09	0.10	0.54	0.25	0.02
Leop.	0.01	0.01	0.02	0.02	0.13	0.77	0.04
Empty scene	0.03	0.03	0.02	0.02	0.01	0.01	0.88

Figure 3. Confusion matrix.

Now, after a session the results of the experiment could be completely described with the aid of a confusion matrix as we see here (Fig. 3).

In the confusion matrix, we have all the responses to the presentations of the different targets. They may be identified correctly. On the diagonal of the matrix we find the correct identification scores, and they may also be confused with all the targets as you may read here in the matrix.

First we see confusions with targets of their own class: jeeps with jeeps, trucks with trucks, and so on. But they may also be confused with other objects. So the confusion matrix really presents all information obtained by the experiment.

What we had in mind was to study the effect of a number of parameters on object recognition, but it would not be practical to follow up all the details of this confusion matrix all the time, so we have decided to look at it in a bit more statistical way: taking the average identification scores, averaged over all objects as the main performance measure.

We can also look at the recognition scores by adding up all numbers here for the confusions within the jeep class, truck class and the confusion class.

Dr. O'Kane: I would be interested in talking to you about this later, because you can put those confusions into a three-dimensional space.

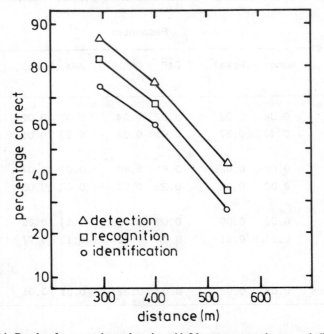

Figure 4. Results of one experimental session with 26 target presentations at each distance.

Dr. van Meeteren: Yes. Sure. Similarities between targets can be derived from this and we may put the targets into a more-dimensional space.

The next slide (Fig. 4) shows our results for the three different distances summarized in the form of identification scores here, recognition scores and detection scores. Note that this really is the sort of frequency-of-seeing curves that we have also seen in the presentation by Kevin Cooke.

Obviously, the recognition data and the detection data run very parallel to the identification data, there is a high correlation, of course; one depends very much on the other. You cannot have identification without detection and recognition first.

Now, if we look at these data, I think it is reasonable to propose that we can just take one number here, the point where we have 50-percent correct identification, and take it as representative for the whole set of data that we have here.

Perhaps we may come back to it later in the discussion, but it seems to be justified to characterize the whole experiment with 76 presentations by just that one number, the 50-percent identification distance. And from now on, that is the thing that I will be talking about.

Dr. Ahumada: But when you varied the distance, the entire background was the same?

Dr. van Meeteren: Yes. It was all scaled.

Dr. Thibos: What is recognition and detection in light of your experiment?

Dr. van Meeteren: Then we will go back to the matrix. Identification is the correct response in the sense that the target is identified correctly.

Recognition, in my terminology (but I may sometimes speak about recognition and really mean identification. I apologize for that) is that the jeep is identified correctly or only confused with the other jeep. And indeed if we didn't know that there were jeeps, trucks and tanks, we could use the matrix and start with the procedure of looking at similarities and then, on the basis of the matrix, define in retrospect that there are classes which we could recognize. All right?

Dr. Menendez: Again, a comment on that: That looks a lot like the Johnson Criteria, the last slide.

Dr. van Meeteren: Yes. There are the same sorts of correlations, of course. And in the Johnson Criteria, it also is assumed that there will be parallel shifts between those three levels.

These (Fig. 5) are the main results of an experiment with image intensifiers, i.e. one particular image intensifier for which we have investigated the effects of luminance level in object space and of atmospheric contrast in object space.

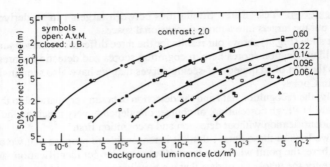

Figure 5. Results of recognition experiments with an image intensifier.

It was all done indoors, because it is, in our opinion, virtually impossible to make such experiments studying the whole parameter space in an outdoor field experiment. It is much better to do it indoors with better control, and have some anchor points for verification in reality.

We have plotted the 50-percent identification distance along the vertical axis, and the results are plotted versus the background luminance along the horizontal axis and the contrast is the parameter.

Contrast was varied in the experiments with the aid of an extra light source superimposing a uniform veiling luminance over the scenery in order to reduce contrast.

The data here refer to two subjects which really come quite close together. And I think that if you would repeat these experiments with more subjects, you would not get exactly the same data, but I think the whole pattern of curves, the whole relation of the data with respect to the variables will be very probably repeated independently of subjects.

The data of course run very much according to expectation in the sense that the identification distance is increasing with luminance, roughly according to a square-root relation. And if you look at one particular luminance they increase with the contrast also roughly according to the square-root relation. You may also see a bit of leveling off at the highest distances where we run into optical resolution limitations.

Now I come to the final objective: Is it possible to predict those data in a much more simple way?

When we first came to this question, the Johnson model was already available, and it is assumed in the Johnson model that the recognition of such complex targets is visually equivalent with the detection of a spatial frequency grating. So that is what we decided we should try out first: Can we compare these data with the detection of spatial frequency gratings?

In order to make that comparison, we have replotted these data in a different way in the next slide (Fig. 6). We have made cross-sections at four different luminance levels and we have plotted here the reciprocal of contrast as a function of distance for each of these luminance levels. In this way we have obtained contrast sensitivity functions for recognition as a function of distance, which can be compared with contrast sensitivity functions for sine-wave gratings as a function of spatial frequency. If you paint a sine-wave grating on a board and look at it from different distances you vary the spatial frequency as it is seen by the eye. The curves here on the slide represent a set of contrast sensitivity functions measured with the same intensifier and with the same subjects and we have shifted this set of curves along the horizontal axis in order to obtain the best correspondence with the data points of the recognition experiment. It now appears that this best fit corresponds with a grating of 1.6 cycles per meter.

Dr. Peli: That is 1.6 cycles per meter at the target scale.

Mr. Kinzly: How many meters is a jeep?

Dr. van Meeteren: A jeep: 1.50.

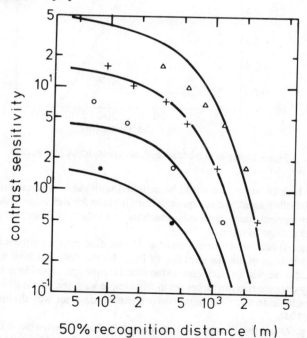

Figure 6. Replot of Fig. 5 (symbols), compared with contrast sensitivity functions for sine wave gratings.

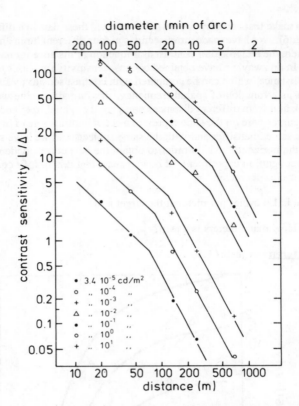

Figure 7. Replot of the Blackwell data (1946; JOSA 36, 624-643).

Now, for lack of better, we could be satisfied with the correspondence we have obtained. On the other hand, we see quite definitely there are deviations. And in fact if we look at the data points, they seem to be much more adequately described by straight lines running under a slope of minus 1.

That brings us back to the detection of a circular disk upon a uniform background, because this reminds us of the classical law of Piper for the description of the detection of a circular disk. So we will be back now to the circular disk upon a uniform background.

If we may characterize our target set in that simple way, the whole literature on this detection is available to us. The most comprehensive data set was the one published by Blackwell in 1946.

Here (Fig. 7) are the Blackwell data also plotted in a somewhat different way than Blackwell did in his original publication. Now we have plotted here what may be called Piper's Law running under a slope of minus 1. And there is another part called Ricco's

Law, mentioned earlier by Kevin Cooke, running under a slope of minus 2.

Both Piper's Law and Ricco's Law can be quite easily understood if we think about contrast detection as a matter of a signal-to-noise ratio, if detection is limited by some sort of spatial noise.

In the Piper domain the targets are bigger than a point source. In that case, you must think of a statistical sample. If you increase the sample in size by a factor of two, the signal-to-noise ratio will improve, by a well-known law of statistics, by a factor of the square root of two. All right?

So if we increase the area of the targets by alpha square, if alpha is the diameter, then the signal-to-noise ratio will be improved by alpha. So the curve will run with a slope of minus 1.

Dr. Cooke: Have you got a breakdown in performance, therefore, in high-brightness, large targets—

Dr. van Meeteren: I will come to that. Sure.

In the case when the targets are so small that their image really cannot be distinguished from the image of an ideal point source, then it is the total energy of the target that matters. Then we run into Ricco's Law with the slope of minus 2.

Now, these Blackwell data can be quite adequately described in this rough way of Piper's Law and Ricco's Law over quite a great part of the parameter space, but there are deviations for higher luminances with bigger targets. I will ask that you keep this in mind, because we will come back to that later on the recognition experiments, as well.

The bending point is interesting. That is the point where the size of the disk is equal to the blur circle of a point source. So this point is determined by the optical quality in this case of the human eye. When we will look through viewing devices, this bending point is characteristic for the optical quality of the device plus the human eye.

This is a rough description, of course, of what really will be a much more gradual transition, but I think this rough description is accurate enough for many of our purposes.

Now, if we go to the next slide (Fig. 8), we make a new comparison of our object recognition data now with a set of curves—these four curves—predicting the detection of circular disks according to Piper's Law and Ricco's Law.

The match here was obtained with an imaginary disk of 0.7 meters at the target scale and is really satisfactory. So we have shown that, when we replace the whole target set by such a 0.7 meter disk, the effects of luminance and contrast, noise in general, upon object recognition are completely reflected in the disk detection.

Now we can normalize all data relative to the distance corresponding with the bending point, and we can normalize all contrast sensitivity data to the same critical signal-to-noise. In this way we can compare all data with one basic prediction curve as is shown in the next slide (Fig. 9). Closed circles refer to the recognition experiments. The open circles refer to measurements of contrast thresholds with a disk, with the same image intensifier.

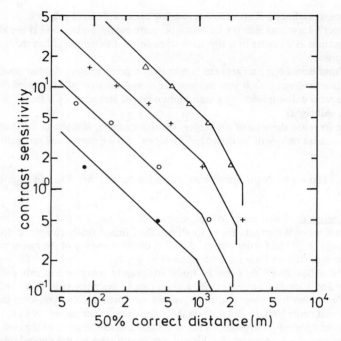

Figure 8. Replot of the results of Fig. 5 (symbols) compared with contrast sensitivity functions for a circular disk upon a uniform background.

Now, note that there is a deviation for very short distances, very big targets, but note that if you look at the mixing of object recognition data and circular disk data, both have the same deviation relative to the basic prediction curve.

So the statement that perhaps object recognition is comparable with disk detection is also correct here, because both deviate from Piper's Law in the same way.

Note that we have completed the prediction curve with an absolute cut-off, a resolution cut-off, but that we do not really have data to verify this. But it is a very logical cut-off, because if you think about the detection of a circular disk, no matter how small you make it, this will always go on. But if you think about object recognition, we will realize that it is not only necessary that we can take just one sample, but in order to distinguish between six targets, you must have a few more samples. And we have assumed here that the distance between the bending point and the absolute cut-off is a factor of two, indicating that we have assumed that it is necessary to be able to distinguish two adjacent samples. But we have no experimental evidence for this here.

Now, this model has been applied by us to very many different image intensifier systems over the last 20 years, and Hans Vos and I have recently given a survey of the applications in the *Journal of Applied Optics*.

I should like to confine myself now to just a few remarks. The first is that specific viewing instruments are characterized by the position of the bending point, so if we really have a specific device and want to use the prediction model, we must first start off finding the bending point. Now, this sounds a lot more easy than it really is. You can see this in the paper I just referred to.

Also, if you think about the reconstruction of contrast in the field from the meteorological conditions, then the model is equally complicated as any other model. There is no way to escape from that.

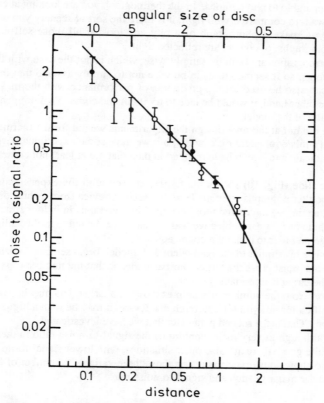

Figure 9. Apparent noise-to-signal ratio at threshold for target recognition as a function of distance (filled circles, data derived from Fig. 5) as well as for disk detection as a function of angular size (open circles, independent measurements).

Additional Experiments with Thermal Viewing Devices

Now, image intensifiers have been superseded by thermal viewing devices in very many conditions. Thermal viewing devices have not completely replaced image intensifiers. If you think about use of night vision goggles, there still is a point for image intensification devices.

In the experiments with image intensifiers we never really came to a resolution limit, because image intensifiers are much more controlled by the atmospheric contrast and luminance conditions than by resolution. But thermal viewing devices may quite well run into a resolution limit.

Now, thermographs are completely different from photographs. Image intensifiers really are comparable to photographs. In the thermograph you are looking at emitted radiation. If you want to compare it with light, it is more the sort of scenery you would have at night when you make a photograph of a city and look at all those self-emitting light sources. Photographs, of course, are reflected light.

Also, thermographs are built up sample-wise, which is not the case with the image intensifier systems, so it seemed to us to be wise not to simply assume that the equivalent disk model can also be used for the prediction of performance with thermal viewing devices. On the other hand, it would be nice to try it out and come to a more general belief in the applicability of the model.

Now, we did not at the time design the experiments we did for the thermal viewing in order to verify this equivalent disk model, but we have some experiments which I would like to just indicate and which have resulted in data that are at least not contradictory with the model.

The next slide (Fig. 10) shows the target set used with the experiments on thermal viewing. The thermographs were made with a special device from a short distance of the target. And, again, we have used those original thermographs in indoor simulation experiments, in which our primary objective was to determine the number of scanlines that must cross the target in order to make it recognizable.

The idea is a bit similar to the equivalent disk model, because if we look at the number of scanlines that must cross the target, our basic idea is that the number of samples that is taken from the target is important.

Now, apart from the number of scanlines crossing a target, you may have also different ocular magnification. If you look through the device, it may be with a bigger or a smaller magnification. That is the second parameter that we have investigated.

Finally, although in very many conditions the signal-to-noise ratio in thermal viewing devices is quite good, there are also other situations, with lower signal-to-noise ratios. So I am going to show some experiments on these three variables: number of lines crossing the target, ocular magnification and signal-to-noise ratio.

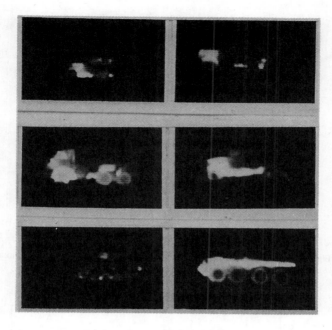

Figure 10. Target set of thermal images.

The next slide (Fig. 11) shows the results of the experiments in which we have kept the number of lines crossing the target expressed in lines per meter constant, and have measured the identification score as a function of ocular magnification. Ocular magnification is expressed here in the width of the scanlines. So two minutes of arc means that the scanlines were two minutes of arc in width, and all the scenery is in scale with this.

Now, what we see is that if we vary from a situation in which the scanlines as seen under an angle of two minutes of arc and then magnify the whole scenery up to 20 minutes of arc—so make it ten times bigger for the eye—then the only thing that changes if you look at the targets is just the size of the whole image, target and scanlines. The information content, the number of samples taken from the target remains the same.

Now, what we see here is that indeed the identification score also remains the same. So it really is much more the number of samples taken from the target than the visual image and its ocular magnification that counts. It is the number of bits taken from the target, so to speak.

Now, with smaller ocular magnification we run into the visual resolution of the human eye, and identification is reduced. Apart from this trivial effect, it is really the number of scanlines that counts.

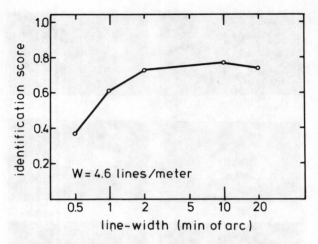

Figure 11. Recognition of thermal images as a function of ocular magnification.

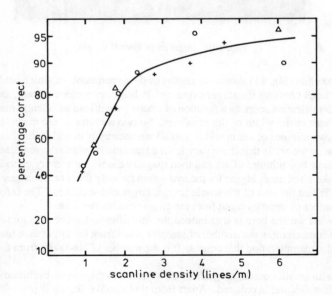

Figure 12. Recognition of thermal images as a function of scanline density.

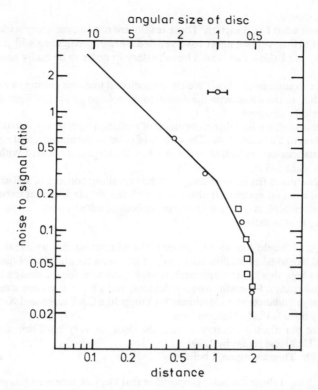

Figure 13. Apparent noise-to-signal ratio at threshold for recognition of thermal images as a function of distance.

In the next slide (Fig. 12) we have measured percentages of correct identification as a function of scanline density, so here we are varying the scanline density, expressed again in lines per meter.

And now we can read at what scanline density we obtain 50 percent correct identification. And if we know the scanline density of a particular device—for instance, a device with 4,000 scanlines per radian—then we may also read distance here, because we can transfer the scanline density of the device into distance.

And, for instance, if we have obtained 50 percent correct identifications here for a scanline density of 1.1 lines per meter on the target and have a device of 4,000 lines per radial, we will obtain an identification distance of 3,600 meters, which really is very satisfactory and not uncommon to have.

Now, in the final slide (Fig. 13) I present some results on 50 percent correct identification distances as a function of the signal-to-noise ratio, determined with thermal viewing simulation devices. These results are compared here again with the prediction curve of the equivalent disk model.

Now, I repeat what I said earlier: These results are not contradictory with the equivalent disk model. However, we never have verified *a priori* predictions with a real thermal device later on, and I think that would be necessary in order to be really and completely happy.

I would like to summarize now. We have concluded that recognition of real objects is more comparable, in our view, with the detection of isolated patches of light than with the detection of periodic structure.

More in particular, we find that recognition of realistic target sets is visually equivalent with the detection of a circular disk. The effects of contrast, luminance, and noise upon the recognition distances are replicated in detail when the targets are scaled with the angular size of an equivalent disk.

And this conclusion fits in, we think, with the prevailing concept of self-similar spatial processing in the visual system. It also fits in with the simple idea that in order to make distinction between objects, you need a certain amount of information.

I would like to stop there.

Dr. Menendez: I would like to take about eight minutes so that we break for lunch at 12:30. I would like to take that time for us to just go over a couple of brief questions.

We can see how this kind of approach is very important for the design in specifying resolution requirements for night imaging devices, and I have also seen similar kinds of things for—image enhancement algorithms for things like CAT scans and X-rays, so there is a wide utility for this kind of information.

I would like our discussants now to take the floor for very brief times, that we may break at about 12:30 and return by 1:30.

Let's see: Dr. Thomas, again, I believe.

Dr. Thomas: Yes. I think the basic proposition that Dr. van Meeteren has put forward is that if we are given discrimination or identification capacity, we can define equivalent detection tasks, and to the extent that this equivalence holds over a range of conditions, it simplifies the prediction problem.

And the other question is what is the range of conditions over which this equivalence holds? There is evidence in the literature that as you vary contrast or fixed viewing distance in set targets, that the relationship between detection and identification remains fixed.

And you have given us some evidence today that as you vary viewing distance plus the veiled magnification factor that it remains fixed.

What I would like to do is suggest some variables that I think need to be investigated, because they may or may not hold up well in this variance. One of them is, of course, the target set. You dealt with a relatively restricted range of targets, and what happens if you use different kinds of targets?

Another one is eccentricity, and I think that is important for the concerns of this particular conference. What experimental work there is in the literature suggests that over a limited range of eccentricities, this fixed relationship between detection and identification will hold, but then it fails.

And the point at which it fails depends upon the size of the objects, the spatial frequency content. So that, I think, is a big area for investigation.

Another one has to do with noise. When you inject external noise—that is, from the atmosphere or from imaging devices—there are ranges of noise over which the relationship between detection and identification is altered.

The studies that are available suggest that as you inject noise, it first has a worse effect on detection than on identification, so that detection drops off faster than identification. And I think this needs more investigation.

Dr. van Meeteren: Yes. I think I could agree with many of those suggestions.

If I may come back first to the question on the target set, it must be clear that in this case—in performing the experiments as we have done them—we start with the target set, and then finally we find out that this target set is well represented by a disk of 0.7 meters.

Now, if you take a different target set, you will find other disk diameters corresponding with that target set. Also, if you have a disk of 0.7 meters, there may be a couple of target sets characterized by that disk size.

So what I really think is that it is really more the size of the disk that is quantifying the difficulty of the target set than in the reverse.

If I would have to start my experiment again, I would never again take as complicated a target set as the one I have now, but it was attractive for us to have jeeps, trucks, and tanks in it.

Once we had discovered this equivalency between simple objects and complicated target sets, it would be much nicer to have uniform target sets—difficult sets and more easy sets—so you could make up a target set with just one jeep, one truck and one tank, which is an easy target set for recognition, but you could also set up a target set all with tanks, which would be a difficult set.

But it would be better to have what I would call uniform target sets, with uniform confusions. Experimentally this would be better, because you could concentrate your data on the same level.

We had 76 presentations. Almost half of the presentations were in the area of unvisible at all or in the area where the tanks were always completely identified.

So if we would go on with these sort of proceedings, thinking about what would really be the best target set is important. I think for the rest I could agree that there is lots of interesting work to be done.

Dr. Thibos: I could follow up on that point. If you had two target sets which had the same equivalent disk diameter—and you might think that merging the two sets together, you would continue to have the same disk diameter, but on the other hand, having twice as big a set size really ought to reduce performance. So doesn't the equivalency then break down? Do you think simple rules will apply, that combining two sets together with the same equivalent disk diameter ought to have the same equivalent disk diameter?

Dr. van Meeteren: If we add two equally difficult target sets, the combination set may be equally difficult, but most probably will not be equally difficult. It all depends on the similarities between objects of the first and the second subset. If it so happens that one or more targets from the first set are more similar to "twin" targets in the second set than to the targets in the first set, the combination set will be a more difficult one. However, this is not necessarily so. If I have a set of six military targets corresponding with 0.7 meters and I also have a set of six animals from the zoo corresponding with 0.7 meters. Then I think adding them probably would be no problem because you would have two sets from completely different parts of space. Do you agree? I didn't think this over very much, I must confess.

Dr. Thibos: But I mean you can see that in the limiting case, the two sets could be identical.

Dr. van Meeteren: Yes.

Dr. Thibos: And then the task would be impossible. You couldn't distinguish them, because now the two sets were the same.

Dr. van Meeteren: Well, if they are identical, there is no need to distinguish.

Dr. Thibos: Right. But I mean they could be arbitrarily close and still be different. So then you have a situation where all of a sudden the performance has to be terrible. It can't be anywhere near.

Dr. van Meeteren: Indeed, if you bring sets with similar differences together and bring objects of one set very close to objects in the other set, you introduce a much more difficult distinction, and you have got a completely new smaller disk size.

Dr. Menendez: Again, we have got to hold the questions. We are going to have discussion panels.
    Mr. Scott, I think you are on line for a comment or discussion question.

Mr. Scott: On one of the probability-versus-range charts you showed—I think where you were referring to the sine-waves, and you had the discrete data—was that the average of all the targets or results for all the targets combined, or were you looking at a specific target.

Dr. van Meeteren: That was the average of all targets.

Dr. Peli: Are you saying that target identification is equivalent to a grating of only 1.6 cycles per meter, i.e. corresponding with only a few cycles covering the target? I know in an early experiment on toy tanks, they needed 28 cycles.

Dr. van Meeteren: You are right. That was a different target set, apparently a much more difficult one.

Dr. Bradley: I just wanted to find out if you thought the correspondence between the distance of recognition data and your disk detection data—is that telling us something about the nature of objects or something about image intensifiers or the visual system? What are we looking at with the correspondence?

Dr. van Meeteren: I think it is telling us something about the nature of objects. The essential features are more patches of light than periodic structure. That is what it is telling us.

Dr. Bradley: I guess my follow-up then would be it seems a strange way to study the nature of objects, but maybe not. I mean, using the image intensifier system and the human eye and a visual system and a detection, all to study the nature of objects. You could imagine simply examining objects, doing a statistical analysis of their properties.

Dr. van Meeteren: Well, I agree with that, but our primary purpose was not the characterization of targets, but the characterization of target recognition. The point is that, if we want to evaluate the use of a viewing device with a realistic observation task, then the nature of the objects comes very much to the fore.

Dr. Menendez: It is quite surprising that this hasn't been done more, that you go out and look at a confusion matrix and do a multi-dimensional scaling analysis to find out what the natural categories and confusions are, what the clusters are, how many dimensions there are.

It is done all the time in the other senses, and for some reason VISION seems to think we can't do that.

I interpret what you have said about—the specular reflections is really what it was. I mean you see that in the camouflage literature. They go like crazy to camouflage the object and then are defeated by specular reflection.

Dr. van Meeteren: More in general, thinking about the visual system and distinctions we make, isn't it all reflecting on the ecology of our environment?

Dr. Menendez: Yes; except these are man-made objects.

VALIDATION OF PREDICTION MODELS
FOR TARGET ACQUISITION
WITH ELECTRO-OPTICAL SENSORS

BARBARA L. O'KANE
U.S. Army Communications Electronics Command
Night Vision and Electronic Sensors Directorate
Ft. Belvoir, VA 22060

This chapter discusses insights into the complex activity of verifying and improving the accuracy of target acquisition models for predicting range performance with thermal imaging devices. Historically, range performance predictions for electro-optical sensors have used an equivalent bar pattern methodology developed at the U. S. Army Night Vision Laboratory in 1959. FLIR92 and ACQUIRE, current models for thermal imagers, continue in this tradition, but are being continuously improved and applied to changing system designs and operational requirements. In redefining parameters of the thermal range performance prediction models to support systems under development, we have chosen an experimental approach employing appropriate users as subject observers. Field tests and laboratory perception experiments using a variety of thermal imagery generation techniques have given us experiences in the improvement and testing of these models. In addition, other organizations have performed experiments with thermal imagers and asked for our participation either before, during or after having conducted a field test to evaluate the applicability of range predictions to their specific sensors and scenarios. All of these experiments are the subject of the pages which follow. While no experiment is perfect, and field tests especially are subject to many uncontrollable circumstances, much can be learned from the errors as well as the successes. Those running field tests are often not versed in experimental design and analysis and may find this present effort helpful when confronted with a question to be answered by means of testing.

1. Introduction

In discussing field experiments to validate models, Dr. Menendez frequently joked that fitting a model to field results merely demonstrates that the model can hit the broad side of a barn created by the envelope of error in field test measurements. This chapter deals with insights into the sources of error in validation efforts supporting modeling and examines such "barnyard" data. While much of the content would apply to most imaging electro-optical sensors, what follows focuses on the thermal spectrum of imagers, which are most commonly used for long range target acquisition.

In the Army regulations, the determination that a performance prediction model is useful and accurate has several components, known as validation, verification and accreditation, or VV&A. Validation is the step in which results from field and laboratory experiments are compared with model predictions. Verification is done to ensure that the equations within the model agree with what is known about the physics and psychophysics of the conditions and hardware. Another step in verification is the determination that the coding of the model into computer software accurately reflects these equations. "Accreditation" of predictive models states the conditions and types of scenarios under which the model should be used to make official decisions, for example, in war games, system development or comparisons among system proposals. This chapter addresses methods to obtain empirical data to support model development, validation, and accreditation.

The concept of "validating a model" is actually illogical and nonscientific since one can never prove that a hypothesis is true, especially for all cases. The scientific method proposes that an experiment be used to reject a null hypothesis (the initial model) and thereby support an alternative hypothesis (a different model). In actual practice, field tests designed to support or reject an integrated model are subject to the whims of nature and represent a snapshot of one or possibly several cases which a model may be used to predict. There may or may not be a suitable or implicit alternative hypothesis waiting in the wings, and the error between predicted and measured performance may not readily indicate in what way the tested model should be changed. Another bold model may be developed from the results, but the error resulting from the next field test may again appear to reject this new and improved model, and so on.

Models are generally based upon either first principles theories or upon previous empirical data. To provide evidence for the model's usefulness for various types of conditions and scenarios, field tests are often conducted. However, as will be shown in the following sections, field tests must be designed carefully, and often field tests alone cannot provide the needed evidence to support a model or to yield data for model enhancement. Other types of experimental data are inevitably required.

We have established, then, that it is against the scientific method to speak of validating a model. However, it is still necessary to determine whether the model can be supported by field test data. If, for the purpose of this discussion, we redefine the term "validation" to mean "obtaining evidence bearing on whether the model is true or not true" then we can ask the question "What is model validation and how does one do it?".

When system developers or modelers decide to do an experiment, they usually have numerous questions about how to actually conduct an experiment, what the critical factors are, as well as basic questions about experimental design. This is often due to the fact that they have not had much background in statistics or the design of experiments. Therefore, they may approach an experimental psychologist, whose background is in these very matters, and ask the following types of questions: "How many subjects should I use? How many trials do I need? How many ranges do I use? How many different targets should there be?" Perhaps they expect an engineering reply in the form, "30, 100, 5, and 9, respectively." But how would one arrive at such rules of thumb? What leads one to any particular set of numbers or ways of deriving them? What are some other rules about running experiments that apply to the validation and testing of models? This chapter will answer these questions by examples and summary of lessons learned through experience.

2. Experimental Methodologies

Frequently, system developers ask questions such as: "Is the model correct with respect to this sensor (or weather condition, or target type)?" Any system test of this nature can in essence be considered part of a larger effort supporting model development and validation. Such experiments, designed and conducted by others, will be discussed here to provide examples of validation efforts (showing what to do, or more often what not to do). The names have been concealed to protect the innocent and guilty alike, and some poetic license has been applied to the facts for illustration purposes.

Partially manipulated or simulated imagery, referred to here as "hybrid", can allow for a more controlled experiment than a field test by including the exact factors and levels desired. Larger numbers of better trained observers are usually available because the experiment can be run virtually anywhere at any time. Such laboratory perception experiments may use field, hybrid or physical terrain board imagery. The imagery can be collected or generated in a variety of ways. First, imagery can be collected in the field with a number of sensors, including calibrated imagers, and then replayed to observers. Second, field imagery of the vehicles on a turntable can be taken at very near range with a calibrated thermal system. The precision and over-sampling in the original imagery can then be manipulated with sensor, atmospheric, and range simulations.[1] Third, quasi-synthetic imagery can be generated by taking video of a physical terrain board. Upon this background are placed target miniatures painted in such a way as to simulate thermal signatures when the video image is reversed.[2] Finally, development efforts are presently underway to provide purely computer-generated imagery which will provide a future source of imagery. For all these methods, great care must be taken to achieve fidelity to the real sensor and scenarios.

All of these methodologies have served experimenters at various times in understanding the performance of observers with respect to finding and identifying targets in thermal imagery. The performance models are run with inputs matching the test situation and the results from the test are compared with the predicted performance. In this way the validity of the model predictions can be assessed. However, few tests give unequivocal results. Like the popular TV show "Jeopardy", an experiment often gives an answer and *post hoc* the exact question is deduced. Knowing the question is absolutely crucial, because unless one does, the answer can be ambiguous. An important consideration is, for example, what the subjects were being asked to do, their expectations about the tasks, and their prior training.

The chapter begins with a description of the traditional Night Vision and Electronic Sensors Directorate (NVESD) models, which are the standard for government and industry in predicting range performance with electro-optical systems. Next, examples of field tests and laboratory perception experiments will be analyzed. These examples are ordered from their origin in respect to the field, i.e., field tests, perception experiments using field imagery, and finally perception experiments using hybrid imagery. The chapter concludes with a summary of lessons learned and recommendations for designing and conducting experiments in support of modeling.

3. NVESD Thermal Range Performance Models (FLIR92/ACQUIRE)

The Army and industry have traditionally used the equivalent bar pattern methodology developed by John Johnson[3] and originally formalized in the Night Vision Static Performance Model.[4] This modeling methodology is based upon the number of cycles which could be resolved at each range if bars encompassing the size of the target at the same temperature difference from the background were actually in the field. This methodology has been used to evaluate sensors and to compare performance among Forward Looking Infrared (FLIR) systems. The system demand portion of the model predicts Minimum Resolvable Temperature Difference (MRTD) relating cycles/milliradian resolvable as a function of targets vs. background temperature. A sensor's sensitivity, noise and resolution characteristics are reflected in the MRTD curves. The input deck for the model is very detailed with respect to the sensor. Both recent[5] and classic books[6,7] can be consulted for a discussion of system characteristics and parameters and their relation to performance.[8]

In NVESD's Image Evaluation Facility and Automated Sensor/Processor Evaluation Center (AUTOSPEC), measurements are made on real systems using four-bar patterns.[9] Thermal bar patterns are produced and stimulate the detectors of the FLIR being tested. An expert observer raises the temperature of the bars until he/she can detect the four bars in the displayed image. [Horizontal and vertical bar patterns are used to obtain vertical and horizontal MRTD curves, respectively.]

The predicted MRTDs compare well to laboratory measurements of MRTD as a function of spatial frequency of the four-bar pattern. A "2-dimensional MRTD" is calculated as the geometric mean of the MRTD for the horizontal and vertical frequencies for a given temperature difference (MRTD). Figure 1 shows generic measured horizontal and vertical MRTD curves and calculated two-dimensional MRTD for a first generation common module-type FLIR. The lower the MRTD curve, the better the sensor's performance is predicted to be.

NVESD measurement methodologies have been accepted as the national standard for the technical charaterization of thermal imagers.[9] FLIR92[10] is the most recent version of NVESD's sensor performance model, which includes an updated sampling and noise methodology for accommodating advanced sensors. [11, 12]

The MRTD curves, along with the target vehicle projected area in meters^2 (A) and apparent temperature (ΔT), produce a range prediction via the ACQUIRE model.[13] The target signature is represented in the traditional ACQUIRE model by:

$$\Delta T = T - B \qquad (1)$$

where T = mean temperature of the target and B = mean temperature of the immediate background. Other signature descriptions which take into account the variance in the tar-

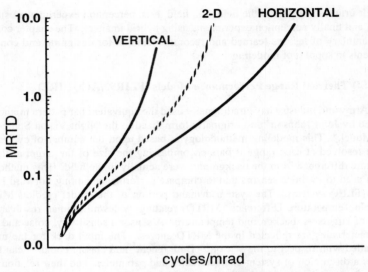

Figure 1. Vertical, horizontal and 2-dimensional MRTD curves for a fictitious first generation system.

get and background have been shown to be useful in the case of detection.[14]

The characteristic dimension of the target is given by $\sqrt{A}$ (meters), where A= target projected area (meters^2). Other metrics for target critical or characteristic dimension are being explored,[15] to account for the size of critical features used by observers in identifying vehicles. The number of resolvable cycles on the target (N) is then calculated as

$$N = \frac{\sqrt{A}}{R} \times f_r \qquad (2)$$

where f_r = the spatial frequency (cycles/milliradian) resolvable from the MRTD curve for the apparent ΔT at the sensor, and R = range (km).

A probability function, known as the Target Transform Probability Function (TTPF), as shown in Figure 2 can then be predicted based upon the following empirically derived formulation:

$$P = \frac{\left(\frac{N}{N_{50}}\right)^E}{1 + \left(\frac{N}{N_{50}}\right)^E} \qquad (3)$$

where

$$E = 2.7 + 0.7\left(\frac{N}{N_{50}}\right) \qquad (4)$$

and N_{50} is the criterion number of resolvable cycles on target required for 50% of an ensemble of trained observers to successfully perform the task of interest. This formulation was developed as part of the 1975 Static Performance Model[4] for sensors based upon the Johnson equivalent bar pattern methodology.[3]   As the acquisition task becomes more difficult the number of bars required would increase. The tasks of interest are normally defined as:

   a. *Detection* -- determination that a target of interest is present

   b. *Recognition* -- determination that a target belongs to a particular functional category (for example, truck, tank or armored personnel carrier)

   c. *Identification* -- correct judgment of the exact nomenclature of the vehicle (T62, M35, M60, etc.)

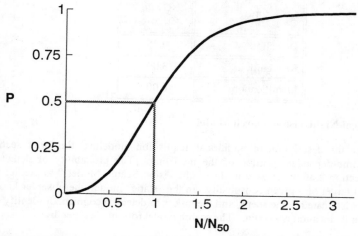

Figure 2. This curve is known as the Target Transform Probability Function (TTPF). The cycles on target, N, is calculated as the product of the resolvable frequency from the 2-dimensional MRTD curve and the square root of the target projected area divided by the range (km). N_{50} is the number of resolvable cycles on target required for 50% of an ensemble of trained observers to be able to perform the task of detection, recognition, or identification. Standard values for N_{50} are 0.75, 3.0 and 6.0 for detection, recognition, and identification, respectively, for an ensemble of targets in low to medium clutter.

Each of these tasks is assigned an empirically derived standard cycle criterion (N_{50}) as shown in Table 1.

The criterion number of cycles on target required for the various tasks of detection, recognition, and identification have been the subject of experimentation which will be described further on in this chapter. The recommendations in the present ACQUIRE[13] model for detection are based upon a low to medium clutter scene (subjectively assessed) and the ensemble of tactical vehicle targets.[15]   There is presently no quantitative parameter which is applied to a scene to measure its clutter level. The analyst or modeler will generally observe the scene and subjectively evaluate whether there appears to be a small amount or a large number of background objects which would make the vehicle more or less difficult to detect. In that light, to account for the detection rate in a "high clutter" scene, the cycle criterion for detection is traditionally doubled. Also, it should be noted that the model predicts range performance against an ensemble of targets. It has long been known that certain targets and aspect angles (such as side views) are relatively easier while others are more difficult even though they belong to the same ensemble class (ΔT, projected area). However, the cycle criteria shown above have served well to predict the FLIR performance against "standard targets." A schematic representation of the stages of military target acquisition along with the required cycles are shown in Figure 3.

Table 1: Recommended Cycle Criteria (N_{50}) for the various tasks.

Task	Cycle Criterion
Detection	0.75
Recognition	3.00
Identification	6.00

4. The Historical Night Vision Search Model

To complete the description of traditional acquisition modeling, this brief section describes the time-dependent portion of the modeling. The probability of detection described in Section 2 above is used in the Night Vision Search Model[16] to predict the time to detect a target of a given conspicuity. In the "static" model, the observer knows where the target is located in the scene, and the task is to detect, recognize, or identify the target given that its location is known. The search model formula is given by:

$$P_d(t) = P_d^\infty [1 - e^{-t/\tau}] \tag{5}$$

where

$$\tau \approx \frac{3.4}{P_d^\infty} \tag{6}$$

and

t = time (seconds) from the first appearance of the scene on the display to the time at which the observer will report a detection

τ = mean time to acquire target (seconds)

P_d^∞ = closely approximated by the probability of detection given infinite time.

The field of view of the sensor, the full field of regard for the search, and the quantity of competing background clutter, among other factors, certainly constitute the possible conditions for search. NVESD has an active program to evaluate search parameters using

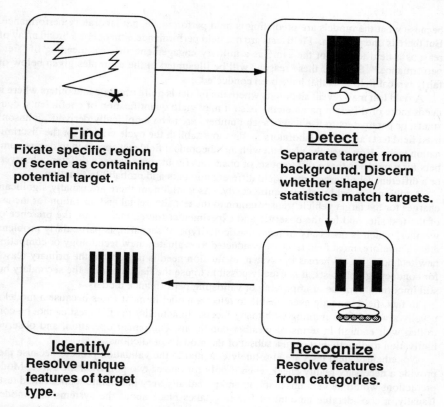

Find
Fixate specific region of scene as containing potential target.

Detect
Separate target from background. Discern whether shape/ statistics match targets.

Identify
Resolve unique features of target type.

Recognize
Resolve features from categories.

Figure 3. This figure shows a schematic drawing of the Johnson [3] equivalent bar pattern methodology. The model assumes that the observer has found the target or that the target has been pointed out and that the task is to detect, recognize, or identify a target at a given location in the field of view. The bar pattern shown above each stylized drawing represents the cycle criterion for the particular task. A search model [16] is used to predict the search time for detecting targets and is based upon the predicted probability of detecting the target given infinite time from the target transform probability function.

the various types of imagery and methodologies discussed in the examples that follow. The experiments discussed below generally focus on the probability of detection, recognition, and identification, rather than on the time required to perform the given task.

5. Field Tests

There is a general impression that a field test is somehow a more "valid" test of a model than an experiment performed in the laboratory. This belief is understandable because what the models are predicting is field performance, not laboratory performance. But there is one problem. Field tests are not field performance either. For a broad array of reasons a field test is not the same as a military engagement, the real meaning of "field performance." Some of these reasons will be illustrated in the examples given below of fairly typical field tests that have been conducted.

A field test may reveal situations where the model is quite accurate and others where it needs more or different parameters. Also it may yield quantification of coefficients, constants, or parameters to use where such numbers are to be empirically derived. Johnson[3] used field tests as well as laboratory studies to establish the cycle criteria for the discrimination tasks. However, the problem with an atheoretical field test approach to derive numbers for a model is that a different set of observers (or in some cases, a different observer) or a different set of targets may yield different numbers and probability function.

Additionally, field trials are quite costly. As a minimum there are usually significant charges for the target vehicle transportation to the test site, rental and operation for the use of the test site, and for the observer and experimenter travel, etc. Then, the presence of weather, which is necessary to test a particular type of scenario, is particularly problematic. Therefore, most field tests are conducted to evaluate a new technology or competing new technologies. Whereas the system evaluation need is most often the primary reason for conducting field tests, it is usually possible to use the field trials for the secondary but still important purpose of improving or validating performance models.

In fact, field tests are even unable to reject a model in most cases because a model is usually a very global framing with many facets. In actuality the field test cannot be controlled well enough in terms of weather conditions, equipment operation, and observer motivation to directly test even a subset of the model's predictions.

Nonetheless, field tests are absolutely essential to the validation process because they provide a necessary reality check, even if only for one or two points on the curve. Model predictions would be very unsatisfying and potentially very inaccurate without field tests. Usually, a considerable amount of learning takes place about the systems and models under test, and also about running field tests.

5.1. Detecting Vehicles with Night Sights

A field test was performed by a system developer using twenty sensors of the same type. (Let's call the sensors "Night Sights.") The fifty observers were to search through a field of regard of approximately 100 degrees and indicate where a target vehicle was, thereby indicating a target detection.

While this seems like a fairly straightforward design that would yield plenty of data to validate a range performance model, it in fact produced lots of virtually useless data. Some of the pros and cons for this test were as follows:

a. The operators in the test were not familiar with Night Sights. Therefore, they did not adjust the gain and level or focus the Night Sights very well as determined by experimenters who viewed through their devices periodically. This less than optimal operation reduced the ability of the Night Sight to display a clear image of the vehicle. Moreover, there was no way to know on any particular scenario how a particular observer had adjusted the controls.

b. Each of the Night Sights was operating at a different level of maintenance and the set of sensors varied in vintage and image quality. Some of the sights were operating well, whereas others were operating with low batteries and other problems. Even though MRTD and other sight measurements were taken during the test, it was impractical to correct for the error due to a particular sensor, since the performance of a particular individual observer was nested within this factor.

c. The field of regard was so large that it is not known whether the observers actually had the target vehicle in their field of view on any particular trial. This is critical data since the model under test assumes that the target is at some point in the field of view.

On the positive side,

d. On each trial, the observers would either detect or not detect the target. The large number of observers in the test allows a resolution of the probability on each trial of 5%. The 95% confidence interval would be relatively small even when at its maximum:

$$95\% \text{ confidence interval} = 1.96 \sqrt{\frac{p \cdot (1-p)}{N-1}} \tag{7}$$

$$\text{and for the 50\% point} = 1.96 \sqrt{\frac{0.5 \cdot (1-0.5)}{50-1}} = 0.14 \tag{8}$$

It is interesting to analyze the error due to the various sensors and observer states and number of subjects. The following questions come to mind. Does the relatively large number of subjects in the experiment compensate for the error in the experiment having to do with uncontrolled factors (e.g., sensor maintenance, observer training)? Let's just speculate that the error in the sensor maintenance and in the subjects are random. The large number of subjects reduces the error in the mean, i.e., its variability. The question is, the mean of what? If one has sampled the subject population appropriately then it would tend to regress towards the mean of the universe from which the subjects were sampled. However, if one has sampled sensors that were not maintained well, then the results would reflect, with great precision, performance expected with poorly maintained sensors.

It is desired to ensure that the sample of observers in the test represents the population being described in the model. The ACQUIRE model predicts the *proportion of trained military observers who would detect (recognize, identify) a target of given* ΔT *(temperature difference from the background) and size (square root of projected area) over an ensemble of targets under the atmosphere encountered.* When seeking to validate this model, one would certainly like to understand the statement *trained military observers.* "Trained in what respect?" one might ask. Possibilities include: trained on the specific targets in the test, trained with the specific sensors in the test, or trained on the specific task (for example, search strategies). One approach to solving this problem is to operationally define "training" as the score an observer achieves on a training program. Such an approach has been developed at NVESD. A detailed training strategy has been developed for the purpose of preparing military observers prior to their participation in laboratory perception experiments. The training package was based in part on *The Infrared Recognition and Target Handbook,*[17] which contains general information on thermal imagery, visible and infrared photographs of the target vehicles, and hints for using specific target cues to recognize or identify them. A criterion performance (90-100%) is required on a self-paced, self-scoring training program.[18] In this manner, one reduces the learning effect which can plague a test by obscuring the effects of the independent variables under test.

If the observer sample is not from the appropriate population (for example, trained military observers) then one has erred. If the experiment has so few observers that one observer has an undue effect on the results of the experiment, then there is such poor resolving power that the results cannot reveal whether the model is working adequately. Because of the relatively poor resolution of the results and the potential for skewing caused by a particularly bad or good observer, there would seem to be no advantage to having a small number of subjects (i.e., less than 10) with dichotomous data (i.e., right/wrong or detect/no detect).

In classical psychophysics experiments in which few subjects, or sometimes only one, participated, there were an extremely large number of trials and the measure was usually thought to be fairly similar over all observers with normal vision. Due to the variations in the skill levels which can come into play when observers perform the discrimination tasks in target acquisition, the representativeness of the sample of observers is critical to a reasonable validation of the model. In fact, the lower level ability of finding potential targets in a scene has been found to be similar across all levels of observer background given similar pre-experimental training. However, the higher level abilities of vehicle recognition, identification, and rejection of false targets are much more variable with observer and training.[14]

5.2. Evaluating a Prototype Sensor Against a Specification

A field test was conducted to determine whether a system was able to meet the specifications required in the operational requirements document. The specifications consisted of a specific probability of detection and recognition for a particular size target (in meters^2) with a given ΔT at a given range for a clear atmosphere.

NVESD learned of these field trials after the test had been conducted when some difficulties arose during the analysis. The individuals and organization which designed and conducted the test were different from those analyzing the test. Those analyzing were in quite a state of despair because they could not make anything out of the results. And what they did find, they did not know whether to believe. Some of the challenges encountered by the analysts of the results were:

a. Between three and six subjects, who were inexperienced in the use of the system, participated on any given trial.

b. The single prototype sensor which served as the only test device was believed to be operating at less than full efficiency.

c. The target, range, and ΔT in the specifications were not explicitly in the design of the test. The ranges were always farther than the specification required, the target was quite a different size, and the ΔT was not known.

Each of these factors in the experiment contributed to a lack of focus for the experiment and an increase in the error. For example, the number of subjects was small and not consistent, causing an increase in the error between trials, and their inexperience reduced the validity of the test with regard to the eventual users.

As for the question under test, if the data were reduced to only that which applied precisely to the specification hypothesis, i.e., probability of detection greater than or equal to specification x (for given range, atmosphere, target size, and ΔT), then there was a small number of trials which could fit approximately into that scenario by compensating for target size by range. When the hypothesis of whether the obtained probability met or exceeded the specification was directly tested, the conclusion was that the hypothesis that the sensor did *not* meet the specification could *not* be rejected.

This experiment more than any other alerted me to shortcomings which can plague field tests that are not designed carefully. For example, the test design should explicitly include the levels of the factors of interest. If the hypothesis being tested concerns a specific range requirement, then the parameters in the experiment should bracket that range. By doing so, the sensitivity of the predictions to a particular factor can also be estimated. For instance, if three ranges are tested including the range of interest along with +/- 1 kilometer and there is no difference between the results for any of the ranges, this gives information as to the sensitivity of the task as a function of range for modeling purposes.

If the models of range performance were believed or known to be accurate and precise, there would be no need to run field tests such as this example. The program manager would simply input an MRTD curve, target signature, projected area, and atmospheric conditions to yield a predicted range performance. Tests like the one above are conducted for a sanity check on the modeling. In this case I believe the managers of the development program returned to the model with a sigh of relief. Previous comparisons between the model and experimental results provided an evaluation of the system with less error and more information than did the field test.

5.3. Detecting Humans with Thermal Devices

A few years ago an opportunity arose to do a field test solely to obtain validation on empirical parameters for the ACQUIRE model (Cooke et al., this volume). The question had been raised as to how many cycles on target are required to detect a soldier in uniform. So off we went to Ft. A. P. Hill for a week to run a field test in the dead of night with 4 sights and 20 observers.[19]

The subjects were divided into four groups of five. Subjects were trained on the operation of the sensor and controls prior to the test and familiarized with the test procedure. Each group used each of the four sensors an equal number of times, thereby removing the nesting of observer effects within the differences among the sensors. There was a strict maintenance schedule for the sensors. A matrix was developed to carefully ensure randomization of trials with respect to range and observer. Complete measurements were made of weather and target ΔT.

On any given trial, zero, one, two or three personnel were standing in one of five range locations within the field of view of the sensor. The task of the observer was to count the number of people in the field of view on each trial. If an observer reported less than the number present, it was assumed that the personnel at the closer ranges were detected.

This experiment was designed well in some respects but suffered from the flaw of not really knowing where the observers were seeing the targets which they counted. For that reason, it is likely that the results were optimistic for the closer ranges and pessimistic for the farther ranges. This flaw could have been averted by a more detailed response system (such as laying out the field of view in a grid with alphanumeric designations). NVESD is also developing an observer-operated laser designator system to provide a search tracking capability.

5.4. Vehicle Recognition

A related set of field trials were conducted to calibrate the cycle criterion with the characteristic dimension (square root of projected area) in the recognition of vehicles. Two sensors, one prototype second generation and another fielded first generation thermal target acquisition system were used. The targets were eight vehicles at two ranges. The task for the observer was to recognize the class of the vehicle (armored personnel carrier, tank, air defense vehicle, or truck).

The test took place over three days and nights with a maximum of four military and three civilian observers on each trial. The three civilians were thermal system engineers who were extremely familiar with the thermal devices and the vehicles. As few as five subjects participated on many of the trials. The best observer, who recognized the vehicles virtually every time, was included on each trial. The results were compared with the model predictions and specifications.

For conclusions to be considered definitive by the highest levels in the Army, all experiments must be performed with appropriately trained military observers. Because one of the FLIRs was required at another test site, it was not possible to retain it in the field long enough to run a sufficient number of appropriate subjects. Therefore imagery was captured digitally from the sensors during the field test. This imagery was then presented (with real-time noise) to a larger number of trained Army aviators. The comparison of the above field trial results with the perception experiment conducted with the field imagery will be discussed in Section 6.1.

5.5. Advantages and Disadvantages of Field Tests

Field tests have certain benefits over other types of experiments as shown in Table 2. However, they tend to be very costly and often cannot be performed with a large sample of observers having the appropriate background.

Table 2: Pros and Cons of Field Tests

Advantages	Disadvantages frequently occurring
Appears "real."	Too much "reality"; too little control over scenarios; any particular scenario cannot be duplicated.
	Usually very expensive.
Capability for observers to adjust the sensor gain and level.	Adjustment of controls not always optimal and levels unknown.
Encompasses many environmental conditions.	Little control over environmental conditions.
Observers are working in real time.	Often difficult to ensure all observers on any particular trial are experiencing the same stimulus.
	May be difficult to have enough observers. More cannot participate if desired after the fact.
	Observers may become fatigued and less motivated, but the test must go on at that time.

6. Laboratory Perception Experiments with Field Imagery

It is often inconvenient to perform a strict field test. All of the most appropriate observers may not be available at the same time, only one sensor is at the site, it is too costly to stay in the field with the targets, and so on. It is much more convenient to seat observers in a clean, darkened laboratory, train them to criterion at their own pace, allow them to take the test with desired breaks, during the day, with a good night's sleep behind them, etc. But the question can be asked, how do these results relate to those which would have been obtained in the field? Clearly, field trials have drawbacks and their results must be used with caution, but how do these laboratory tests rank in veracity?

If calibrated thermal imagery is available that was taken simultaneously with imagery from the tactical sensor under investigation, then the "inherent" signatures (i.e., unaffected by atmospheric transmission in the path) of the target vehicles and the terrain are known. In combination with the laboratory evaluation measurements of the FLIR, which give the RMS noise of the system, appropriate presentation of the imagery to the observer can be achieved. For example, simulated frames of noise with the same characteristics as the measured noise can be added to the calibrated imagery. The computer then displays the frames in real time allowing for a realistic simulation.

The fidelity of imagery is extremely important when performing experiments in the laboratory using field imagery. The recording methods must be carefully chosen in accordance with the method of playback and the type of imagery being stored. When sensors have a digital port from which to record imagery, this is generally convenient, if one has a system for storing the frames of data. The chance of contamination by intermediate noise sources is virtually eliminated. Some systems, however, produce 12-bit data and perform various digital corrections which complicate optimal display of the information when a fixed calibration is desired. A great deal of research and development is being performed to determine the best way to display such information.[20]

Capturing first generation FLIR imagery is much more difficult since the imagery is normally not digital. If one uses hi-8 mm, VHS, 22-track tape recorders, or some other tape medium, recording itself can add a new source of noise. This noise source can be avoided by digitizing the analog imagery, averaging frames, and then synthesizing noise. Digitizing the imagery also more easily allows an interface with the subject in the experiment, which is not normally practical with video.

6.1. Vehicle Recognition

This example is the perception test derived from the Section 5.4 field trials. The digital imagery was captured from the sensor by a high bit-rate recorder and downloaded onto an optical disk for use with personal computer observer stations. Via an EPIX image processing card, sixteen frames of each image were stored. During the time allotted for observers to view each image, the sixteen frames were displayed sequentially in a loop at 30 Hz in order to represent real time noise present in FLIR systems. In fact, we took the observer stations to the military post via a trailer truck and presented the images to them in their backyard parking lot. A comparison of the results from the field and laboratory tests for the two ranges and two systems is shown in Figure 4. While in every case there was a reduction in performance in the laboratory test, the difference is not statistically significant, as can be seen by noting that the error bars for the field results overlap the corresponding value for the laboratory tests.

This experiment is one of the few that allow a comparison between the results from a field test with the same imagery brought into the lab and presented to observers in a controlled setting. The pattern of results is clearly the same for the laboratory and field, with a slight reduction for each condition in the laboratory setting. There are two plausible post-hoc explanations for the slight, though consistent, reduction in performance in the laboratory imagery. At the time that this experiment was conducted,[21] our methods for recording imagery were still being developed. There may have been a slight degradation of the imagery due to the recording process.

A look at the statistical nature of the results may be enlightening. The field test was performed with six (6) observers. One observer was virtually 100% correct so this puts a plateau for each trial of approximately 17-20% due to the small number of observers. The performance for a particular trial would never fall below that rate. One observer performing at 100% among 19 other observers would only put a 5% cushion on the bottom of the

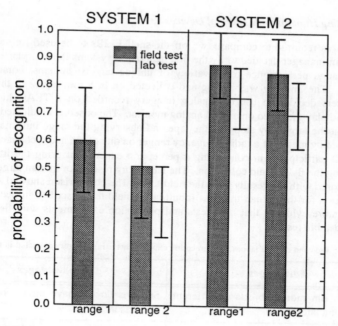

Figure 4. A field test was performed with six observers varying widely in ability. A second experiment was performed using the field imagery in a laboratory setting with 19 trained aviators. In every case the error bars (standard error of the mean) overlap, indicating that the means are not significantly different.

data. This is a good reason to have a reasonable number of observers. The effect of one particularly good or bad observer would not thereby skew the data to any appreciable degree. Even as few as ten observers allows a substantial shift (10%) due to one outstanding observer. Therefore, whenever field tests are run with 5-10 observers, the results may be questionable. Usually when there are few observers, the sample cannot reflect the population of interest due to the potential for one observer who happens to be "experiment-wise" to skew the mean.

In the field the observers can reverse the polarity from "black=hot" to "white=hot" and back as desired to obtain a clear image of the particular target. Unfortunately, during the time that the experiment described in Section 6.1 was conducted, the capability for the observers to reverse polarity and adjust the gain and level of the sensor did not exist. Such capabilities are being developed for real-time application in perception experiments. This improvement in laboratory methodology will allow the experience with the imagery to be more similar to field experience.

6.2. Detecting Humans with Thermal Devices

A test was required to compare two off-the-shelf FLIRs to be used for surveillance. The program manager decided to fly the first generation systems in an airplane and determine the range performance for a variety of unique targets: humans, horses, canoes, trucks, etc. The imagery was analog and collected on hi-8 mm tape. In this case the experimenters decided to use the analog imagery recorded on a TEAC hi-8mm tape recorder and play the video on a good analog monitor. The observers indicated when they could detect the targets by stopping the tape and observing the range information which was recorded by means of a radio frequency ranger on one of the audio channels.

NVESD participated in conducting a perception experiment using the imagery collected during the fly-by field collection. The laboratory results for human target detection were compared with the results from the field tests. The comparison showed an identical cycle criterion for the human that was found in the field test described in Section 5.3, [19] providing more evidence that field tests and perception experiments with field imagery yield comparable results.

Table 3: Pros and cons of laboratory perception experiments using imagery collected in the field.

Advantages	Disadvantages
Ability to run more subjects or different subjects at a later time.	Subjects do not have direct control over the sensor.
Ability to test various hypotheses.	Validation of imagery may be an issue.
Considerably less expensive than field tests. Initial outlay for equipment is compensated by repeated use.	No acceptable method for capturing non-digital FLIR imagery.
Consistent and known stimuli.	Minor differences in stimuli from exactly what is seen in the field.
Virtually total control over the conditions of the experiment.	Lack of face validity since the subject is not in the field in front of the device.

6.3. Advantages and Disadvantages of Perception Experiments using Field Imagery

In general, perception experiments using field imagery are convenient and more easily managed than the same test conducted in the field, as shown in Table 3. More observers are available, and the imagery is constant. The disadvantages generally have to do with the fact that the observers are not directly operating the sensor, and therefore there is not the real-time interaction with the scene that is a part of real field performance. However, this disadvantage did not seem to change the actual results, since there was generally no significant difference between the results when the experiment was performed in the laboratory vs. in the field. The advantages in control and number of subjects may outweigh the cost of bringing the soldiers to the field. However, the necessity for field data collection is not obviated. The imagery to be used must nevertheless be obtained. Field data needs would include calibrated and tactical sensor imagery and well-documented ground truth.

7. Perception Experiments with "Hybrid" Imagery

Often we wish to evaluate the effects of certain features of a sensor which is under development to perform sensitivity analysis or to validate the model for new types of sensor features. When the task of interest does not require a realistic background, the simulation can be performed with vehicles segmented from the backgrounds to remove background cues which could be useful for identification of the targets when a target is shown repeatedly in a particular place in the background. To perform simulations, imagery greatly exceeding the sampling rate and detector size is required. Therefore, we frequently use thermoscope imagery which was taken with the target very close up, allowing the simulation to be performed on the most pristine image possible. By degrading the thermoscope imagery with the NVESD sensor, atmosphere, and range simulation,[1] observers can be presented with the target in any atmospheric environment seen through any sensor at any range. In this way the stimulus is controlled and manipulated to meet the needs of the experiments.

Experiments using manipulated imagery are very useful for modeling purposes. The experiment is not at the whim of any environment, system breakdown, or range restriction. Specific target, aspect, atmospheric, sensor and range requirement issues can be directly addressed. The subjects can be trained at their own pace. If it is determined that more observations are required, more observers can be run or more trials added to the experimental design and a follow-up experiment conducted.

7.1. Effects of Sampling on FLIR Performance

With the advances in technology culminating in 2nd generation FLIR concepts, modeling questions arose as to the quantitative and qualitative effects of certain detector parameters on recognition and identification range performance. For example, the advanced sensors can sample at various rates relative to the detector size, whereas first generation thermal sensors were not sampled in the horizontal direction and vertical sampling was standardized in the model. Issues that arose included whether or not the model adequately accounted for increases in image quality due to sampling at greater than one sample per detector dimension.

In order to evaluate the effects of sampling on performance it was essential to be able to simulate a variety of potential sensor parameters, including varying the sampling rate of the system and the detector size independently. Of course, the cost which would be incurred in acquiring sensors for an experiment which vary in their sampling rates and detector sizes is prohibitive. However, simulation can provide imagery similar to what would be cseen through the sensors.

A series of experiments on sampling[22] and resolution[23] conducted at NVESD was able to provide valuable information on the relative effect of various sensor parameters in range performance. It was verified, for example, that with high contrast targets and a system with a realistic detector size, sample spacing is the most important factor in performance, and that reducing the sampling rate below one sample per detector dimension results in severely degraded performance due primarily to the aliased information in the image.[22] Also confirmed was that within realistic engineering limits, vertical and horizontal resolution are of equal importance for the tasks of interest but that departures from this equality do not appreciably affect performance as long as the 2-dimensional sampling density is held constant.[23] When one has established a groundwork for the modeling and performed enough of the designed experiments with simulations to understand the processes to be modeled, then one can build a definitive model, testing again with other methodologies to verify the robustness of the modeling approach and any empirical constants.

7.2. Validating Projected Area as Characteristic Dimension for Modeling

The original Static Performance Model[4] used the minimum dimension, normally the height, as the critical dimension against which the horizontal MRTD was the measured system function for calculation of "cycles on target." When ACQUIRE was enhanced to include the 2-dimensional MRTD, taking into consideration both horizontal and vertical resolution, a decision was made to use the square root of the target projected area as the dimensional input to the model. The need to validate this formulation for the characteristic dimension arose in time and a focused experiment was performed to do so for the tasks of target recognition and identification.

The methodology chosen was to use imagery captured with a thermoscope, which has the qualities of being oversampled, virtually noiseless due to frame averaging, and available for many vehicles and orientations. Upon this imagery, sensor effects corresponding to an idealized second generation FLIR were added using standard downsampling and digital convolution techniques[1,24] and noise frames. In addition, the target signature histogram was modified to produce defined signatures with means and standard deviations that spanned the MRTD at three specific points. In order to obtain full probability curves at each of these points on the MRTD curve, ranges were introduced which were predicted to produce on average 25%, 50% and 80% performance for each of the points on the MRTD curve reflected in the target ΔTs. Thus there were nine cells resulting from three ranges for each of three ΔTs.

Observers were trained using the standard perception lab training package, which is self-paced and self-scored[18,24] and were required to reach 100% criterion performance on the training imagery prior to participating in the experiment.

The results from the test for each target were compared to the predictions using three and six cycles on target for recognition and identification, respectively. What was learned from this experiment for model validation is that the square root of the target projected area is an improvement over the vertical dimension for the side aspects of targets, but that some significant residual error remains which cannot be accounted for by the number of pixels on target. This result has led to a new direction in modeling thermal vehicle identification to include feature structure and spatial relations among hot spots. At present other concepts are being evaluated, such as the Recognition-by-Components theory of Biederman[25] which postulates orientation invariant geometric primitives (for example, spheres, cones, bricks, etc.) as the basis of object recognition. Therefore, whereas the validation was considered to be successful in that it demonstrated over the ensemble of vehicles the average error to be less than 10%, the study led to the evaluation of new directions for the model, to include more specific target configuration effects.[26]

7.3. Finding Targets in Clutter

NVESD's physical terrain board provides another form of controlled imagery. The terrain board is a scale background model that resembles all major landscape types, mountains, forest, high and low desert. It contains man-made features such as airports and towns. Miniature vehicle models (1/285 scale) are meticulously painted with pigment of known reflectivity to represent thermal signatures when the captured digitized video imagery is reversed in polarity. This technique produces a likeness of thermal imagery and allows an economical and feasible way to include a variety of backgrounds and target signatures in the stimulus set for experimentation with human observers.[27]

A series of experiments was performed to evaluate modeling metrics to describe the target signature. Terrain board imagery of targets in various background clutter levels was used as the stimuli following the process shown in Figure 5. The video imagery was digitized and five frames were averaged to yield a frame of imagery without visible noise. An atmospheric simulation was added based upon 90% transmission for the first kilometer and a pixel-by-pixel apparent range map of the terrain board. Then sensor simulations of one first generation and two second generation sensors were added to the frames. Nineteen noise frames were created for each sensor simulation and added to the scenes to yield an apparent real-time noise stimulus when played in a loop at frame rates of approximately 30Hz.

While being timed, observers searched through the scenes and indicated areas in the scene where a target might potentially be present. After indicating all regions in a particular scene which would require a further look, the observers then went on to interrogate each of the "found" areas and chose a level of discriminability from a menu for each area of interest. The choices included "area of interest only", "probably a target," "definitely a target," the various names of the targets (i.e., T62, BMP, etc.), "probably not a target," and "definitely not a target." The results from the observers included: time to find the targets, the (x, y) location where targets were found, and the menu choice. The menu choices produced a measure of the degree of confidence that the observer had in whether a target was actually present.

Finally, these results (search time, hits, and confidence) were evaluated against a thorough image analysis. Each target was segmented from the background and the histogram of the pixel values was statistically analyzed for a variety of first and second order statistics, edge strength measures, and many other contrast and resolution metrics. The background was analyzed by a variety of global and local background clutter metrics. The

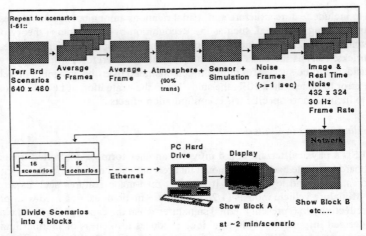

Figure 5. Method of generating imagery typical of thermal scenes from digitized video imagery of a physical terrain board with painted target miniatures.[2]

results from the observers for each target and scene were then analyzed with respect to the image analysis of the scenes. All of the results are stored in a database that can be shared with other model developers and validators.

This study has provided an enormous wealth of modeling resources for a variety of organizations studying aspects of target acquisition. One of the reasons is because the imagery, observer results, ground truth, and 50 statistical metrics on the scenes and targets are stored in a usable database that can be queried to provide tables for any number of analysis issues. The confidence level of the observer, measured in the menu choice, provides a path for studying false alarms as well as target findings, detections and identifications.

7.4. Advantages and Disadvantages of Using "Hybrid" Imagery

Performing experiments with imagery that has been manipulated to simulate a variety of sensors, atmospheres, and ranges is an efficient technique, as shown in Table 4. It avoids the difficulty encountered with field tests and field imagery in that to some extent one is confined to the available targets, atmospheres, range restrictions, and sensors that already exist. It is impossible to investigate the effects of small changes in the sampling rate, resolution, or noise of the sensor in a field imagery collection. The freedom to explore designed experiments with simulations has begun to burgeon. The development of computer-generated imagery, as stated in the introduction, is sure to allow even greater latitude with experimental design since it will be possible to manipulate and control backgrounds as well as targets. Also, the collection of high resolution, low noise imagery with calibrated sensors having uniform detectors will enable the performance of informative and controlled experiments and should be possible within the next few years.

Table 4: Pros and cons of laboratory perception experiments using manipulated or simulated imagery.

Advantages	Disadvantages
Ability to run many subjects or different subjects at a later time.	-
Stimuli are consistent and known.	Stimuli may not be exactly the same as what is actually seen in the field.
Ability to specifically test various hypotheses.	No acceptable method for simulating non-digital FLIR imagery.
Nearly total control over the conditions of the experiment.	Validation of simulation may be an issue.
Stimuli can be generated to directly manipulate the parameters of interest.	Methodology for inserting targets in backgrounds is not yet perfected.

8. Criteria for Accepting a Model

Establishing criteria for whether a model is accurate enough is a much overlooked task. Typically, there is a desire for an improved model, but the degree of improvement desired or possible is not specified. The error in the prediction is certainly going to be related by mathematical necessity to the region of the performance prediction curve, since it will necessarily be smaller as one approaches 0 and 100% and largest at 50%.

Historically, the Static Performance Model[4] gave a range performance error associated with the model of +/- 20%. This error is assumed to be unsystematic and not related to any presently modeled factors. NVESD has found approximately this amount of error in performance due to the motivation, background or training of observer groups.[22]

Before pursuing a validation effort it would be wise to determine what the exit criteria will be for the model at different parts of the performance prediction curve. A possible method is to use a root mean square error calculation in various probability bins. Due to the statistical nature of the error on different regions of a cumulative binomial distribution, the error in the tails will be smaller than the error in the middle part of the curve. For example, a 0.10 RMS error or less may be acceptable for the 0.4-0.6 probability region, and 0.05 or less elsewhere. Since no model involving human performance will ever be without variance, some approach to deciding when a model has achieved an adequate level of accuracy is clearly necessitated.

A method brought to our attention by Jim Silk[28] for assessing the goodness of fit of a predictive model is the log likelihood ratio (LLR) described in Hosmer and Lemeshow.[29] This method is used for dichotomous data. Since detection, recognition, and identification data are generally dichotomous with respect to an observer on a particular trial, the log-likelihood ratio is computed by the following formula where the sum is over all targets i in the test:

$$LLR = N \cdot \sum_i P_i \log \Pi_i + \left(1 - P_i\right) \log\left(\left(1 - \Pi_i\right)\right) \qquad (9)$$

and P=probability obtained in the experiment and Π=probability predicted by the model.

If Π is replaced by P, the resulting log-likelihood ratio represents the best a model can do, known as the "saturated model." The deviance, D, is defined as twice the difference between the LLR of the fitted model and that of the saturated model. The distribution of D is assumed to be chi-squared, with degrees of freedom equal to the number of data entries minus the number of free parameters of the model. The significance level for the hypothesis test is related to the distance between the LLR for the saturated vs. the predicted model in number of σ from the chi-squared distribution.

Similarly, one computes the "minimal" model analogous to the saturated model by assuming a single constant probability. Comparison of the resulting distribution of the G statistic, defined as the deviance D above but using the single probability LLR, shows the improvement resulting from the model.

Dr. Silk used this method to evaluate modeling formulations to predict the results of the experiment described in Section 7.2 for finding targets in a scene. The LLR of the saturated model was -4200 and of the minimal model -7400. The analysis showed that whereas the results were significantly different from the saturated model, they were nevertheless a great and significant improvement over the minimal model. This analysis was very helpful in evaluating modeling progress. The model cannot do better than -4200 and no model would be -7400. Thus, this type of analysis gives a feeling for how much closer to an accurate model the improvements have brought one. A modeling user's committee can define a criterion level for the model to be considered useful by the community.

9. Recommendations for Designing Experiments in Support of Model Improvement and Validation

The various methodologies for supporting model development and validation each play important but different roles. Careful analysis of these methodologies enable an assignment of purpose to each type of experiment. Figure 6 shows the various methods and the reasonable expectations for their results.

A modeling and simulation experiment can be used to test concrete hypotheses about the effects of certain parameters (e.g., sampling, resolution, atmospheric conditions, target signature) on observer performance. Once these results are assimilated into the model, a perception experiment using field imagery will generally provide data which can indicate how well the model works for realistic imagery in real backgrounds. There will be sources of error introduced which were not a concern in the pure simulation. Examples of such error are the wider variation in the target signature and the background, adding a degree of clutter to the scene. Finally, a full-blown field test may be desired to ensure that the model provides reasonable agreement with a field experience. However, a field test

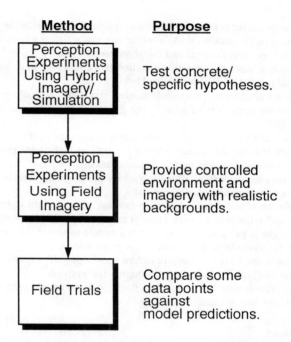

Figure 6. The methods of experimentation discussed in this chapter are each valuable for supporting model development and validation. Expectations for the methods should be in accordance with what is achievable given the limitations and possibilities of each.

should not be expected to validate an entire model, but rather points on the curve.

To summarize, below is a list of ten lessons learned regarding the design and conducting of field trials and laboratory perception experiments.

1. Explicitly define the question to be answered as a basis for designing the experiment. Simplify the question to the most basic hypothesis, thereby becoming attuned to the significant factors to include in the test structure.

2. Based upon the hypothesis developed, ensure that the target characteristics and range(s) of interest are explicitly in the experimental design. If possible, bracket these specific target characteristics and ranges to obtain a sensitivity measure from the results. If the need is to validate a whole curve, try to ensure that the ranges in the design extend to where virtually no observers will perform and as close as possible to the range at which nearly 100% of observers will perform. Ensure that some data points are obtained where the curve is steep. Spanning the whole psychometric curve in this way will prove to be a very useful design for validating models.

3. If the experiment is to be performed in the field, familiarize the observers with the operation of the sensor(s). As a minimum, this training would include focus, gain and level, polarity reversal and threshold techniques.
4. Be sure that there is some way to calibrate the imagery to determine the temperature and ground truth of targets and backgrounds.
5. Develop a strategy to ensure information about the setup of the systems is known to allow the capability of relating the ground truth to the uncalibrated field imagery.
6. Ensure that there is enough statistical power through number of observers and trials, such that the confidence interval is small enough at the probability of interest to allow adequate precision for decision-making.
7. Train the observers to a criterion level on the target signatures to eliminate a disruptive learning curve during the test.
8. Sample the observer population of interest. If the sight is being developed for pilots and helicopter gunners, attempt to use these military personnel. Conversely, if the sight is to be used in coast guard cutters to search for personnel overboard, select observers from the nearest coast guard station.
9. Develop a database architecture before conducting the experiment and then populate the database carefully and thoroughly for analysis.
10. Define criteria which will enable a decision as to whether the model is achieving desired predictive capability.

10. Conclusions

Validation of models is a complex function and one that can be approached from a variety of angles. It is possible to use field tests, perception experiments with field imagery, and laboratory experiments to obtain converging evidence for model development and validation. Which method is appropriate will be based upon the desired level of control over the experimental variables, the financial cost, the availability of observers and systems, and the power of the method to answer the question at hand.

Acknowledgements

Luanne Obert, John D'Agostino, Dr. Clarence Walters, Marnita Crenshaw and Kathy Ayscue offered many helpful comments upon reviewing the first draft of this chapter. Luke Scott, the designer and maintainer of FLIR92 and ACQUIRE, was always gracious with his time and effort in technical discussions and documentation. Sherry Harding was invaluable during the preparation of the manuscript for publication. Beth Nystrom has consistently provided competent and responsive support in the daily operations of the perception laboratory. The author would be sorely amiss not to acknowledge with gratitude all of the observers whose hard work supplied the data for the field and laboratory tests.

References

1. J. D. Horger, "Image generation for perception testing using computer FLIR simulation", in *Proceedings of SPIE International Symposium on Optical Engineering and Photonics in Aerospace Engineering* (1990).

2. C. Walters, "Removing the automatic target recognition performance evaluation bottleneck: The C2NVEO AUTOSPEC Facility", *Optical Engineering* 30 (1991).

3. J. Johnson, "Analysis of image-forming systems", in *Proceedings of the Image Intensifier Symposium* (1958), p. 249.

4. J. A. Ratches, "Static performance modeling for thermal imaging systems", *Optical Engineering* 15 (1976) 525.

5. G. Waldman & J. Wootton, *Electro-Optical Systems Performance Modeling* (Artech House, Boston, 1993).

6. M. Lloyd, *Thermal Imaging Systems* (Plenum, New York, 1975).

7. R. D. Hudson, *Infrared System Engineering* (John Wiley, New York, 1969).

8. J.D. Howe, "Electro-optical imaging system performance prediction", in *The Infrared & Electro-Optical Systems Handbook: Vol. 4, Electro-Optical Systems Design, Analysis, and Testing*, ed. M.C. Dudzik (Infrared Information Analysis Center, Ann Arbor, 1993).

9. C. W. Hoover and C. M. Webb, "What is an MRTD and How do I get one?" in *Proceedings of SPIE* 1488 (1991), p. 280.

10. L. Scott & J. D'Agostino, *FLIR92 Thermal Imaging Systems Performance Model* (NVESD, Ft. Belvoir, VA, 1992).

11. J. D'Agostino, "The modeling of spatial and directional noise in FLIR90. Part I: 3-D noise analysis methodology", in *Proceedings of the IRIS Symposium on Passive Sensors* I (1991), p. 193.

12. C. M. Webb, "The modeling of spatial and directional noise in FLIR90. Part II. Methodology", in *Proceedings of the IRIS Symposium on Passive Sensors* I (1991), p. 347.

13. D. Tomkinson, *ACQUIRE* (NVESD, Ft. Belvoir, VA, 1990).

14. B. O'Kane, C. Walters, J. D'Agostino, and M. Friedman, "Target signature metrics analysis for performance modeling", in *Proceedings of the IRIS Symposium on Passive Sensors* II (1993), p. 161.

15. M. Friedman, D. Tomkinson, L. Scott, B. O'Kane, and J. D'Agostino, "Standard Night Vision thermal modeling parameters", in *Proceedings of SPIE* 1689 (1992), p. 204.

16. W. R. Lawson, T. W. Cassidy, and J. A. Ratches, "A search model", in *Proceedings of the IRIS Specialty Group on Imaging* (1978).

17. J. Palmer, J. D'Agostino, and T. J. Lillie, *Infrared Recognition and Target Handbook* (NVESD, Ft. Belvoir, VA, 1982).

18. R. LaFollete, J. Horger, and B. O'Kane, "PC-based system for thermal identification training", in *Proceedings of the Human Factors Soc.* 2 (1991), p. 1512.

19. B. O'Kane, M.Crenshaw, J. D'Agostino, and D. Tomkinson, "Human target detection using thermal devices", in *Proceedings of the IRIS Symposium on Passive Sensors* (1992).

20. J. Silverman and V. E. Vickers, "Display and enhancement of infrared images", in *Electro-Optical Displays*, ed. M.A. Karim (Marcel Dekker, New York, 1992).

21. B. O'Kane, "Vision I perception experiment", *Proceedings of the IRIS Symposium on Passive Sensors*, (1990).

22. J. D'Agostino, M. Friedman, R. LaFollette, and M. Crenshaw, "An experimental study of the effects of sampling on FLIR performance", in *Proceedings of the IRIS Symposium on Passive Sensors* I (1990), p. 193.

23. L. Obert, J. D'Agostino, B. O'Kane, and C. T. Nguyen, "An experimental study of the effects of vertical resolution on FLIR performance", in *Proceedings of the IRIS Symposium on Passive Sensors* I (1990, p.) 235.

24. J. D. Howe, "Thermal model improvement through perception testing", *Proceedings of the IRIS Symposium on Passive Sensors* II (1989), p. 11.

25. I. Biederman, "Recognition-by-Components: A theory of image understanding", *Psych. Rev.* **94** (1987) 115.

26. B. O'Kane, I. Biederman and E. Cooper, "Modeling thermal target vehicle identification: Beyond resolution and noise", in *Proceedings of the IRIS Symposium on Passive Sensors* II (1994) , p. 225

27. B. Blecha, H. Do-Duc, M. Crenshaw, and B. O'Kane, "A search experiment to increase our understanding", in *Proceedings of the IRIS Symposium on Passive Sensors* I (1991) p. 207.

28. J. Silk, unpublished manuscript (Institute for Defense Analysis, Alexandria, VA, 1993).

29. D. W. Hosmer and S. Lemeshow, *Applied Logistic Regression* (John Wiley, New York, 1989).

APPLYING HUMAN SPATIAL VISION MODELS TO REAL-WORLD TARGET DETECTION AND IDENTIFICATION: A TEST OF THE WILSON MODEL

SHARI R. THOMAS

Optical Radiation Division, Occupational and Environmental Health Directorate,
Armstrong Laboratory, 8111 18th Street
Brooks Air Force Base, TX 78235-5215, U. S. A.

and

NORMAN BARSALOU

The Analytic Sciences Corporation, 750 E. Mulberry Street, Suite 302,
San Antonio, TX 78212, U. S. A.

Human detection and identification thresholds were measured using real-world targets to test Wilson's[1] spatial vision model. The Wilson[1] model was installed on an image-processing system along with a digitized image of a B-1B aircraft target (i.e., airplane image target (AIT)). The computerized version of the Wilson[1] model was used to filter the AIT and determine the magnitudes of the responses of the individual basis filters within the model to the AIT. Two targets were generated by combining the response outputs from three basis filters contained within the computer-implemented Wilson[1] model. The first filter target (FT1) was generated from the combined outputs of the three basis filters that had highest response magnitudes to the AIT. The second filter target (FT2) was created from the response outputs of three basis filters whose response magnitudes to AIT were at one-half of the overall maximum level of all of the filters contained within the computer-implemented Wilson[1] model. To obtain detection and identification thresholds for three subjects, AIT and FT1 were presented on a homogeneous photopic background and photopic backgrounds containing either static or dynamic Gaussian "white" noise. Detection and identification thresholds measured for AIT and FT2 only used the homogeneous background. The mean detection and identification thresholds for AIT and the two filter-generated targets were compared to determine if the information contained within the filters' outputs is that which is required for detection and identification of the AIT. Mean AIT and FT1 detection and identification thresholds were only statistically significantly different when measured using dynamic Gaussian noise backgrounds. Mean AIT detection and identification thresholds were statistically significantly different from mean FT2 thresholds. The results indicate that applications of Wilson's[1] model can be used to predict the spatial information contain within real-world static targets that is required for detection and identification. Dynamic noise results provided information about the temporal sampling rate of the human visual system.0

1. Introduction

Psychophysical and neurophysiological data collected on humans and higher primates over the last two decades have indicated that spatial information (i.e., orientation, location, spatial frequency) within a scene is processed by the visual system in discrete neurophysiological channels.[2] These channels can be grouped into psychophysically defined mechanisms (pathways) depending on their spatial frequency tuning characteristics. Only a limited number of mechanisms (e.g., 6 - 8) are believed to encode the entire range of spatial frequencies that can be resolved by the human eye.[1-2] The tuning bandwidths of these mechanisms have been reported to be approximately 1-2 octaves.[1-5] The orientation tuning of the mechanisms is dependent on their spatial frequency tuning. Mechanisms tuned to higher spatial frequencies have smaller orientation tuning bandwidths associated with them[6-7] and, therefore, are tuned to a larger number of orientations.[1] Sampling at the Nyquist frequency and adherence to nearest neighbor response pooling are proposed to be the mechanisms by which high spatial frequencies (e.g., 30 cycles per degree (cpd)) can be encoded in the visual system using channels tuned to only low and medium spatial frequencies (e.g., 0.5 - 16 cpd).[1] Temporal parameters of the stimulus are processed through a different set of channels that interact and influence the sensitivities of the spatial vision mechanisms.[1-2] Although there is some debate over the number of temporal frequency-tuned mechanisms that process information, there is evidence that indicates that there may be as few as two or three of these different channels.[2-8] Because the spatial and temporal stimulus properties are very infrequently covaried within the same experiment, the interactions between the spatially and temporally tuned mechanisms is not thoroughly understood.

Campbell and Robson[9] were the first to demonstrate that information from only the channel most sensitive to the target (i.e., fundamental component) is required to signal threshold detection of simple grating targets. If any of the channels responsible for encoding the spatial information of a compound grating target are at threshold, the grating can be detected, regardless of whether the other channels are below threshold.[4] Furthermore, if the frequency components of the compound grating differ by at least a factor of two, psychophysical performance can be described by assuming independence between the detection mechanisms.[10] Because detection by the mechanisms is independent, the phase relationship between them does not influence the results.[4] However, more recent studies report interactions between mechanisms that are tuned to widely separated spatial frequencies.[11-12] For example, inhibitory interactions may exist between pathways that respond to spatial frequencies that are separated by a factor of three or more.[2] Campbell and Robson's[9] results have been replicated by many investigators using a variety of experimental paradigms[1-2] and using simple and compound gratings and other relatively simple[a] targets (e.g., chevrons and other targets common to vernier acuity studies).[1] However, empirical evidence that supports these results for the detection or identification of real-world targets (e.g., airplanes) that contain many different spatial frequencies and orientations is not available.

Several models have emerged over the past decade to explain how the human visual system processes information about spatial structure and detail.[1-2,13] Many of these models have common features. Most models consist of a set of mathematical filters (e.g., difference of Gaussian (DOG) or Gabor) selectively tuned to several different spatial frequencies, orientations, and spatial locations. Other properties, including sampling densities, response pooling, and filter sensitivity weightings, are also contained in the models. Unlike many models, which compare and contrast the human observer to an ideal detector, the model proposed by Wilson[1] was developed to explain and predict results

---

[a] The term "simple" here is used in relation to real-world targets and real-world scenes, where the visual information contained within an object may have a multitude of spatial frequencies and orientations.

obtained from psychophysical and physiological experiments performed on human and non-human primates. Wilson's model has been successfully demonstrated to make these predictions.[1]

The spatial tuning of the six mechanisms within the Wilson[1] model is produced by combining either two or three (for low spatial frequency tuned mechanisms) DOG filters.[b] The DOG filters of the Wilson[1] model have similar response properties as classically defined for neurons in the primate retino-geniculo-cortical pathway[14-17] and their sensitivities are weighted in accordance with the human spatial contrast sensitivity function. The spatial frequency and orientation tuning of the Wilson[1] model filters have been shown to correspond to that of neurons recorded in area 18 of the primate visual cortex.[1,6] A basic underlying assumption of the Wilson[1] model and other detection models of spatial vision is that at detection and identification threshold, information from only a small number of the spatial channels, which are most sensitive to the target, is required for processing. This basic underlying assumption of the Wilson[1] model has never been directly tested using complex, real-world targets.

This report describes the results from a set of experiments designed to directly test whether this underlying assumption of the Wilson[1] model holds for real-world target detection and identification. Our basic goal was to determine whether a human spatial vision model, such as Wilson's[1] could be used to successfully predict detection and identification contrast thresholds for real-world targets that have military operational relevance. The results from these experiments provide some preliminary information on how few spatial channels are required for threshold detection of a real-world military airplane target. The results also provide some preliminary information on how temporal information processing within the human visual system compares to that predicted by the ideal signal detector theory.

2. Methods

2.1. Experimental Rational

A general hypothesis of the Wilson[1] model and other models based on linear analysis[c] is that a target will be detected by the visual system if the responses from a small number of spatially tuned mechanisms[d] to which the visual system is most sensitive is above threshold. If this general hypothesis is correct, then it follows its rationale that the visibility of a target at threshold may be predicted from the visibility of a second target, which is a linear combination of a small subset of the individual components within the original target's elementary basis function to which the visual system is most sensitive.

---

[b] See Wilson (1991) for a more complete description of the model, the rationale and data upon which it is based, and its predictive capability.

[c] Spatial vision models based on linear analysis characterize the output of a filter by the convolution of the luminance distribution of the stimulus with the sensitivity of the filter's channel to the stimulus as a function of its spatial or temporal processing. The luminance distribution of the stimulus and the sensitivity of the filter's channel can be specified in terms of spatial and temporal frequency by performing a Fourier transform of the luminance and sensitivity functions. This process produces filter spatial frequency and orientation selectivity.

[d] The population of spatially tuned mechanisms form the elementary basis function of the system.

These components essentially correspond to the neurophysiological responses of spatially tuned mechanisms within the visual system. Furthermore, if a small number of neurophysiological mechanisms are signaling when a low-contrast target of arbitrary complexity is at threshold, that target will be indistinguishable from another, simpler target (composed of fewer frequencies and orientations) provided that it produces the same response from the neurophysiological mechanisms at threshold. If the filters within the Wilson[1] model are comparable to the neurophysiological spatially tuned mechanisms within the visual system, then these two targets will be indistinguishable if they produce the same response from the Wilson[1] model filters when they are at threshold.

If the hypotheses given above are indeed correct, and the general underlying assumption of the Wilson[1] model is true, we predict that detection and identification thresholds measured for a complex, real-world target will be equivalent to those measured for a second target that is generated from the combined visual outputs of a small number of the implemented Wilson model basis filters, provided that only the basis filters having the highest responses to the real-world target are used to generate the second target. To test this prediction, a digitized computer image of a B-1B aircraft, which we called the aircraft image target (AIT), was selected to represent a real-world target. The AIT was filtered using our computer implementation of the Wilson[1] model, and two filter targets were created from the linear combination of the basis filters' responses to the AIT. The first filter-output target (FT1) was created by using the combined outputs of the three Wilson[1] model basis filters that had the highest response magnitudes to the AIT after filtering it (i.e., filters #1 - #3). The second filter target (FT2) was created from the visual output of three Wilson[1] model basis filters whose response magnitudes to AIT fell within the middle region of those calculated for all of the basis filters contained within the implemented model. Given our prediction that detection and identification thresholds measured for FT1 should be statistically equivalent to those measured for AIT because FT1 contains the spatial information within AIT to which the visual system is most sensitive, then it follows the same logic that detection and identification thresholds measured for FT2 should be statistically different from those measured for AIT. Although FT2 contains a subset of the spatial information that is within AIT, it is not the spatial information to which the visual system is most sensitive. Therefore, additional contrast will be required to detect FT2 than is required to detect either AIT or FT1.

We designed a series of six experiments on real-world, complex target detection and identification to test these predictions that were derived from the underlying assumption of the Wilson model. This assumption, that only the information from a few neurophysiological channels which carry spatial information within a complex target to which the visual system is most sensitive is required for detection and identification, is based on the original findings of Campbell and Robson.[9] Military operations require the detection and identification of complex targets in visually rich (i.e., highly structured), low-contrast, or camouflaged environments. An application of an established model of human spatial vision, as describe above, to determine the information within a real-world target that is required for visual detection and identification, and then subsequently predict their contrast thresholds, could potentially be used to improve military operational capability. However, verification of the basic assumptions of these types of models must be confirmed using real-world targets of military significance.

2.2. Experimental Design

In Experiments 1 and 2, the contrast of AIT and FT1, or FT2, respectively, was systematically lowered until detection thresholds were obtained. Theoretically, as contrast is reduced to detection threshold, the number of activated neurophysiological channels should be minimized so that only those channels most sensitive to the target will be signaling at a level which is above threshold. Likewise, as contrast is lowered to detection threshold, only those Wilson[1] model filters having the highest response magnitudes to the AIT will be signaling. If the model's underlying assumption and our predictions are correct, we would not expect FT1's thresholds to differ significantly from those measured for AIT. Thresholds measured for FT2 would be expected to be significantly different from those measured for AIT.

In Experiments 3 and 4, a Gaussian "white" noise inset was superimposed onto the image to degrade visibility, and target contrast within the noise inset was systematically reduced to obtain detection threshold measurements. By definition, "white" noise, which has no structural correlation between each pixel, should activate all of the spatial frequency-tuned neurophysiological channels equally. As target contrast is reduced to detection threshold, only the channels with the highest sensitivity to the target should respond with enough strength to produce a signal-to-noise ratio (SNR) that is above threshold. Likewise, under the Gaussian noise/reduced-contrast conditions, only the Wilson[1] model filters with the strongest response magnitudes to AIT should produce an SNR of sufficient strength to signal threshold.[e] Detection thresholds obtained for FT1 and AIT in these experiments would not be expected to differ significantly. Variations of the root-mean-squared (rms) levels of the noise would be expected to only change the relative adaptation of the visual system and not affect which filters (or channels) are signaling at detection threshold. Therefore, we predict that increasing the noise rms level would only result in raising the contrast threshold. If AIT and FT1 thresholds are not found to differ significantly when measured under low rms noise conditions, we would not expect them to differ significantly from each other when measured under a higher noise rms condition.

In Experiment 4, we sought to determine whether adding a temporal component to the Gaussian noise would lower detection thresholds similarly to what would be predicted from the ideal detector theory. The ideal detector theory predicts that dynamic noise thresholds should be lower than their corresponding (i.e., same noise rms level) static noise thresholds by the inverse of the square-root of the temporal integration frequency of the Gaussian noise if the human visual system is a perfect temporal integrator. We tested how the human visual system compared to an ideal integrator by measuring AIT and FT1 thresholds using the same experimental conditions utilized in Experiment 3 except that a dynamic Gaussian noise inset, instead of static noise inset, was used to degrade target visibility. The rms levels of the dynamic noise used in Experiment 4 were the same as those used for the static noise in Experiment 3. Thresholds obtained from the static and dynamic noise experiments were directly compared.

[e] If the neurophysiological channels of the visual system have constant amplitude and constant bandwidths in octaves, the noise energy in each channel would be expected to increase with spatial frequency. The bandwidths of the Wilson model filters decrease with spatial frequency. However, because the gains of the filters are weighted in accordance with the human contrast sensitivity function, the noise energy in each filter should be relatively constant for Gaussian noise.

Finally, in Experiments 5 and 6, target identification thresholds were obtained for AIT and FT1, and for AIT and FT2, respectively, using a method similar to that used in Experiments 1 and 2. If the model's hypothesis and our assumptions are correct, identification thresholds measured for AIT and FT1 should not differ significantly from each other, but identification thresholds for AIT and FT2 should be significantly different.

2.3. Subjects

Six adult observers between 25-41 years of age served as subjects in these experiments. All subjects had corrected visual acuity of 20/20 or better, and normal stereopsis (line D or greater on the Air Force VTA-ND test) and fundus appearances upon ophthalmological examination. Subject populations differed slightly between the earlier and later experiments performed; therefore, not all of the subjects that participated in the detection experiments using FT1 participated in the detection experiments using FT2. All subjects met the visual criteria for a Flying Class II physical examination.[1] In all experiments, one-third of the subjects were female. All subjects gave signed, informed voluntary consent prior to experimentation, which met with the approval of the U. S. Air Force Advisory Committee on Human Experimentation per Air Force Regulation 169-3.

2.4. Model Implementation and Noise Generation

The DOG filters of the Wilson model, illustrated in Figure 1, were programmed on an image-processing system consisting of a microVAX computer with a Parallax frame buffer and PV~WAVE image-processing software. The different orientation tunings of the filters, as described by Wilson,[1] were accomplished by rotating each basis filter into the desired orientation, translating the rotated basis filter to the selected location, and performing the fast Fourier transform (FFT) of the rotated and the translated filter. This procedure produced approximately 16,000 filters, as shown in Table 1. The filters were installed in a rectangular sampling grid to represent the central 0.3° x 0.5° of the fovea. The corners of the rectangular grid were tapered in order to allow the circular DOG basis filters to fit within the rectangular sampling grid without overflow. The spatial resolution of the total sampling grid approximated the Nyquist frequency of the human fovea.[18]

A photograph of an B-1 bomber airplane was imaged by an Hamamatsu CCD camera, and subsequently digitized by the image-processing system. The resulting digitized image of the airplane (AIT, see Figure 2) had an angular extent of 0.50° x 1.75° image in azimuth and elevation, respectively, at the 57-in viewing distance.

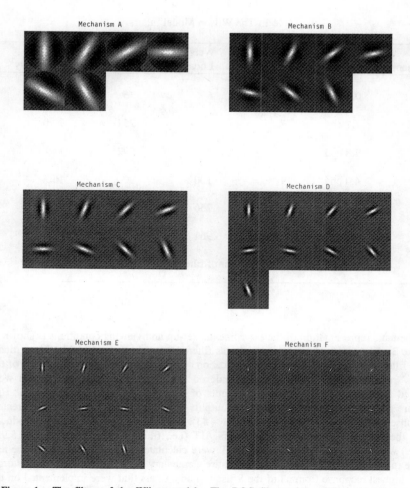

Figure 1. The filters of the Wilson model. The DOG filters of the Wilson model were implemented on an microVAX-based image-processing system using PV~WAVE software. The six mechanisms (A-F) are tuned to different spatial frequencies and orientations. Orientation tuning for the filters was produced by rotating the filters to the desired orientation and taking the FFT of the filter. The number of orientations to which each mechanism was tuned was chosen by dividing 360° by the orientation tuning bandwidth of the mechanism, as determined from Figure 3.5 (p. 67) of Wilson.[1] The filters were evenly spaced within a rectangular sampling grid representing the central 0.3° x 0.5° of the fovea to approximate the Nyquist frequency[18] luminance of 50cd/m². Noise presentation, when used, was always identical to target presentation. The two noise rms levels that were used in Experiment 3 and Experiment 4 represented easy-to-detect (35 rms) and difficult-to-detect (15 rms) conditions. Dynamic noise different from static noise in that the pixel values were varied as a Gaussian function.

Table 1. The Wilson Model Filters.

Peak Mechanism	Basis Frequency	Number of Orientations	Weighted Locations	Number of Filters	Filter Sensitivity[f]
A	0.8 cpd	6	6	36	30.0
B	1.7 cpd	7	36	252	70.0
C	2.8 cpd	8	49	392	140
D	4.0 cpd	9	100	900	150
E	8.0 cpd	11	256	2816	76.7
F	16 cpd	12	961	10,532	18.4
			Total number of filters	15,928	

A schematic representation of the experimental set-up and viewing conditions is shown in Figure 3. The digitized airplane image was filtered by each of the 15,928 Wilson model basis filters via frequency domain multiplication. The absolute magnitudes of each of the filters' responses were determined and indexed for later use. Two filter targets were created from the recombined, stored outputs of select Wilson model basis filters. FT1 (Figure 4, top) was generated using the outputs from the three filters with the greatest response magnitudes to the AIT (filters #1 - #3). FT2 (Figure 4, bottom) was produced from the combined outputs of three filters AIT (i.e., filters #300 - #302 of the 15,928 filters) whose response magnitudes to AIT were calculated to be approximately one-half of the maximum level calculated for the entire elementary basis function. In other words, if the highest response from all of the Wilson[1] model filters that were implemented on the image processing system after filtering the AIT was normalized to 1.0, the response magnitudes of the three basis filters that were used to generate the FT2 were approximately 0.5. The shape of the function relating the response magnitude to AIT to the individual basis filters was used to determine the which three basis filters were selected to produce the AIT, FT1, and FT2 images that were stored in the computer for use during the experiments.

[f] The Wilson model filters are weighted in sensitivity in accordance with the spatial contrast sensitivity function. See Wilson (1991) for further explanations.

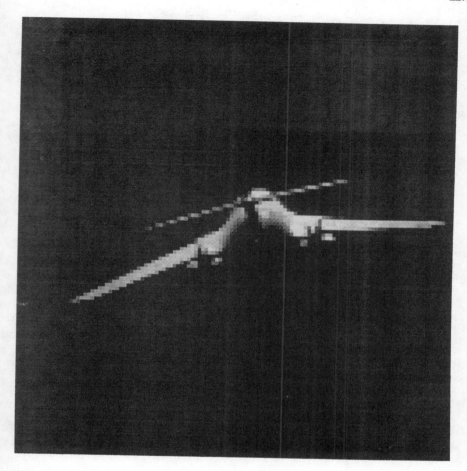

Figure 2. The airplane image target. A picture of the back view of a B-1 bomber aircraft was digitized on the image-processing system and displayed as an image on a CRT. At the experimental testing distance, this target subtended 0.50° x 1.75° of visual angle over subsequent frames as well as across the pixels within the noise inset. The integration frequency of the dynamic noise was 30 Hz. All noise patterns were randomly generated for each subject testing session and, therefore, differed for each experimental run.

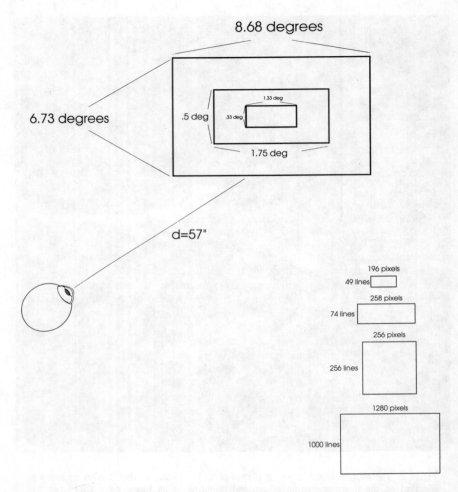

Figure 3. Schematic diagram of the experimental set-up and viewing conditions. The distance between the CRT screen on which the targets were presented and the subjects eyes was 57 inches. The 1280 pixels x 1000 lines CRT screen (see inset) had a photopic (50 cd/m^2) "white" background, which subtended 8.68° x 6.73° on the retina. The targets were always presented in the center for the CRT screen. The size of the AIT was 196 pixels x 49 lines (see inset), which subtended 1.75° x 0.50° on the retina. For experiments using Gaussian "white" noise, the Gaussian noise was presented in a 256 pixels x 256 line inset (see inset), which correspond to a 1.79° x 1.79° retinal image. The Gaussian noise had no spatial structure associated with it, and the AIT and FT1 were superimposed upon it at varying contrasts across trials. The rms of the static and dynamic Gaussian noise was set at either 15 (difficult to see) or 35 (easy to see). The temporal integration frequency of the dynamic Gaussian noise was set at 30 Hz.

During the experiments, AIT was displayed on a color cathode-ray tube (CRT) monitor (1024 x 1280 pixel resolution) as a 0.50° x 1.75° target on a 6.73° x 8.68° white background (see Figure 3 inset). The luminance of the "white" (C.I.E. coordinates x = 0.28, y = 0.32) background was maintained at 50 cd/m^2 throughout the experimental sessions. Gaussian "white" noise was generated using PV~WAVE and displayed as a 1.79° x 1.79° inset (128 x 128 pixel image zoomed by a factor of two) superimposed upon the targets (see Figure 3 inset). Gaussian noise was clipped at plus or minus 2.5 standard deviations and displayed over subsequent frames as well as across pixels within the noise inset. The Gaussian noise which was added to the visual scene had no associated spatial structure (i.e., no correlation from one pixel to another). The integration frequency of the dynamic noise was 30 Hz. All noise patterns were randomly generated for each subject testing session and, therefore, differed for each experimental run.

2.5. Procedure

A two-alternative forced choice procedure was used for the detection experiments. Following an initial 3-min light adaptation period to the 50 cd/m^2 background, a computer signaled the beginning of the trial, paused for 2 s, and then signaled each of the two subtrials within a trial using different audio cues. In one of the two subtrials, either the AIT or one of the filter targets was ramped up in contrast for 0.5 s, held at a fixed contrast for 3 s, and ramped down in contrast for 0.5 s. At the end of the second subtrial, the computer signaled the subject to respond. The subject indicated which subtrial contained a target by pressing the appropriate computer key. Immediately following the subject's response, the computer signaled the next trial. In Experiments 3 and 4, Gaussian noise was ramped up for 0.5 s, held at one of the two rms levels for 3 s, and ramped down for 0.5 s in both of the two subtrials (with or without the target present).

The procedure for the identification experiments varied somewhat from that used in the detection experiments. In each trial, either the AIT or one of the two filter targets was ramped up in contrast for 0.5 s, held at a fixed contrast for 1 s, and ramped down in contrast for 0.5 s. The computer randomly selected which target was presented during each trial using the ML-TEST adaptive staircase procedure.[19] Following each trial, the computer displayed one of two questions, which asked the subject if either the AIT or one of the filter target had been seen (i.e., "Did you see the airplane target?" or "Did you see the filter target?"). The computer randomly selected which of the two questions was displayed after the individual presentation trials so that the coupling between which target and which question were presented for each trial did not follow any specific pattern. The subject responded to the question by pressing the appropriate computer key. Subjects were told to always respond correctly to the question. Therefore, if a target was not seen (i.e., it was below threshold), the subject responded by pressing the "NO" computer key. The subjects were shown the AIT and the filter targets several times prior to beginning the experimental session.

The ML-TEST adaptive staircase procedure[19] was used to control target contrast, as well as which target was presented on each trial. Six staircases (three per target) were randomly intermixed within an experimental session. Therefore, three thresholds were obtained for each target during every experimental session. Subjects completed three

230

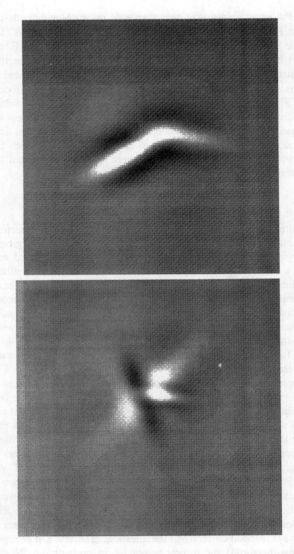

Figure 4. The filter targets. The filter targets were produced by multiplying the FFT of the AIT shown in Figure 2 with the FFTs of the Wilson model filters shown in Figure 1. The absolute response magnitudes of the filters was computed, subscripted, and stored for identification. FT1 (top) was generated from the combined visual outputs of the three filters with the highest response magnitudes. FT2 (bottom) was generated from the combined outputs of three filters with one-half of the maximum response magnitude. Filters 300 - 302 were used to generate FT2.

experimental sessions for a total of nine thresholds per target for each of the six subjects. The ML-TEST software ended the experimental session when a 95% confidence interval had been obtained about each staircase threshold. The confidence interval was set at 0.20 contrast. Because a Weibull function (slope of 3.5) was used to fit the frequency-of-seeing curves, threshold corresponded to 82% correct response.

2.6. Data Analysis

For Experiments 1 and 5, the Weber contrast thresholds obtained for AIT and FT1 were compared using a three-way analysis of variance (ANOVA) statistical test. For Experiments 2 and 6, the three-way ANOVA statistical test was used to compare the Weber contrast thresholds obtained for AIT and FT2. Independent variables of target type (i.e., AIT or FT1, or AIT or FT2), subject, experimental session, and their interactions were analyzed to determine the significance of their effect on the Weber contrast thresholds.

For Experiments 3 and 4, the Weber contrast thresholds calculated from ML-TEST were converted to scaled luminance-based rms values (corresponding to the standard deviation of the space-averaged luminance) using the CRT's gamma correction. This conversion was done to better characterize the target contrasts against the Gaussian noise. The three-way ANOVA test (explained above) was performed to compare the luminance-based rms thresholds obtained in Experiment 3 and in Experiment 4. Thresholds obtained under the 35-rms and 15-rms noise levels were analyzed in separate ANOVA tests.

3. Results

Mean contrast thresholds obtained for AIT and FT1 in Experiment 1 (Figure 5, left panel) are very similar for all subjects except one. Subject BJ's AIT and FT1 thresholds are similar to each other but much higher than those obtained for the other five subjects. ANOVA test results indicated no significant difference between the overall mean FT1 and AIT thresholds (all subjects, all sessions, n = 54). Furthermore, no other significant main effects (i.e., subject or experimental session) were found for the mean data from Experiment 1. When the data were analyzed within subject, a significant effect of experimental session was found for Subject BJ ($p < 0.02$). Post-hoc t-test analysis indicated that this difference was due to Subject BJ's thresholds for one experimental session being much higher than those obtained in the other experimental sessions. However, even for BJ's experimental session with the abnormally high thresholds, the mean AIT threshold was not significantly different from the mean FT1 threshold.

Very little inter-subject variability is found for FT2 and AIT contrast thresholds measured in Experiment 2 (Figure 5, right panel). However, FT2 and AIT thresholds are significantly different from each other ($p < 0.01$). ANOVA test results (all subjects, all sessions, n = 54) did not indicate significant effects of subject, experimental session, or any interactions of the independent variables on the contrast thresholds, even though Subject WR's data appear considerably different from the other five subjects' data.

DETECTION THRESHOLDS

(ALL SUBJECTS, ALL SESSIONS)

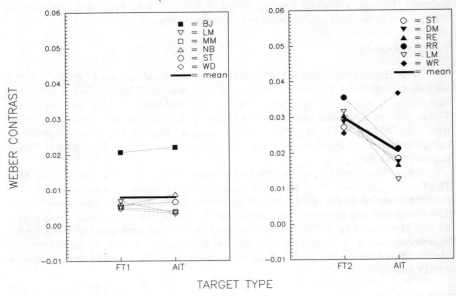

Figure 5. Contrast detection thresholds on a homogeneous background. Mean Weber contrast thresholds for the individual subjects (n = 9 per subject) are represented by different symbols connected by dotted lines. The mean contrast thresholds for all of the subjects are represented by thick solid lines. The lines connecting the filter and airplane thresholds are shown to ease visual comparisons between AIT and filter target thresholds and do not represent any type of curve-fitting to the data. Detection thresholds for AIT and FT1 are shown in the left panel and detection thresholds for AIT and FT2 are shown in the right panel.

Within subject ANOVA testing indicated that although Subject WR's mean FT2 threshold is lower than his mean AIT threshold, they are not significantly different. If the data collected for Subject WR's third experimental session are removed from the analysis, the mean FT2 threshold is not lower than his mean AIT threshold. Because removing Subject WR's data does not change the overall mean data result (i.e., the significant difference between mean FT2 and AIT thresholds), we did not exclude it from the data analysis. Within subject analysis for all other subjects indicated that FT2 thresholds were higher than AIT thresholds. However, the difference in these thresholds was only significant ($p < 0.05$) for Subject RE. Thus, the significant effect of target type found for the overall mean data is only consistent with the individual data obtained from subject RE. This result may be due to the small sample size used in these experiments, and definitely warrants further investigation before firm conclusions can be made from these data.

Mean thresholds obtained for the static noise experiment (Experiment 3) are considerably more variable (Figure 6)˙than those obtained in Experiment 1 (Figure 5). Threshold variability is higher for the 35-rms noise condition (Figure 6, right panel) than for the 15-rms noise condition (Figure 6, left panel), which is not surprising given the increased difficulty of the visual task under the 35-rms static noise condition. As expected, luminance-based rms thresholds obtained under the 35-rms noise condition are generally higher per subject than those obtained under the 15-rms noise condition. However, under both the 15- and 35-rms static noise conditions, the overall mean FT1 threshold is not significantly different than the overall mean AIT threshold. ANOVA results (all subjects, all sessions, n = 54) indicated no significant main effects on mean rms thresholds obtained in the static noise experiment. When the data were analyzed within subject, a significant effect of target was found for Subject BJ under the 15-rms condition. No significant effects of target type were found by within subject analyses of the 35-rms data, even though these differences are implied from the graphical representation of the data (Figure 6, right panel). Significant effects of experimental session ($p < 0.05$) found by the within subject analyses of many of the subjects' 35-rms data may explain why no significant effects of target type were found.

The variability of the thresholds measured under the dynamic noise condition (Experiment 4, Figure 7) is similar to what was found under the static noise condition (Figure 6). Thresholds measured under the dynamic noise condition are approximately one-half of those measured under the same rms level static noise condition (note the difference between the scales on Figure 6 and Figure 7). The dynamic noise thresholds are much higher than what we would expect to obtain if the human visual system was behaving like an ideal integrator. Ideal detector theory predicts that the dynamic noise thresholds should be equal to approximately 18% of luminance-based rms static noise thresholds (i.e., the inverse of the square-root of 30 is 0.183). In addition, the overall mean FT1 threshold (all subjects, all sessions, n = 54) is significantly lower than the overall mean AIT threshold under both the 15-rms (left panel, Figure 7) and the 35-rms (right panel, Figure 7) noise conditions ($p < 0.05$). No other significant main effects were found from the ANOVA for the 15-rms data. A significant main effect of subject ($p < 0.05$) was found for the overall ANOVA of the 35-rms data.

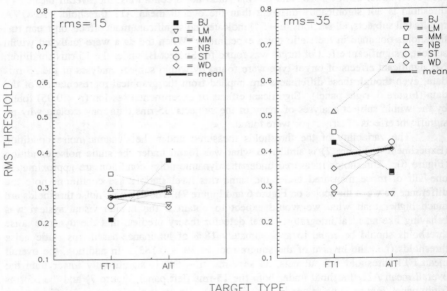

Figure 6. Detection thresholds obtained under static noise conditions. Root-mean-squared (rms) thresholds for AIT and FT1 obtained under the 15-rms (left panel) and 35-rms (right panel) dynamic Gaussian noise conditions are shown. Symbolic representations are the same as described for Figure 5.

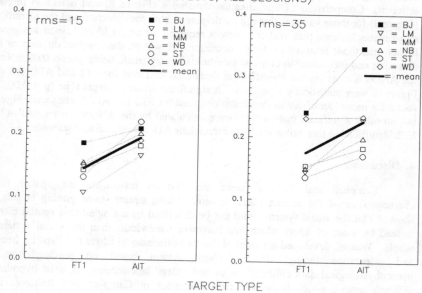

Figure 7. Detection thresholds obtained under dynamic noise conditions. AIT and FT1 rms detection thresholds obtained under the 15-rms (left panel) and 35-rms (right panel) are shown. Symbolic representations are the same as described for Figure 5.

Within subject ANOVA testing of the subjects' data indicated significant main effects and interactions for three of the subjects under the 15-rms condition. Significant main effects of target ($p < 0.05$) and session ($p < 0.05$) were found for Subject ST and Subject LM. Significant effects of the interaction between target and session ($p < 0.05$) were found for Subject LM and Subject WD. No significant main effects or interaction effects were found from within subject ANOVA of the 35-rms data from Experiment 4.

Contrast thresholds obtained in the identification experiments (Experiments 5 and 6) are very similar to those obtained in the detection experiments (Experiments 1 and 2) even though the subject populations for the detection and identification were slightly different. Comparisons of identification thresholds (Figure 8) and detection thresholds (Figure 5) for those subjects that did participate in both the detection and the identification experiments indicate that Weber contrasts required for target identification are generally higher than those required for target detection. However, the absolute differences in the detection and identification contrast thresholds is very small, being within 0.02. None of the ANOVA tests on the identification thresholds obtained for FT1 and AIT (left panel, Figure 8) were statistically significant. A significant effect of target type ($p < 0.002$) was found for mean identification thresholds obtained for FT2 and AIT (right panel, Figure 8), but no other significant main effects were calculated by the ANOVA tests. All subjects' FT2 identification thresholds are higher than their AIT identification thresholds.

4. Discussion

Campbell and Robson[9] were the first to investigate the spatial filtering characteristics of the human visual system. Using square wave grating targets, they showed that the visual system could not be described by a single linear spatial filter, but instead by a set of filters which had narrower bandwidths than the visual system as a whole. Wilson[1] developed a model of the two-dimensional filters (i.e., spatial frequency and orientation tuning) of the visual system based on psychophysical and neurophysiological data collected in his and others' laboratories. A basic hypothesis of Wilson's model, which is derived from the work of Campbell and Robson[9], is that detection and identification thresholds of a complex target (i.e., containing many spatial frequencies and orientations) can be predicted from the responses of the model's filters to the target. Following the logic of this underlying assumption of the Wilson[1] model, if threshold detection is signaled by only those neurophysiological channels having the highest sensitivity to the complex target, then a simpler target, comprised of only the information from those channels, will produce the same thresholds as the original complex target. If the basis filters in the Wilson[1] model are equated with the receptive field properties of the neurons in these neurophysiological channels,[1] thresholds for a complex, real-world target would be expected to be equivalent to those obtained for a second target generated from the combined visual output a small number of basis filters with the highest response to the real-world target. Thresholds obtained for a target composed of the combined visual output of basis filters with significantly lower response magnitudes would be expected to be significantly different from those measured for the real-world target. This result would be expected because more sensitive channels would reach threshold and signal detection of the real-world target prior to the less sensitive channels reaching threshold and signaling detection of the second filter target.

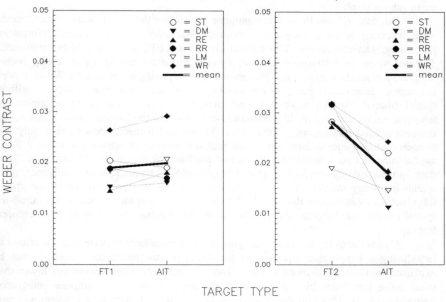

Figure 8. Identification thresholds obtained on homogeneous backgrounds. Threshold contrasts required to identify AIT and FT1 (left panel) and AIT and FT2 (right panel) are shown. Symbolic representations are the same as described for Figure 5.

Our data support this fundamental hypothesis of the Wilson[1] model and Campbell and Robson's theory[9] using real-world targets. We have shown that both mean detection and mean identification thresholds obtained for an airplane target and a target generated by combining the outputs of three Wilson model filters with the highest responses to the airplane target are not significantly different. These results were obtained when target visibility was degraded by reducing contrast alone, thereby minimizing the number of neurophysiological channels signaling detection threshold, and by superimposing static Gaussian noise and reducing target contrast. By superimposing Gaussian white noise, which has no structural correlation between the pixels within the noise, all neurophysiological channels should have been equally stimulated, and only those most sensitive to the target should have produced a high enough SNR to signal detection at threshold. In addition, we demonstrated that overall mean thresholds obtained for a filter target generated from the outputs of three filters with responses that were one-half of the maximum value were significantly different from those obtained for the airplane target. However, within subject analysis indicated that although this latter significant effect was obtained for the overall subject mean thresholds, the effect was only significant for one subject's data. We recommend that this latter experiment be repeated using a larger sample size and superimposing the static and dynamic Gaussian noise to verify the overall mean subject result.

Our data indicate that our assumptions concerning the theory of the Wilson[1] model were incorrect when a temporal component was added to the spatial information processing. Detection thresholds obtained for AIT and FT1 were found to be significantly different when the Gaussian noise was dynamic; in other words, noise having both a temporal and spatial component. This result is not surprising given that the Wilson model[1] is a spatial vision model that does not specify the temporal bandwidths associated with its spatial filters. Further experiments are planned in our laboratory to determine the temporal tuning and bandwidths associated with each of the Wilson model's[1] six spatial frequency-tuned mechanisms. Data from Watson and Robson[8] indicate that only two temporally-tuned mechanisms exist, and that the number of spatially frequency tuned mechanisms that are associated with the two mechanisms is considerably different. Their data[8] indicate that the mechanism tuned to high temporal frequencies only influences three spatial frequency mechanisms, which are the ones that are tuned to the lowest spatial frequencies. Watson and Robson's[8] data also indicate that all of their seven purported spatially-tuned mechanisms are influenced by the mechanism tuned to low temporal frequencies.

Comparisons of the static and dynamic noise thresholds indicate that the effects of introducing a temporal component to the visual processing of the targets cannot be explained by the ideal detector theory. Dynamic noise thresholds were not lower than static noise thresholds by the inverse of the square-root of the temporal integration frequency (i.e., 30 Hz). Instead, the data indicate that the human visual system was only integrating over approximately 2.2-3.4 Hz (respectively for FT1 and AIT) even though 30 Hz information was available.[8] This is approximately the same temporal frequency at which the human spatial contrast sensitivity function has been found to change from bandpass to lowpass.[21] Because the human observer has been previously shown to differ from an ideal detector,[22,23] we were not surprised to find that our dynamic noise thresholds could not be predicted by the ideal detector theory.

In addition, the spatial frequency tuning of the Wilson model basis filters that were used to create FT1 were all tuned to 2.8 c/d (i.e., Mechanism C in Table 1 and Figure 1), and therefore, should have been within the three lowest spatially frequency tuned mechanisms. If Watson and Robson's[8] predictions are correct, these basis filters should have been subserved by the high temporal frequency mechanism, and therefore, should have been capable of being temporally integrated at a higher sampling rate. However, it is possible that the lower frequency-tuned temporal mechanism is more sensitive to 2.8 c/d spatial frequency stimuli and mediated detection under the dynamic noise viewing

---

[8] The 3-4 Hz integration frequency was derived by using the ideal detector theory to determine the temporal integration frequency which corresponded to the difference in threshold contrasts obtained under the static and dynamic noise conditions.

condition. Because the differences in the dynamic and static noise contrast thresholds for detecting of FT1 and AIT were essentially the same under the 15 rms and the 35 rms conditions, we do not believe that the 30 Hz dynamic noise stimulation selectively adapted the high frequency-tuned temporal mechanism, thereby making the low frequency-tuned temporal mechanism more sensitive for mediating detection. If this selective adaptation had occurred, we would expect that the differences in the dynamic and static noise detection thresholds for FT1 would be greater under the 35 rms conditions than under the 15 rms conditions.

Our data indicate that as few as three of the filters with the highest response to the AIT can signal detection and identification at threshold. Again, if the Wilson model filters are equated to the spatial-filtering neurophysiological channels in the visual system,[1] this result indicates that information from as few as three of the neurophysiological channels is required to signal real-world target detection and identification. We chose to use the outputs from three filters to generate our filter targets for the following reason. If the most sensitive filters to a grating target differed only in their spatial location tuning (i.e., had the same spatial frequency and orientation tuning), information from at least three filters would be required for the subject to identify the target as a grating. We did not determine if thresholds for a filter target generated from the most sensitive filter, after convolution with the AIT, were significantly different from those measured for the AIT. We also did not determine thresholds from the visual outputs of each of the filter components within FT1 or FT2 independently. Therefore, our interpretation of the data does not consider the effects of probability summation on the results. However, we believe the effects of probability summation on the results are not dramatic, especially for the FT1 target, where the three filters had the same spatial frequency tuning and varied only slightly in orientation and location tuning. Given that the three filters used to produce FT1 had the same spatial frequency tuning, it is possible that the information from only the most sensitive filter is required to signal target detection and identification. Further experiments investigating this possibility, as well as the effects of probability summation on our results should be conducted before firm conclusions from our data are made.

Two subjects in our study had considerably different performance from the rest of the subject population. We believe these differences are due to poor attention to the experimental task by the subjects rather than an inconsistency between the data from these two individual subjects and our general interpretations of the group data. First, for both subjects, the unusual mean thresholds they produced can be eliminated by removing data from one peculiar experimental session from the analysis. This is true for Subject BJ's high thresholds in Experiment 1 and Subject WR's AIT thresholds being significantly higher than his FT2 thresholds in Experiment 2. The other factor which indicated that these subjects' idiosyncratic data were due to their poor attention to the experimental task comes from laboratory notebook comments made during each subject's experimental session. Laboratory notebook comments consistently reported poor attention, stress, and fatigue for Subject BJ throughout the study. They also indicated that Subject WR stated that he kept trying to determine how ML-TEST was working during his experimental sessions in Experiment 2. After he was instructed to attend only to the experimental task during the session, his data more closely matched that obtained for the other subjects.

By using the visual outputs of the Wilson[1] filters convolved with the AIT as targets, the information contained within FT1 and FT2 was double passed through the observers' visual systems. If the filtering nonlinearities of the visual are multiplicative, this double passing of information could reduce the signal strength of the less sensitive channels more than the stronger channels. Because our paradigm did not account or control for the double passing of the filter targets' information, we cannot rule out the premise that a multiplicative process such as this does not account for why FT2 thresholds were found to differ significantly from AIT thresholds. Experiments using correlated (i.e., spatially structured) noise might be one approach to investigate the possible effect of double passing on the results. If filtering nonlinearities in the visual system do reduce the signal strength of the less sensitive channels more than the stronger channels, selectively adapting the different channels using correlated noise should allow us to determine these effects. Multiplicative filtering nonlinearities would produced more significant reductions in AIT, FT1, and FT2 thresholds obtained using different types of correlated noise than would be predicted from simple selective adaptation. The relative significance of the differences in the orientation and spatial position tuning of the FT1 filters to AIT detection could also be examined using noise that is correlated for spatial frequency but not orientation or spatial location.

Although the overall mean thresholds we obtained for FT1 and AIT (averaged across all the subjects) were not significantly different, some subjects did show a statistically significant effect of target on within subject ANOVA tests. If a relatively small average difference between FT1 and AIT does truly exist, an experiment of this relatively small sample size (i.e., six subjects) might not be powerful enough to detect it. We recommend that all of these experiments be repeated on a larger population before drawing conclusions on the use of the Wilson model to predict human detection or identification performance for real-world targets.

Within subject ANOVA tests for the data found significant main effects of session for some of the subjects. Many of these subjects were highly motivated and highly experienced psychophysical observers. In fact, in some instances, these subjects were those who had the most training on the experimental task (i.e., the authors). The significant effect of session was not consistently found for any of the subjects across the six experiments. Therefore, we do not believe that the significant effect of session found for some of the subjects on within subject ANOVAs was due to a training effect. The discovery of these effects does help justify our recommendation that additional testing on a larger populations should be conducted before more firm conclusions about the data and its implications are reached.

The data presented here only represent a limited attempt to validate the use of Wilson's[1] model to predict and describe real-world complex target detection. Numerous other investigations and analysis procedures are required to verify these results. For example, we did not attempt to predict detection thresholds for AIT from the responses of the Wilson model filters to AIT after they had been weighted by the individual subjects' empirically determined spatial contrast sensitivity functions. We had several reasons for not attempting to implement the Wilson model in this manner. First, and of most practical significance, was that these procedures were not practical for us to include in our experiments due to the amount of computer memory and time that they would have required. Also, "personalizing" our implementation of the Wilson model for each individual subject was contrary to the overall final goal of this project. Our overall purpose of this study was to provide preliminary data to determine whether an established model of human spatial vision could be implemented and used to predict the spatial information contained within complex, real-world targets of military significance that is required for detection and identification. We would eventually like to be able to use an existing (or slightly modified) spatial vision model to improve military target detection and identification in operational environments. Several military incidents have occurred because friend and foe identification of targets by aircrew members was reduced due to visual clutter in a cockpit weapons system display. If the display scene could be decluttered using a human spatial vision model so that only the information required to detect, identify, or discriminate a target was presented on the display, the likelihood of these types of occurrences might be reduced. This type of visual display decluttering could also reduce the visual task workload of the pilot (which is extremely high for fighter pilots), and improve overall flight safety and operational capability. Although using model generated targets that were tailored to the individuals' own contrast sensitivity functions may remove some of the individual variability found in our results and improve the data's interpretation from a theoretical sense, we seriously doubt that this type of "personalized" application of would be implemented in the field (fulfilling our overall objective).

We also did not measure discrimination thresholds for AIT and the two filter targets, or attempt to determine if very similar targets (e.g., two different types of airplanes) identification and discrimination thresholds could be predicted by analyzing the responses of the model's filters. According to Wilson,[1] predictions of this sort should be possible by analyzing the difference of the model's filters to each target. These differences could be plotted as vectors in a filter response magnitude space, where the length of the vector would represent the magnitude of the differences in the two targets spatial contents. The differences could also be represented as a difference response function for the two targets. The combined visual outputs of the basis filters with the highest response magnitudes in this difference function could then be displayed to the subject to facilitate target discrimination and identification. Correlated noise experiments could also be included to determine whether selectively reducing the sensitivity of these highest responding filters would degrade target discrimination and identification. This latter type of information would be of extreme importance in determining how to better camouflage military targets.

Olzak and Thomas[24] demonstrated that using certain experimental paradigms, discriminating the single frequency components of a compound grating stimulus can be performed more efficiently (i.e., at lower contrasts) than detecting the compound grating. This result was found for compound gratings whose components were of considerably different (e.g., 3 and 12 c/d) but not widely separated (i.e., 3 and 18 c/d) spatial frequencies. When the components spatial frequencies were very similar (i.e., 3 and 6 c/d), the thresholds obtained for compound grating stimulus detection were similar to those obtained for discriminating the individual component frequencies. This latter finding is consistent with the theory that if a single channel provides the critical information for target detection and identification, then detection and identification thresholds will be equivalent. Olzak and Thomas[24] found that when the spatial frequencies of the components were widely separated (i.e., 3 and 18 c/d), detection thresholds for the compound grating and identification thresholds for the component gratings were essentially identical. These data support other reports that discrimination of the components of a compound grating is, in general, easier if the component spatial frequencies are detected by different spatially tuned channels.[1-2, 8] Olzak and Thomas[24] suggested that the data indicate that the different spatially tuned mechanisms of the visual system might not be independent. Inhibitory interactions between the mechanisms might enhance discrimination performance if activity in one set of mechanisms curbs the noise levels in other mechanisms, which might otherwise be mistaken for stimulus response signals. The detection and discrimination experiments we have proposed using AIT and our implementation of the Wilson model might provide an interesting method by which to validate Olzak and Thomas' results using more complex, real-world targets. Superimposition of structural noise, which is correlated to varying spatial frequencies within two targets' discrimination difference function, could provide insight as to how interactions between different spatial frequency-tuned channels can influence human detection and identification performance.

Finally, our dynamic noise data showed that FT1 produced significantly lower detection thresholds than AIT. The additional spatial information within AIT, as compared to FT1, which is processed by different spatial frequency channels might influence the sensitivity of the temporally tuned mechanism which is mediating detection under 30 Hz dynamic Gaussian noise viewing conditions. This finding suggests that image compression by an appropriate set of filters may improve real-world target detectability. The ability to enhance target detection and identification performance in noisy visual environments would be a great benefit in a variety of medical and military applications and is another line of investigation we plan to pursue in the future.

Acknowledgments

James C. Brakefield was responsible for the development of the software used in this study. We thank Denise Varner for her many helpful discussions on the preliminary design of several of these experiments. We thank Phelps Crump and Capt Erik Neilsen for their support on the statistical analysis of the data. We also thank Hugh Wilson for providing us with a prepublication copy of his model and his many helpful discussions on our experiments and the implementation of his model. Finally, we thank Dianne Mirro, Marta Myers, and Janet Pinnix for their excellent technical assistance. This work was supported by Contract F33615-88-C-0631, let by the U.S. Air Force Armstrong Laboratory, Brooks Air Force Base, Texas, to KRUG Life Sciences Inc., and by an Independent Laboratory Investigative Research Award to Norman Barsalou by the U. S. Air Force Armstrong Laboratory.

References

1. H.R. Wilson, "Psychophysical models of spatial vision and hyperacuity", in *Vision and Visual Dysfunction: Spatial Vision*, **10**, ed. D. Regan (CRC Press, Boca Raton, 1991), pp. 64-68.

2. L.A. Olzak & J.P. Thomas, "Seeing spatial patterns", in *Handbook of Perception and Performance: Sensory Processes and Perception*, ed. K.R. Boff, L. Kaufman, and J.P. Thomas (John Wiley and Sons, New York, 1986), pp. 7-1 to 7-56

3. C. Blakemore & F.W. Campbell, "On the existence of neurons in the human visual system selectively sensitive to the orientation and size of retinal images", *J. Physiology* **203** (1969) 237-260.

4. N. Graham & J. Nachmias, "Detection of grating patterns containing two spatial frequencies: A comparison of single-channel and multiple-channel models", *Vision Res.* **11** (1971) 251-259.

5. C.S. Furchner, J.P. Thomas, & F.W. Campbell, "Detection and discrimination of simple and complex patterns at low spatial frequencies", *Vision Res.* **17** (1977) 827-836.

6. R.L. DeValois, D.G. Albrecht, & L.G. Thorell, "Spatial frequency selectivity of cells in macaque visual cortex", *Vision Res.* **22** (1982) 545-559.

7. G.C. Phillips & H.R. Wilson, "Orientation bandwidths of spatial mechanisms measured by masking", *J. Opt. Soc. Am. [A]* **1** (1984) 226-232.

8. A.B. Watson & J.G. Robson, "Discrimination at threshold: Labelled detectors in human vision", *Vision Res.* **21** (1981) 1115-1122.

9. F.W. Campbell & J.G. Robson, "Application of Fourier analysis to the visibility of gratings", *J. Physiol.* **197** (1968) 551-566.

10. M.B. Sachs, J. Nachmias, & J.G. Robson, "Spatial-frequency channels in human vision", *J. Opt. Soc. Am.* **61** (1971) 1176-1186.

11. J. Hirsch, R. Hylton, & N. Graham, "Simultaneous recognition of two spatial frequency components", *Vision Res.* **22** (1982) 365-375.

12. L. Olzak, "Inhibition and stochastic interactions in spatial pattern perception", doctoral dissertation, University of California, Los Angeles (1981).

13. N.V.S. Graham, "Visual Pattern Analyzers", (*Oxford Univ. Press*, New York, 1989).

14. F.M. deMonasterio, "Properties of concentrically organized X and Y ganglion cells of macaque retina", *J. Neurophysiol.* **41** (1978) 1394-1417.

15. F.M. deMonasterio, "Center and surround mechanisms of opponent-color X and Y ganglion cells of retina of macaques", *J. Neurophysiol.* **41** (1978) 1418-1434.

16. D.H. Hubel & T.N. Wiesel, "Receptive fields and functional architecture of monkey striate cortex", *J. Physiol.* **195** (1968) 215-243.

17. V.H. Perry, R. Oehler, & A. Cowey, "Retinal ganglion cells that project to the dorsal lateral geniculate nucleus in the macaque monkey", *Neurosci.* **12** (1984) 1101-1123.

18. U.S. Air Force Regulation 160-43, "Medical examination and medical standards", *Headquarters U.S. Air Force*, Washington, D.C., October 24, 1986.

19. D. Williams, "Aliasing in human foveal vision", *Vision Res.* **25** (1985) 195-205.

20. L.O. Harvey, Jr., "Efficient estimation of sensory thresholds", *Behav. Res. Meth., Instr. Comp.* **18** (1986) 623-632.

21. J.G. Robson, "Spatial and temporal contrast sensitivity functions of the visual system", *J. Opt. Soc. Am.* **56** (1966) 1141-1142.

22. W.W. Geisler, "Physical limits of acuity and hyperacuity", *J. Opt. Soc. Am. [A]* (1984) 775-782.

244

23. A.B. Watson, "Detection and recognition of simple spatial forms", in *Physical and Biological Processing of Images*, ed. O.J. Braddick and A.C. Sleigh (Springer-Verlag, New York, 1983) pp. 100-114.

24. L.A. Olzak & J.P. Thomas, "Gratings: Why frequency discrimination is sometimes better than detection", *J. Opt. Soc. Am.* **71** (1981) 64-70.

A VISUAL DISCRIMINATION MODEL
FOR IMAGING SYSTEM DESIGN AND EVALUATION

JEFFREY LUBIN
David Sarnoff Research Center
201 Washington Road, Princeton, NJ 08540-6449

ABSTRACT

This report describes the structure, performance, and some applications of the Sarnoff Visual Discrimination Model. The model has been designed for physiological plausibility as well as speed and simplicity of operation, and has been shown to be highly accurate in predicting performance in a large number of visual discrimination and image quality rating tasks. The model can be used to assess the visual effects of variations in imaging system parameters, and is thus well-suited for applications in the design and evaluation of imaging systems and their components.

1. Introduction

1.1. Bridging the Communication Gap Between Designers and Users

Designers and manufacturers of imaging systems are accustomed to specifying the performance of their systems in terms of physical parameters that are easy for them to measure. As shown in the right hand side of Figure 1, these typically include display parameters such as brightness, contrast, resolution and, if the image is to be transmitted, various parameters of the compression/reconstruction process as well (e.g., bit-rate).

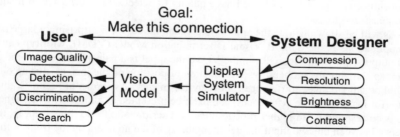

Figure 1. A modeling approach to imaging system optimization.

However, the end user of the imaging system is not directly interested in these physical parameters, but is instead concerned with the visual performance that can be expected with the system, as indicated on the left side of Figure 1. For example, a radiologist wants to know whether a tumor that is visible on standard film media will also be visible in the softcopy display system under consideration. On a more subjective level, a home television consumer wants to know whether the receiver will produce visually pleasing images, without obvious artifacts or distortions.

Thus, the user speaks a language of *visual* performance requirements, while the manufacturer speaks of *physical* performance specifications. The center of Figure 1 shows how a sequence of two models – a display system simulator and a vision model – can translate between these two languages. By using the physical display parameters to render simulated display images (in the display system simulator), and then feeding these images to a model of human visual performance, the effects of physical parameters on visual performance can be directly assessed.

1.2. The Appropriate Structure for a Vision Model

The input/output structure of an appropriate display system simulator is conceptually simple. Based on the input display specifications and imagery, the simulator should produce a map of the display surface that indicates light output as a function of position; i.e., a map that simulates the response of a photometer as it steps across the display surface. The difficulties in display simulation occur not in determining the appropriate input/output structure, but instead in addressing questions of accuracy – e.g., how closely does the model output at each sampled point need to match the photometer reading of the real display, how does one set up the model to achieve this desired level of accuracy, and how many sample points per unit of display surface are needed to render the display in question.

The difficulty of these questions should not be minimized, but their complexity does not hide the simplicity of the underlying model input/output structure: i.e., parameters in, images out. However, the structure of an appropriate vision model is not as obvious. The question is: how does one generate a model that takes rendered display model images as input and returns useful predictions of human visual performance on measures ranging from subjective ratings of esthetic image quality to detection performance in medical or reconnaissance tasks.

As will be shown below, the appropriate vision model for a surprisingly large number of applications is the Sarnoff Visual Discrimination Model (VDM), with typical inputs and outputs shown in Figure 2. In the VDM, the input is a pair of images and the output is a map showing the probability, as a function of position on the images, that an observer would be able to detect differences between the images. As shown in Figure 2, this *JND Map* (for just noticeable differences) can itself be presented as an image, with higher gray levels corresponding to higher probabilities of discrimination. So, for example, the difference between the two input images in legibility of the numbers on the front of the tram is indicated by a bright area in the JND map at the corresponding location.

The actual probability values on the JND maps are calibrated in terms called JNDs, where 1 JND corresponds to a 75% probability that an observer viewing the two images multiple times would be able to see the difference. JND values above 1 are then calculated incrementally. For example, if Image Y is 1 JND higher in contrast than Image X, and Image Z is 1 JND higher in contrast than Image Y, then Image Z is 2 JNDs higher in contrast than Image X. In probability terms, this 2 JND difference corresponds to 93.75% probability of discrimination ($0.75 + 0.75 \times (1 - 0.75)$), and a 3 JND difference corresponds to 98.44% probability. Although probability of discrimination asymptotes quickly as a function of JNDs, the units are useful because they correspond to roughly linear magnitudes of subjective visual difference, as will be shown in Section 3 below.

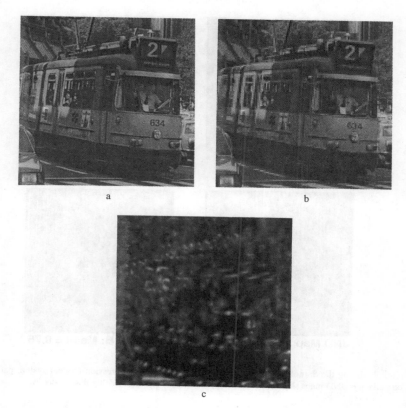

a

b

c

Figure 2. Typical inputs (a, b) and JND map output (c) for the Sarnoff Visual Discrimination Model.

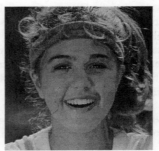

Input Image

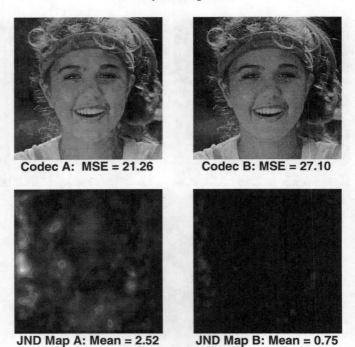

Codec A: MSE = 21.26   **Codec B: MSE = 27.10**

JND Map A: Mean = 2.52   **JND Map B: Mean = 0.75**

Figure 3. Using the Sarnoff VDM to compare compression/decompression (codec) system parameters. Comparison of JND maps shows that Codec B produces better image fidelity than Codec A.

1.3. Applications to Image Fidelity

A discrimination model with the i/o structure outlined above has some obvious applications in assessing the fidelity with which a display system can reproduce input imagery. For example, Figure 3 shows an image fidelity application of the Sarnoff VDM in a comparison of image compression/decompression (codec) schemes.

The codec images shown in Figure 3 are the outputs of two hypothetical compression/decompression schemes (A and B). The mean squared error (MSE) values indicated for each codec image are the current standard measure of codec image fidelity, with lower values indicating a closer match between the original and codec image. For example, a codec designer using MSE to decide between codecs A and B would choose A, since the MSE value of 21.26 for codec A is lower than the value of 27.10 for codec B. Unfortunately for this designer, visual inspection of codec images A and B shows that this design choice would be incorrect, since the artifacts in codec image A are much more perceptually noticeable than are the artifacts in codec image B. On the other hand, a codec choice based on the JND measure of image fidelity produces much better agreement with perception: the lower average JND value from codec B (0.75) than from codec A (2.52) indicates that the image from codec B is *perceptually* closer to the original, even though its MSE value is higher.

This demonstration shows that the JND image fidelity metric is useful in comparing competing codecs. By the same logic, it can also be used to compare different parameter settings within a single codec, allowing applications within an encoding loop, as shown by the example in Figure 4. In this hypothetical application, a JND map is computed between the original source image and a codec image as generated by the algorithm's first guess of a good set of quantization parameters. The JND map then feeds back into a controller that modifies the quantization parameters based on the desired level of image fidelity and the number of available bits. Iteration continues until the JND criterion has been achieved, or until available bits have been used up.

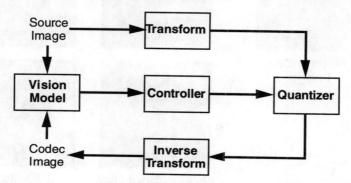

Figure 4. An application of the Sarnoff Visual Discrimination Model within a DCT encoding loop.

Currently, most encoding algorithms assume that image fidelity is directly proportional to quantization sampling density. This assumption is often erroneous, with the result that bits are squandered where they have little impact on image fidelity. An advantage of the vision model-based approach to encoding shown in Figure 4 is that image fidelity as a function of quantization parameters is actually measured, instead of being assumed. The result can be higher, more uniform image fidelity for a fixed bit rate, or better bit rates for a desired level of fidelity. The approach in Figure 4 is obviously incomplete as an algorithm; it is presented here simply as an example of future developments in encoding that could take strong advantage of a workable image fidelity metric such as the Sarnoff VDM.

Image fidelity applications of the VDM are not restricted to image compression. In display design, just as in image compression, various parameters must be adjusted to render images with acceptable fidelity to the source imagery. Figures 5 and 6 show how a display model followed by the VDM can be used to optimally adjust one such parameter, CRT spot size.

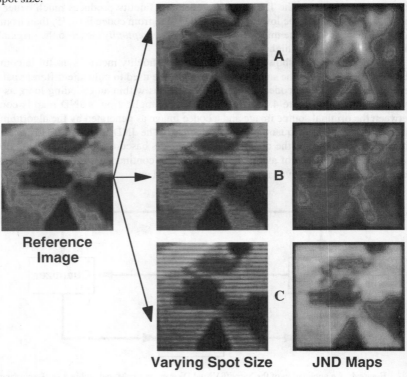

Figure 5. An application of the VDM to the display design problem of optimizing CRT spot size.

As illustrated in Figure 5, Sarnoff's Display System Simulator (DSS) was used to render, from a single reference image, simulated CRT images with a range of different spot sizes. Then, a JND map was computed for each comparison of the reference image with one of the rendered images. Inspection of the rendered images and corresponding JND maps gives an intuitive feel for the nature of the optimization. For a display with a spot size that is too large, images can look blurry (as in rendered image A in Figure 5), while for a spot size that is too small, the visibility of the scan line structure becomes objectionable (as in rendered image C). These two problems are manifest in different ways on the corresponding JND maps. For image A, bright spots on the JND map at positions corresponding to edges in the original image indicate that high frequency information is being lost in the rendered image, while for image C, the bright regions in the JND map show the visibility of the scan line structure in the background regions of the rendered image.

In Figure 6, these effects of spot size are quantified graphically to show how an optimal spot size can be chosen. In this figure, average JNDs for each comparison of a rendered image with the original are plotted against the spot size used for the rendered image. The plot shows a minimum at a spot size corresponding to image B, indicating that this spot size produced the image that was perceptually closest to the original.

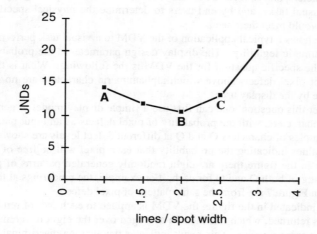

Figure 6. A plot of average JNDs vs. spot size, for the example illustrated in Figure 5. The labels A, B, and C refer to the images of the same labels in Figure 5.

The utility of this model-based approach to display design optimization is especially significant when one considers the alternative; i.e., construction and visual evaluation of hardware prototypes. Considering the large amount of money and time that goes into prototype construction and testing, the model-based approach illustrated in Figures 5 and 6 represents a much more economical alternative to display design. It is also generally a more reliable approach, since the VDM represents a standard observer, without the biases or large variances of human evaluators.

1.4. Applications to Visual Task Performance

The VDM applications described in the previous section were all based on the assumption that the best measure of imaging system performance is the fidelity with which input imagery is rendered at the output. In most cases this assumption is valid, especially for applications like home entertainment, in which displays are generally judged on subjective measures of image quality. However, in other applications, displays are often used for specific visual tasks such as reading or target detection, for which more objective measures of visual performance can be applied. In these cases, the VDM can generate predictions of the expected level of visual performance as a function of imaging system parameters, and so it can be used by manufacturers to help design systems tailored to specific visual tasks, and by end users to determine the physical specifications of a display that would meet their needs.

Figure 7 shows a typical application of the VDM to a visual task performance; in this case, alphanumeric legibility. The display design parameter is the probability of pixel defect, and the specific question for the VDM is the following: What is the maximum probability of pixel defects above which alphanumeric characters are no longer easily discriminable by the display user?

To answer this question, one can first use a simple display model to generate images of different characters, with the probability of pixel defects as an input parameter to the model. Examples of characters O and Q at different defect levels are shown in Figure 7, with the p values indicating the probability that each pixel will be free of defects. For each p value in the figure there are eight randomly generated patterns of pixel defects, and a rendering of both O and Q for each. For example, the renderings at the tails of the two arrows in Figure 7 are from the same pattern of pixel defects.

Next, as indicated in the figure, the VDM is applied to each pair of renderings, and a JND value is returned, which can then be averaged over the eight different pairs of renderings at the same p value. This result indicates the average discriminability between characters at a specific probability of pixel defects. This average can then be plotted as a function of p, to determine the minimum p value at which characters are sufficiently discriminable to produce legible text on the display.

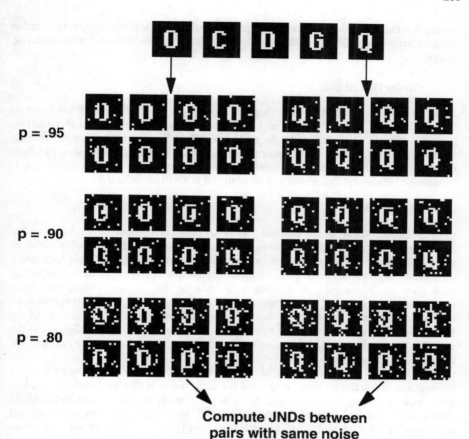

Compute JNDs between pairs with same noise

Figure 7. An example of VDM application in determining display requirements for a specific visual task; in this case, alphanumeric legibility as a function of pixel defect probability. See text for details.

This example shows the basic difference between the two discussed modes of VDM application. In the case of image fidelity applications as described in Section 1.3 above, the model is used to help find a minimum of discriminability between two images, since this minimum represents a maximum of image fidelity between input and output. In the case of visual task performance applications discussed in this section, the visual task is first expressed in terms of a discrimination between two input signals (e.g., two easily confusable characters, or a pair of regions from a medical image, one with a tumor present and one without). Then, each signal is put through the display model, and the visual discrimination model is applied to the pair of outputs. In this case, the design goal is to ensure that the discriminability between the two images is sufficiently *high*, as opposed to the goal in the image fidelity applications of minimizing the discriminability between two images.

2.   Model Description

In the previous section, a wide range of applications of discrimination modeling to questions of imaging system design and evaluation were discussed. In this section, Sarnoff's Visual Discrimination Model will be described in some detail, after establishing the historical context for its development. Physiological and/or psychophysical justification for the individual model components will not be offered here, but the prediction performance of the model as a whole will be analyzed in detail in Section 3 below.

2.1.   Background

The Sarnoff Visual Discrimination Model has direct antecedents in an earlier vision model developed at Sarnoff, the Carlson and Cohen (1980) JND Model. In this model an input image is decomposed by partitioning its one-dimensional power spectrum into a number of discrete adjacent frequency bands. The integral of the amplitude values within each band is then subject to a static non-linearity that is accelerating for small input values and compressive for large values. Changes in the output of this process from one member of a pair of images to the other provide a simple perceptual measure of the visibility of differences between the two images. This model can successfully predict the visibility of changes in edge sharpness and of various display artifacts, for example the seam visibility data to be described below.

However, the model is somewhat complicated to compute, among other reasons because a noise parameter must be adjusted for each change in display parameters such as luminance or display size. A similar but computationally simpler model is the SQRI (square root integral) Model of Barten (1987, 1990), which has been successfully applied to a number of different display evaluation problems. In this model, the separate frequency-selective bands are replaced by a single integral over spatial frequencies. This integral is:

$$J = \frac{1}{\ln 2} \int_{0}^{v_{max}} \sqrt{\frac{M(v)}{M_t(v)}} \, \frac{dv}{v}$$

(1)

where J is the visibility (in JNDs) of the displayed signal, v_{max} is the maximum spatial frequency displayed, $M(v)$ is the modulation transfer function of the display, and $M_t(v)$ is the threshold modulation transfer function of the human visual system; i.e., the threshold contrast for grating detection as a function of the spatial frequency of the grating, as expressed by an arithmetic curve fit to data from van Meeteren and Vos (1972). This model, like the Carlson and Cohen model, is spatially one-dimensional, and Barten himself does not generally give details on how the second dimension is handled for specific model applications.

Similar models have been introduced into the basic psychophysics literature by Wilson and his colleagues (e.g., Wilson, McFarlane, and Phillips, 1983; Wilson and Regan, 1984; Wilson, 1991), based on the threshold model of Wilson and Bergen (1979), and by Legge and Foley (Legge and Foley, 1980; Foley and Legge, 1981). These models successfully predict human performance in simple psychophysical tasks such as grating contrast detection and discrimination. In all of these models, the input image is first decomposed into independent spatial frequency channels by a set of linear filters. The output of each filter is then put through a sigmoid non-linearity, the shape of which matches very closely that of the non-linearity imposed by the noise and squaring steps of the Carlson and Cohen JND Model.

These basic psychophysics models, like the Carlson and Cohen and Barten models described above, are spatially one-dimensional; that is, they predict sensitivity to spatial variation in one dimension only. Watson and his colleagues (Watson, 1983; Ahumada and Watson, 1985; Nielsen, Watson, and Ahumada, 1985) have implemented a model that generalizes the linear filtering stage of these models to two dimensions. Each filter is a two-dimensional Gabor function, with a number of different scales, orientations, and phases of filtering at each point in the two-dimensional visual field, and an increase in the overall scale of filtering as a function of eccentricity. The model has been validated on some detection and discrimination data.

One limitation with the Watson *et al* model is that it is only accurate at stimulus levels near detection threshold since, unlike the other models described above, there is no point non-linearity after the linear filtering stage. This limitation has been addressed in a more complicated model by Daly (1993a), who used a similar linear filtering stage – the Watson (1987) Cortex Transform – followed by a non-linear masking function. The Daly model, like the Sarnoff model, produces maps of the visibility of differences between pairs of input images. It has been shown to produce reasonable fits to a number of different data sets (Daly, 1993b), but only when a free parameter is readjusted from one data set to the next.

The design of the Sarnoff model as an engineering tool has been motivated by considerations of speed and accuracy, and as such combines many of the positive features of earlier engineering tools such as the models of Barten and Carlson and Cohen. Additionally, the Sarnoff model design is motivated by considerations of mechanistic accuracy; i.e., so that components of the model have the same functional response as physiological mechanisms in the visual pathways of the brain. This second consideration becomes especially important when one attempts to further develop the model beyond its original scope of stimulus or task domains. For example, the Barten model may work well on the simple detection applications for which it was designed, but its lack of mechanistic structure becomes a distinct disadvantage when trying to predict such effects as some of the super-threshold interactions between different signal components reported by Tolhurst and Barfield (1977), Sagi and Hochstein (1983), Olzak (1985), Lubin (1992), and Lubin and Nachmias (1990), among others. These effects can be modeled by assuming gain-setting interactions between neural mechanisms differing in frequency and orientation selectivity, and are thus relatively easy to implement in a model in which the appropriate neural mechanisms are already represented. However, for the Barten model, incorporation of these effects would require a significant restructuring of the calculation, with the new model probably bearing little similarity to the old.

2.2 Model Statement

The flow diagram in Figure 8 represents the architecture of the Sarnoff Visual Discrimination Model. As mentioned above, the model design was motivated primarily by considerations of speed and accuracy. As will be discussed in detail below, speed is accomplished primarily by the use of a contrast pyramid to generate the bandpass contrast responses, while accuracy is accomplished by the use of physiologically plausible mechanisms at each stage, and by a robust parameter setting procedure that obviates the need (from which the Daly model suffers) to readjust parameters from one data set to the next.

The first stage in Figure 8, labeled *stimuli*, refers to the model inputs. These are entered as two digitized images, representing sampled luminance distributions on a planar surface; i.e., as would be returned from a photometer sampling from a uniform grid of closely spaced points on the output surface of a display device. In addition to the two images, four other input parameters can be entered, all of which are set to reasonable default values unless over-ridden.

These parameters are:

1. The physical distance between sample points on the input images (in mm)
2. The distance of the modeled observer from the image plane (in mm)
3. Fixation depth (in mm)
4. Eccentricity of the images in the observer's visual field (in degrees).

Of these four parameters, the first two are most likely to vary between model runs, since they depend on the type of display and application. The last two are only used in applications such as cockpit display visibility prediction, in which, for example, it is important to know the extent to which information on a display is legible when the observer is fixated on some other point in the visual field.

Next, at the stage labeled "optics" in Figure 8, the input images are convolved with a function approximating the point spread by the optics of the eye. This function, from Westheimer (1986) is:

$$Q(\rho) = 0.952 \exp(-2.59|\rho|^{1.36}) + 0.048 \exp(-2.43|\rho|^{1.74}) \tag{2}$$

where ρ is distance in minutes of arc from a point of light, and $Q(\rho)$ is the intensity of light at a distance ρ, relative to the maximum.

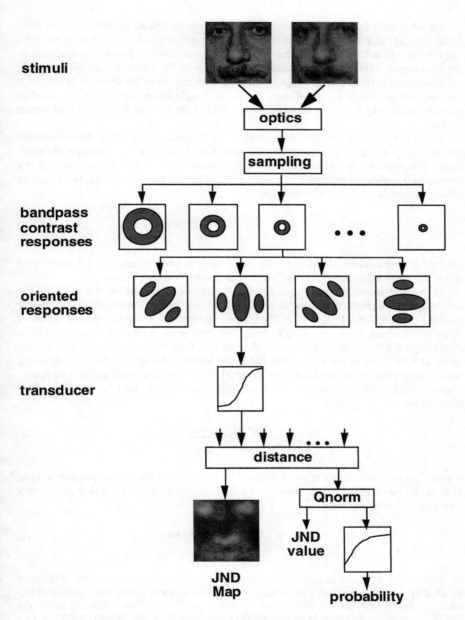

Figure 8. Flow diagram for the Sarnoff Visual Discrimination Model.

An additional operation is performed at this stage of the model when the fixation depth does not match the image depth. In this case, geometrical optics is used to calculate the size of the blur circle, and then the image is convolved with this disk-shaped convolution kernel. This calculation requires knowledge of the distance from the exit pupil to the imaging surface (i.e., the retina), taken as 20.3 mm from Westheimer (1986). It also requires an estimate of pupil size. For this, a simple interpolation routine is used to estimate pupil size at any light level, from a table published in Hood and Finkelstein (1986).

At the next model stage, labeled "sampling" in Figure 8, sampling by the retinal cone mosaic is simulated by a Gaussian convolution and point sampling sequence of operations. The result for foveal viewing is a *retinal image* of 512×512 pixels, sampled at a density of 120 pixels per degree of visual angle. For non-foveal viewing, the sampling density is calculated from the expression

$$d = \frac{120}{1 + ke}, \tag{3}$$

where d is the calculated density, e is the eccentricity in degrees, and k is a parameter set at 0.4, the value estimated from psychophysical data by Watson (1983).

In the next model stage, labeled "bandpass contrast responses" in the diagram, the raw luminance signal is converted to units of local contrast as follows, using a technique similar to that of Peli (1990). First, the image is decomposed into a Laplacian pyramid (Burt and Adelson, 1983), resulting in seven bandpass levels with peak frequencies from 32 through 0.5 cycles/degree, each level separated from its neighbors by one octave. Then, at each point in each level, the Laplacian value is divided by the corresponding point upsampled from the Gaussian pyramid level two levels down in resolution. Mathematically, this *contrast pyramid* operation can be expressed (in the continuous domain) as:

$$\hat{c}_k(\vec{x}) = \frac{I(\vec{x}) * (G_k(\vec{x}) - G_{k+1}(\vec{x}))}{I(\vec{x}) * G_{k+2}(\vec{x})}, \tag{4}$$

where $\hat{c}_k(\vec{x})$ is the contrast at pyramid level k, $\vec{x}$ is a two-dimensional position vector, $I(\vec{x})$ is the input image (after optics and sampling operations), and where $G_k(\vec{x})$ is a Gaussian convolution kernel

$$G_k(\vec{x}) = \frac{1}{(\sqrt{2\pi}\sigma_k)^2} e^{-(x^2+y^2)/2\sigma_k^2} \tag{5}$$

for which $\sigma_k = 2^{k-1}\sigma_0$. The result of this contrast pyramid operation is a local difference divided by a local mean; i.e., a local measure of contrast, localized in both space and frequency. For a sine grating within the frequency passband of one pyramid level, the resulting contrast measure is approximately equivalent to the Weber contrast; i.e.,

$(L_{max} - L_{min})/L_{mean}$, where L_{max}, L_{min}, and L_{mean} refer respectively to the maximum, minimum, and mean luminance of the grating pattern.

In the next stage, marked "oriented responses" in the diagram, each pyramid level is convolved with four pairs of spatially oriented filters. Each pair consists of a directional second derivative of a Gaussian (in one of the four directions indicated in Figure 8) and its Hilbert transform. These filters have a log bandwidth at half height of approximately 0.7 octaves, a value within the range of bandwidths inferred psychophysically (e.g., Watson, 1982). The orientation bandwidth of these filters (i.e., the range of angles over which filter output is greater than one half the maximum) is approximately 65 degrees. This figure is slightly larger than the 40 degree tuning of monkey simple cells reported by DeValois *et al.* (1982), and the 30 to 60 degree range reported psychophysically by Phillips and Wilson (1984). However, smaller bandwidths would require more filters to uniformly cover the range of orientations, which would lead to a computationally expensive, slower model. Four orientations was thought to be a reasonable compromise, although prediction accuracy on some orientation masking data is somewhat degraded. For convenience and speed of operation, the filters are implemented as the steerable filters of Freeman and Adelson (1991).

After oriented filtering, corresponding Hilbert pairs of filter output images are squared and summed, resulting in a phase-independent energy response:

$$e_{k,\theta}(\vec{x}) = \left(o_{k,\theta}(\vec{x})\right)^2 + \left(h_{k,\theta}(\vec{x})\right)^2 \tag{6}$$

where θ indexes over the 4 orientations, k is pyramid level, and o and h are the oriented operator and its Hilbert transform. This operation is used to mimic a widely proposed transformation in the mammalian visual cortex from a linear response among simple cells to an energy response among complex cells. The phase independence resulting from this operation has some useful properties; e.g., it makes the model less sensitive to the exact position of an edge, a property exhibited in human psychophysical performance as well.

At the "transducer" stage shown next in Figure 8, each energy measure $e_{k,\theta}(\vec{x})$ is first normalized by a value M_t, which is close to the square of the grating contrast detection threshold for that pyramid level and local luminance. (The adjustment of these normalization factors is described in the section on model calibration below.) The result of this normalization process is

$$\hat{e}_{k,\theta}(\vec{x}) = \frac{e_{k,\theta}(\vec{x})}{\left(M_t\left(v_k, L_k(\vec{x})\right)\right)^2} \tag{7}$$

where v_k is the peak frequency for the pyramid level k, and L is the local luminance value used in the contrast calculation described above. Next, each normalized energy measure is put through a sigmoid non-linearity of the form

$$T\left(\hat{e}_{k,\theta}(\vec{x})\right) = \frac{2\left(\hat{e}_{k,\theta}(\vec{x})\right)^{n/2}}{\left(\hat{e}_{k,\theta}(\vec{x})\right)^{(n-w)/2} + 1} \tag{8}$$

which is needed to reproduce the dipper shape of contrast discrimination functions, first reported by Nachmias and Sansbury (1974), as will be discussed in more detail in the section below on model calibration, together with a justification of the threshold normalization described above. This function has a number of interesting properties when one considers a grating stimulus input of contrast c and frequency v_k. For small values of c, the maximum transducer output from pyramid level k accelerates as c^n, where n is a real number around 2, while for large values of c, the function is compressive as c^w, where w is a real number less than one. For an intermediate value of c at the contrast detection threshold for frequency v_k, the transducer output is 1.

The oriented filters described above have the property that, for a single filter at a single spatial position given a sine grating to which it is optimally tuned, the output as a function of number of cycles in the patch will asymptote at little more than one cycle. In contrast, foveal human sensitivity continues to improve as the number of cycles in the patch continues to increase to around 5 (Hoekstra et al., 1994). To account for this effect, the model includes a pooling stage that, for foveal inputs, averages transducer outputs over a small neighborhood by convolving with a disc-shaped kernel of diameter 5.

For stimulus eccentricities outside the fovea, the diameter dp of this kernel increases as a linear function of eccentricity, according to the expression

$$d_p = d_0\left(1 + \frac{e}{k_p}\right) \tag{9}$$

where d_0 is the foveal diameter (5.0), e is the eccentricity in degrees, and k_p is a scaling factor. This eccentricity dependent increase in pooling is needed to model an eccentricity dependent loss in performance, beyond that attributable to a loss in contrast sensitivity, on tasks requiring accurate relative localization of stimulus features, such as character discrimination. See Lubin (1993) for a more complete description and justification of this eccentricity dependent pooling stage in the model.

After this pooling operation, each image's model output for each spatial position can be thought of as an m-dimensional vector, where m is the number of pyramid levels times the number of orientations. In the box marked "distance" in the diagram, the distance between these vectors for the two input images is calculated as follows. First, the smaller pyramid levels are upsampled to the full 512×512 size, the result being a set of m arrays $P_i(\vec{x})$ (where i indexes from 1 to m) for each input image $\vec{x}$. From these, a distance measure D is calculated as follows:

$$D(\vec{x}_1, \vec{x}_2) = \left\{\sum_{i=1}^{m}\left[P_i(\vec{x}_1) - P_i(\vec{x}_2)\right]^Q\right\}^{1/Q} \tag{10}$$

where $\vec{x}_1$ and $\vec{x}_2$ are the two input images, and Q is a parameter currently set at 2.4. (For $Q=2$, this expression corresponds to the Euclidean distance between the two vectors.) The result of this model stage is a spatial array of distance values; i.e., the JND map output of the model.

As indicated in Figure 8, other model outputs are also available. From the box labeled "Qnorm", the values across the JND map can be combined according to a similar distance metric as described above. In practice, one of two different combinations are used: the average across the map, or the maximum. For threshold discrimination tasks, the latter is the more useful statistic; for rating tasks, it is the former, as will be shown in the later section on model predictions. This single JND value output can then be converted to a probability value, according to the technique described in the introduction to this report.

Figure 9 illustrates the processing that an image undergoes as it passes through the various stages of the model. The input image, called a *zone plate*, is a circular cosine function whose frequency increases linearly with radius. It is a useful test image to examine the orientation and frequency decomposition by the model, since it contains a wide range of spatial frequencies and orientations that vary continuously by position on the image. For example, the frequency selectivity of the different levels of the contrast pyramid is illustrated by the fact that, for each successively smaller contrast pyramid image in the figure, the radius of the brightest bands of rings decreases, thus indicating a lower frequency passband. The orientation and spatial frequency tuning of the oriented filters in the model is illustrated by the kidney-shaped bright regions in the images of oriented responses, with the arc of each region showing the range of orientations to which the filter is tuned and the width in the radial direction showing the frequency tuning. The JND map at the bottom of Figure 9 shows the discriminability between the zone plate input image and a uniform field of the same mean luminance.

2.3. Model Calibration

The model predictions to be shown in Section 3 were all generated without any readjustment of model parameters. To achieve this robustness, model calibration is performed in a two step procedure, illustrated in Figures 10 and 11. This procedure is based on the assumption that the shape of the transducer function is independent of pyramid level or orientation channel, except for a scale factor that sets the gain as a function of frequency band.

The first model calibration step is based on a fit to the spatial *contrast sensitivity function*, as first measured by Schade (1948). In a contrast sensitivity measurement, the contrast of a grating pattern of a fixed spatial frequency is adjusted until the grating is just detectable. This *threshold contrast* measurement is repeated at a number of different spatial frequencies, so that the results can be plotted as a function of spatial frequency. The bold curve in Figure 10 shows a typical set of such results.

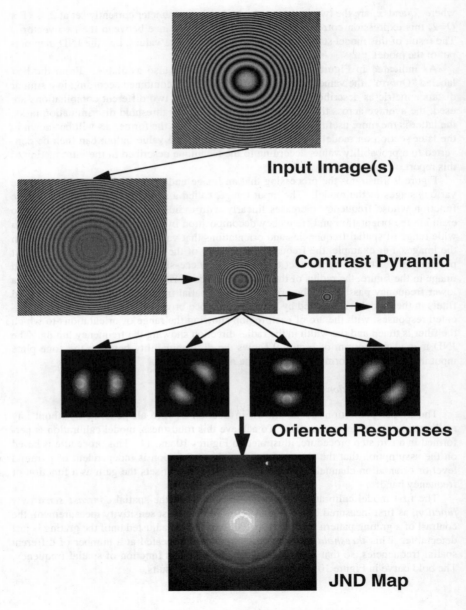

Input Image(s)

Contrast Pyramid

Oriented Responses

JND Map

Figure 9. Model throughput for zone plate test image.

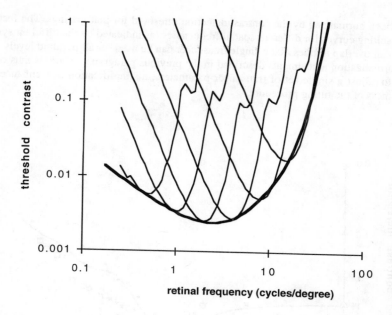

Figure 10. Spatial frequency decomposition by the Sarnoff VDM, showing sensitivity adjustment of pyramid levels to achieve fit to contrast sensitivity function.

One can also plot the results of such an experiment run on a reduced version of the model which contains only one contrast pyramid level, and no transducer. For each spatial frequency, the contrast of the grating is adjusted until the maximum response from the oriented filter stage for that pyramid level is exactly 1. The results of such a computational experiment for each pyramid level are shown by the set of thinner lined curves in Figure 10. The important point to note here is that these curves can be shifted up and down by changing the value of the contrast normalization term M_t for each pyramid level. So, in this step of the calibration procedure, the values of M_t are adjusted to shift each curve up and down until their combined envelope produces the best possible fit to the overall contrast sensitivity function. The fit shown in Figure 10 is the result of such an optimization procedure.

The second stage of calibration is based on the contrast discrimination results of Bradley and Ohzawa (1986) shown by the plotted symbols in Figure 11. In a contrast discrimination experiment, a just detectable change in grating contrast is measured as a function of the starting contrast of that grating. For the results plotted in Figure 11, both the threshold contrast change (ordinate values) and starting contrast (abscissa values) have been normalized by the contrast detection threshold for that grating. The fact that the resulting curves for different spatial frequencies (as indicated by the different symbol types) all overlap implies that a single transducer can be used for all pyramid levels, after the normalization adjustments described in the previous paragraph. There is thus only a need to adjust a single set of transducer parameters, a simplification that enhances the robustness of the fitting procedure.

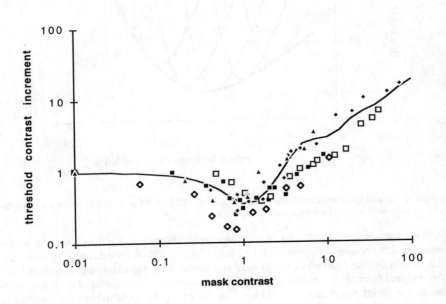

Figure 11. Predictions of the Sarnoff VDM on contrast discrimination data of Bradley and Ohzawa (1986), showing fit of transducer parameters. Different symbol types indicate different spatial frequencies. Plotted discrimination thresholds are normalized on both axes by the contrast detection threshold for that grating.

3.   Model Predictions

After calibration by the procedure outlined in the last section, the model accurately predicts a large amount of human visual performance data, both in detection and discrimination tasks and, perhaps more surprisingly, in rating tasks in which the observer is asked to estimate a magnitude of subjective image quality. In this section, many of the experiments on which the model has been tested to date will be described. For each experiment, a plot showing data vs. model predictions will be presented.

3.1. Detection and Discrimination Data

The model has been tested against contrast detection data involving three different types of broadband stimuli. As summarized in the plots of Figures 12, 13, and 14, these three stimuli are:

1. Small luminous disks, from a study by Blackwell (1971)
2. Checkerboard patterns, from an unpublished study at Sarnoff
3. Thin luminous lines, from Alphonse and Lubin (1992).

In the Blackwell (1971) experiment, threshold contrast ratios between a small disk and its surround were measured as a function of disk diameter, as shown in Figure 12. These data were in fact collected to advance the Allied effort during the Second World War, as a means of measuring the visual requirements for the detection of incoming enemy aircraft. The plotted points of two different symbol types in Figure 12 show results for two different background luminances, as indicated in the legend, with the two lines showing model predictions in these same conditions. The predictions are good, with no systematic deviation in either direction from the measured thresholds.

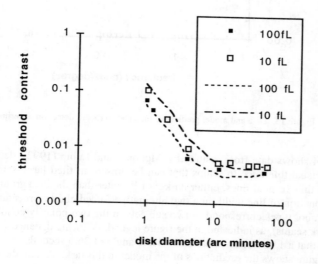

Figure 12. Model predictions on disk detection data from Blackwell (1971).

In Figure 13, the stimulus was a 5 × 5 black/white checkerboard pattern, which could vary in size and contrast. (This pattern is of interest to some users because of its prevalence in display test patterns.) Contrast detection thresholds were measured in a two alternative spatial forced choice staircase paradigm, as a function of checkerboard size, and are plotted (with four replications per data point) as open squares. Mean luminance was approximately 8 fL. Model predictions are shown by the solid curve in the plot. Here again, there is no obvious disparity between data and model predictions.

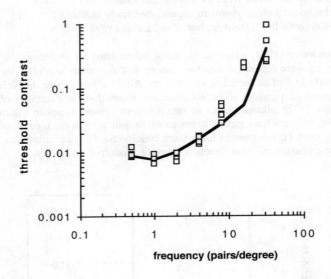

Figure 13. Data and model predictions on a checkerboard detection experiment.

Figure 14 shows data from a study by Alphonse and Lubin (1992), designed to test the human visual tolerance to seams that can be present in tiled large-screen displays. Visibility of thin vertical lines, either darker or brighter than the background, was measured as a function of line width in a two alternative forced choice procedure. The four different symbol types correspond to two subjects in the two polarity conditions (bright seams or dark seams), as indicated in the figure legend. Viewing distance was 5.6 meters (18.5 ft), so that a 1 mm seam subtends a visual angle of 36.5 seconds of arc. The thick line in the figure shows the predictions of the model in this task. Again, the quality of the predictions is quite good.

Figure 15 shows data and model predictions for a character discrimination task performed at a range of visual eccentricities, from Lubin and Bergen (1991, 1993). This study was run in support of a NASA effort to assess aircraft cockpit display designs for conditions such as those in which the pilot may be fixating at a point outside the aircraft, but needs to retrieve information from an alphanumeric display at the same time. The stimuli were uppercase characters adapted from the Macintosh Helvetica 14 point font to accurately replicate the size and bitmap pattern of the Size A characters described in the Apache Longbow Crew Systems Interface Document (1989).

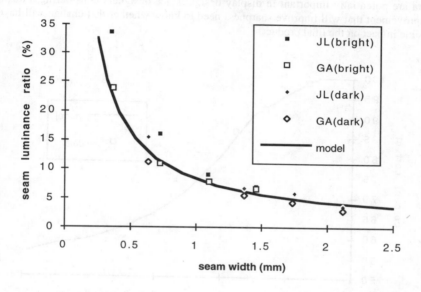

Figure 14. Model predictions on seam visibility data from Alphonse and Lubin (1992).

A small fixation mark (+) was continuously present at the center of the screen. During each trial a single character was flashed on for 167 msec, at an eccentricity *e* either to the right or to the left of the fixation point. This direction, as well as the identity of the character, was randomly varied from trial to trial. The eccentricity *e* remained constant within a session, as did the luminance of the characters and background. The subject's task was to identify, with a keypress, which of two possible characters was presented. A session ended when each of the four possible combinations of character identity and position had been presented *n* times, where *n* is typically 50.

The open squares in Figure 15 show data for one subject in an O vs. Q discrimination task, under lighting conditions of 10 fcd illuminance, and 6 fL average screen luminance. The solid curve shows the predictions of the model. The model performance is quite good in this test of the model's ability to predict changes in performance as a function of position in the visual field.

Figure 16 shows data and model predictions for an edge sharpness discrimination task of Carlson and Cohen (1980). In this task, observers were asked to discriminate a change in sharpness of an intensity edge as a function of the base sharpness of that edge. These data are potentially important in display design, since designers considering a display improvement that will improve sharpness need to know whether that change will have a visible impact on the final product.

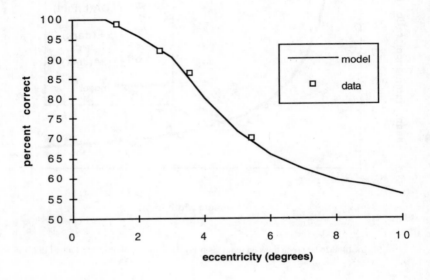

Figure 15. Data and model predictions for character discrimination as a function of eccentricity. From Lubin and Bergen (1991, 1993)

In this task, the stimuli are vertical edges, with a horizontal cross-section that can be described as an error function (erf):

$$\text{erf}(x) = \frac{2}{\sqrt{\pi}} \int_0^x \exp\left(-t^2\right) dt. \tag{11}$$

The sharpness of the edge in this expression is controlled by the following parameterization for x:

$$x = \frac{d\pi f_c}{\sqrt{\log(2)}} \tag{12}$$

where d indexes the distance across the edge image in degrees and f_c is the frequency at which the modulation transfer function for the edge has fallen to one half its maximum. Plotted in Figure 16 against starting values of f_c (labeled f1 in the figure), are normalized values for the threshold change in f_c, plotted as (f2-f1)/f1, where f2 is the value of f_c for an edge that is just discriminable from an edge with an f_c value of f1. Different symbol types are for different observers and viewing distances. The curve through the data points shows the predictions of the model and indicates good predictive power for the model in this task.

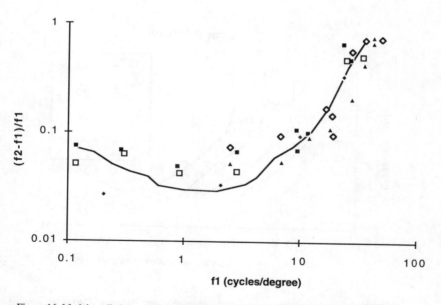

Figure 16. Model predictions on Carlson and Cohen (1980) edge sharpness discrimination data.

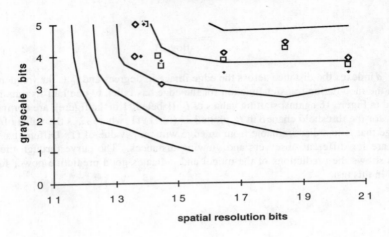

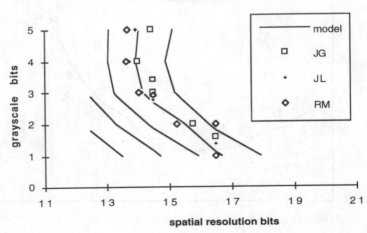

Figure 17. Visibility of quantization artifacts, with and without error diffusion. Curves are iso-JND contours from the model, with JND value indicated next to each contour. From Gille *et al.* (1994).

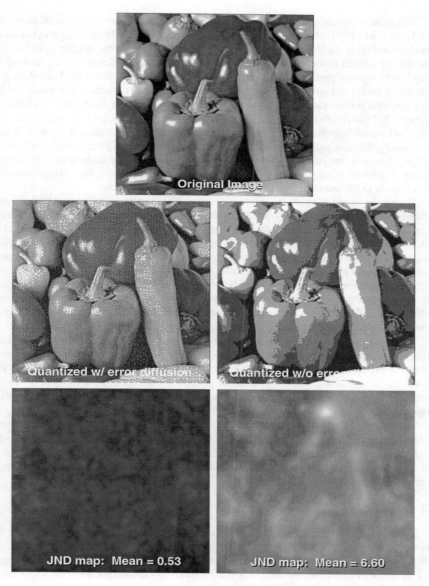

Figure 18. Sample images and JND maps from resolution/greyscale tradeoff experiment (Gille *et al.*, 1994). Input image has been quantized with and without error diffusion. Corresponding JND maps show the relative visibility of artifacts from each.

The final experiment to be reported in this set of detection and discrimination results is a Gille *et al.* (1994) study designed to assess visibility trade-offs between grayscale and pixel resolution in the design and manufacture of displays. In some display systems, it is possible at a fixed manufacturing cost to trade-off grayscale resolution (i.e., number of gray levels) against pixel resolution (i.e., number of pixels per unit area). Therefore, it is extremely useful to know the design point along this trade-off function that produces the best possible image quality. One way to answer this question is to plot, as shown in Figure 17, "iso-JND" contours in a two dimensional resolution vs. grayscale design space, where each contour represents the set of grayscale and resolution degradations that are equally discriminable from an "ideal" (high resolution, high grayscale) reference image. Because one can also plot the "iso-cost" contour in this same space, the design choice is reduced to the simple task of choosing the point along the iso-cost contour that corresponds to the minimum value from the underlying JND surface.

To test the model's ability to produce accurate JND contours in this two dimensional design space, Gille *et al.* (1994) collected data in which discrimination thresholds were measured between an original reference image and an image that had been degraded in resolution and/or grayscale, in order to determine empirically the location of the 1 JND contour. As shown by the two panels in Figure 17, this experiment was performed both with and without *error diffusion*, a dithering technique illustrated in Figure 18.

The plotted points in each panel of Figure 17 show the experimental results for each dithering condition, with the different symbol types for three different subjects, as indicated in the legend. In both plots, the grouping of these data points along the 1 JND contour indicates excellent predictive performance by the model.

It is also interesting to note the overall improvement in image quality that results from error diffusion, as seen by the shift of all JND contours to the lower resolution/grayscale corner of the error diffusion plot in the bottom panel of Figure 17, compared with the results in the top panel. This improvement is demonstrated in Figure 18, both by visual comparison of the two quantized images, and by inspection of the accompanying JND maps that show a much lower average JND value for the error diffused image.

The plots in Figure 17 show that the model can accurately predict discrimination performance even among complex images that are undergoing complex sets of distortions. In the next section, it will be shown that the model's ability to handle complex images is not limited to discrimination predictions, but extends to predictions of subjective image quality ratings as well.

3.2.   Rating Data

The first set of rating data to which the model was applied was from a study by Snyder *et al.* (1982) in which trained government image analysts were asked to rate the quality of aerial imagery as a function of distortions in both noise and blur, as illustrated in Figure 19. These analysts are extensively trained to rate images according to a functional quality scale called NIIRS (National Image Interpretability Rating Scale) which assigns a number from 1 to 10 to an image, based on the level of detail that they estimate would be visible on objects of interest. For example, by assigning a NIIRS rating of 5 to an image, an analyst is estimating that discriminations would be possible between objects such as different kinds of railroad cars (e.g., gondola vs. flat). With a NIIRS rating of 6, the analyst would be able to identify an automobile as either a sedan or a station wagon, while at a NIIRS 8, the windshield wipers on that vehicle would be visible.

For each of several images, 15 trained analysts NIIRS-rated the original image, as well as 25 degraded versions of that image (five noise levels × five blur levels). These ratings for each degraded image can be described in terms of the difference in NIIRS rating between that degraded image and the original image, a difference referred to here as the ΔNIIRS value. In Figure 20, the ΔNIIRS value for each degraded image is plotted against the average of the JND map between that degraded image and the original. If it is the case that this JND value is capturing the difference in rated image quality between the two images, then there should be a strong correlation in this scatter plot. This is in fact the case, as shown by the highly linear, tight clustering between ΔNIIRS and JNDs over most of the plot's range.

The last two experiments in this set of image quality rating studies were designed to test the extent to which the model can predict the perceptual magnitude of typical distortions introduced by processes of image compression and reconstruction. As illustrated in Figure 21, images in the first experiment were distorted by the addition of grayscale errors varying along two dimensions – noise range and block size. For each block size, the same randomly chosen grayscale error was added to each square block of pixels, with block sizes set at 1, 2, 4, 8, or 16 pixels on a side. (For clarity, only three of these block sizes are shown in the figure.) The random error for each block was generated by sampling uniformly from a grayscale noise range $\pm r$, where r could take on values 3, 4, 5, 6, or 7. (Again, only three of these are shown in the figure.) The result of these stimulus manipulations is, for each source image, a set of 25 (5 block sizes × 5 noise ranges) different distorted versions of that image.

Four different source images were used in the experiment. Figure 21 shows a small piece of one of the four, a portrait of a woman. Other source images included a view onto a city house, a harbour scene, and a still life with wine bottles. This set of images was chosen to span a wide range of typical television subject matter. In each session, there was free viewing of each pair of images (i.e., an undistorted image vs. one of the distorted versions of that image) for each of the 25 distortion conditions and each of the four images. Presentation order of the distortion conditions was random within each original image, but blocked by original image. There were four replications of each rating judgment, where each subject rated 1 (best) through 5 (worst), after a pre-screening in which each subject saw all versions of each image to establish a quality range.

Increasing Blur

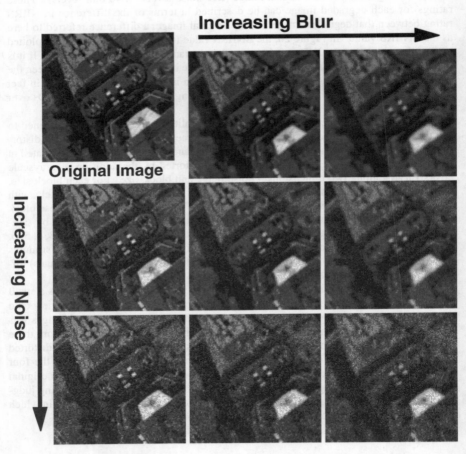

Original Image

Increasing Noise

Figure 19. Demonstration of stimulus manipulations for Snyder *et al.* (1982) NIIRS rating study.

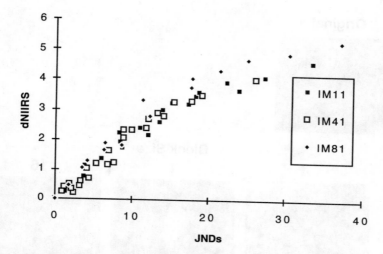

Figure 20. Delta NIIRS ratings vs. model JNDs for Snyder *et al.* (1982) data set. Different symbol types correspond to three different source images.

Figure 22 shows the results of this rating experiment, as compared against model JNDs and mean squared error. Each plotted symbol represents the rating data for one of the 25 distortion conditions, averaged across two subjects, four images and four replications per condition. Different symbol types correspond to different block sizes, as indicated in the plot legends.

The top plot in Figure 22 shows these rating results compared against the average JNDs from the model, as calculated by computing an average from the JND map between each distorted image and its undistorted source, and then averaging this JND value across the four images for each distortion condition. The correlation plot in the top panel of Figure 22 is then constructed by plotting the rating average against this JND average for each distortion condition. The excellent linear correlation shown between these two measures in the top panel of Figure 22 indicates that the JND measure is an excellent linear predictor of the subjective image quality ratings collected in this study.

The quality of this correlation is dramatized further by comparing the top panel of Figure 22 with the bottom panel, where the JND map for each comparison has been replaced by a map of the simple squared difference between the two comparison images. Here, the change in rating with block size is obviously not predicted, as indicated by the vertical spread of points for different block sizes at each of five MSE values corresponding to the five different noise ranges. These results give strong evidence that the model JND metric is much more suitable than MSE for assessing subjective image quality for imagery distorted by typical codec artifacts.

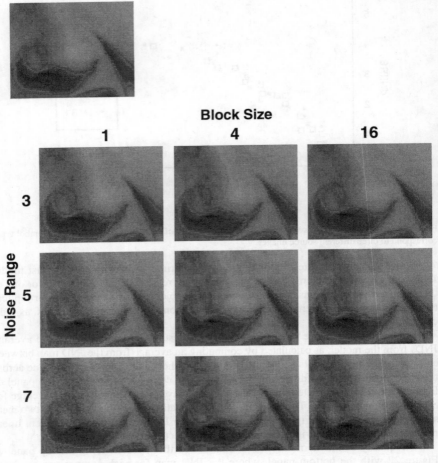

Figure 21. Demonstration of stimulus generation for block size vs. noise range rating experiment. From Lubin (1994).

In the last experiment of this series, a similar rating study was performed, except that the artificially introduced block distortions were replaced by distortion from actual JPEG compression. Figure 23 shows a typical source image from this study, together with codec images compressed at two different JPEG rates. Four source images consisting of aerial views were used in this experiment, to simulate the type of imagery that is returned from a remotely piloted reconnaissance vehicle.

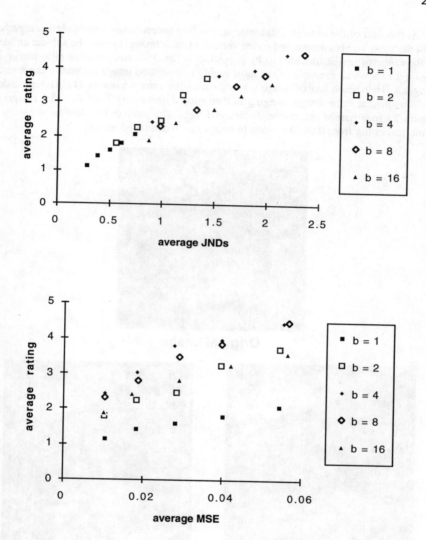

Figure 22. Rating results and model predictions from block size vs. noise level experiment (Lubin, 1994). Top plot shows ratings vs. model JNDs, bottom plot shows ratings vs. mean squared error.

278

At the start of the experimental session, the four source images were shown together with the most highly compressed codec version of each image, to give the subject an idea of the range of image qualities to be presented. (The 35:1 compression ratio image in Figure 23 shows an example of the most highly compressed image for one of the source images.) Then, each source image was shown on the same screen as 11 different codec versions of that same image, ranging in distortion detectability from the 35:1 image in Figure 23 to a barely detectable distortion level. The subject's task was to assign a numerical rating from 0 to 100 (worst to best) to each displayed image.

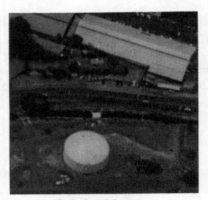

Original Image

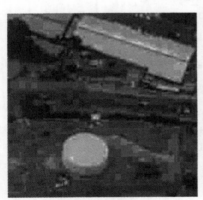

35:1 Compression

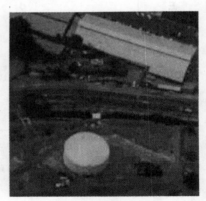

20:1 Compression

Figure 23. Sample source image and JPEG compressed stimuli for JPEG rating experiment.

Eight different subjects participated. The rating values on the abscissa of Figure 24 show averages across subjects for each image and compression level. The JND values on the ordinate of Figure 24 were calculated in the usual way; i.e., by computing the average from the JND map for each comparison between an original and distorted image.

It is interesting to observe in Figure 24 the extremely tight correlation between JNDs and ratings, even over the four different source images, as indicated in the figure and legend by the four different symbol types. The correlation is highly linear over most of the range, with some saturation in ratings at higher JND values, a feature that was also observed in the JND vs. ΔNIIRS results of Figure 20. As in that case, this saturation effect indicates increasing subjective indifference to increasingly large distortions in the images.

The plots in Figures 20, 22, and 24 all show excellent linear correlation between JNDs and ratings for different rating methodologies, source imagery and types of distortions. This success recommends the Sarnoff Visual Discrimination Model as a metric not only for the threshold discriminations for which it was calibrated, but also as a general image quality metric for subjective super-threshold evaluation of distorted images. It is especially useful when one considers that the standard alternative, mean squared error, is often easily fooled into predicting higher quality for images that in practice receive lower ratings.

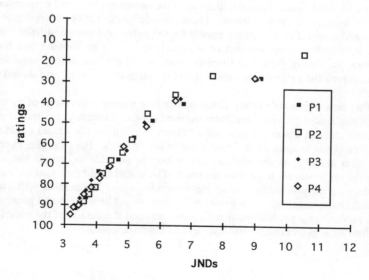

Figure 24. Ratings vs. model JNDs for JPEG rating experiment. Four different symbol types correspond to four different source images.

4. Future Directions

The visual discrimination model described in this report has been designed and tested to predict visibility of luminance differences between static input images. Working versions of the model have also been implemented that predict differences along two additional dimensions: time and color. The temporal extension of the model is especially useful for MPEG compression work, since it allows prediction of the visibility of temporal artifacts between an input and an output image sequence. These two model extensions will be described in future reports.

In addition to these extensions to additional stimulus dimensions, there are various model refinements planned that will help improve performance even with the static luminance model. Primary among these is the modeling of interactions between the different pathways in the model. There is abundant evidence, summarized in Lubin (1992), that inhibitory interactions exist between different orientation and motion channels. These are relatively simple to implement in the existing model architecture, and would help improve discrimination predictions for some kinds of complex stimuli.

In addition to these model enhancements, it is also important and interesting to consider some model simplifications, especially considering the computational burden associated with a multi-frame, multi-colorplane, complete discrimination model. For example, parametric studies are planned to determine the decrement in model performance as a function of increasing simplification. These include: removal of separate orientation channels, and removal of everything except for the optics and sampling front end, to be replaced by a simple mean squared error calculation. It is anticipated that for many applications, the first of these two simplifications would produce little noticeable decrement in accuracy for a significant imporvement in computation speed, and should thus be pursued.

Another area of possible future development is to augment the range of visual tasks for which the model provides performance predictions. Currently, the model predicts performance only in discrimination tasks. Future versions of the model could include performance predictions in identification and/or search tasks. For example, to create an identification model from this architecture, it may be possible to include internal templates in the set of stimuli to be discriminated. The model could then return a confusion matrix showing the probability that an input stimulus would be confused with each possible match in the target set. This model refinement would help the model generate more accurate performance predictions that take into account the details of the visual task in applications such as reconnaissance and medical image diagnosis.

Acknowledgement

This research was supported in part by NASA and by the National Information Display Laboratory (NIDL).

References

1. A. Ahumada, Jr. and A. B. Watson, "Equivalent noise model for contrast detection and discrimination," *J. Opt. Soc. Am. [A]* **2** (1985) 1133-1139.
2. G. A. Alphonse and J. Lubin, "Psychophysical requirements for seamless tiled large-screen displays,"*Society for Information Display International Symposium Digest of Technical Papers* **23** (1992) 941-944.
3. P. G. J. Barten, "The SQRI method: a new method for the evaluation of visible resolution on a display," *Proceedings of the Society for Information Display* **30** (1987) 253-262.
4. P. G. J. Barten, "Subjective image quality of high-definition television pictures," *Proceedings of the Society for Information Display* **31** (1990) 239-243.
5. O. M. Blackwell and H. R. Blackwell, "Visual performance data for 156 normal observers of various ages" *J. Illum. Engr. Soc.* **61** (1971) 3-13.
6. A. Bradley and I. Ohzawa, "A comparison of contrast detection and discrimination," *Vision Res.* **26** (1986) 991-997.
7. P. J. Burt and E. H. Adelson, "The Laplacian pyramid as a compact image code," *IEEE Transactions on Communications* **COM-31** (1983) 532-540.
8. C. Carlson and R. Cohen, "A simple psychophysical model for predicting the visibility of displayed information," *Proceedings of the Society for Information Display* **21** (1980) 229-245.
9. *Crew Systems Interface Document for the Apache Longbow*, Volume 5, Revision A, Controls and Displays Management, 22 December 1989, McDonnell Douglas Helicopter Company, Mesa, AZ.
10. S. Daly, "The visible differences predictor: an algorithm for the assessment of image fidelity," in *Digital Images and Human Vision*, ed. A. B. Watson (MIT Press, Cambridge, MA, 1993), pp. 179-206.
11. S. Daly, "Quantitative performance assessment of an algorithm for the determination of image fidelity," *Society for Information Display International Symposium Digest of Technical Papers* **24** (1993) 317-320.
12. R. L. DeValois, E. W. Yund, and N. Hepler, "The orientation and direction selectivity of cells in macaque visual cortex," *Vision Res.* **22** (1982) 531-544.
13. J. M. Foley and G. E. Legge, "Contrast detection and near-threshold discrimination in human vision," *Vision Res.* **21** (1981) 1041-1053.
14. W. T. Freeman and E. H. Adelson, "The design and use of steerable filters," *IEEE Transactions on Pattern Analysis and Machine Intelligence* **13** (1991) 891-906.
15. J. Gille, R. Martin, and J. Larimer, "Spatial resolution, grayscale, and error diffusion trade-offs: impact on display system design,"*Conference record of the 1994 International Display Research Conference*, Oct. 10-13, 1994, Monterey, CA.
16. J. Hoekstra, D. P. J. van der Goot, G. van der Brink, and F. A. Bilsen, "The influence of the number of cycles upon the visual contrast detection threshold for spatial sinewave patterns,"*Vision Research* **14** (1974) 365-368.

17. D. C. Hood and M. A. Finkelstein, "Sensitivity to light," in *Handbook of Perception and Human Performance*, ed. K. Boff, L. Kaufman, and J. Thomas (Wiley and Sons, New York, NY, 1986).

18. G. E. Legge and J. M. Foley, "Contrast masking in human vision," *J. Opt. Soc. Am* **70** (1980) 1458-1470.

19. J. Lubin, *Interactions among motion-sensitive mechanisms in human vision*, Unpublished doctoral dissertation, University of Pennsylvania, 1992.

20. J. Lubin, "The use of psychophysical data and models in the analysis of display system performance," in *Digital Images and Human Vision*, ed. A. B. Watson (MIT Press, Cambridge, MA, 1993), pp. 163-178.

21. J. Lubin, "A practical vision model for the evaluation and optimization of image compression schemes," Invited talk, 1994 Optical Society of America Annual Meeting, Dallas, TX.

22. J. Lubin and J. R. Bergen, "Pattern discrimination in the fovea and periphery," *Investigative Ophthalmology and Visual Science Supplement* **32** (1991) 1024.

23. J. Lubin and J. R. Bergen, "Cockpit display visibility modeling," *NASA Contractor Report 177623* (NASA/Ames Research Center, Moffet Field, CA, 1993).

24. J. Lubin and J. Nachmias, "Discrimination contours in an f/3f stimulus space," *Investigative Ophthalmology and Visual Science Supplement* **31** (1990) 409.

25. J. Nachmias and R. V. Sansbury, "Grating contrast: Discrimination may be better than detection,"*Vision Res.* **14** (1974) 1039-1042.

26. A. van Meeteren and J. J. Vos, "Contrast sensitivity at low luminances,"*Vision Res.* **12** (1972) 825-833.

27. K. Nielsen, A. Watson, and A. Ahumada, Jr., "Application of a computable model of human spatial vision to phase discrimination," *J. Opt. Soc. Am. [A]* **2** (1985) 1600-1606.

28. L. A. Olzak, "Interactions between spatially tuned mechanisms: converging evidence," *J. Opt. Soc. Am. [A]* **2** (1985) 1551-1559.

29. E. Peli, "Contrast in complex images," *J. Opt. Soc. Am. [A]* **7** (1990) 2032-2040.

30. G. C. Phillips and H. R. Wilson, "Orientation bandwidths of spatial mechanisms measured by masking," *J. Opt. Soc. Am. [A]* **1** (1984) 226-232.

31. D. Sagi and S. Hochstein, "Discriminability of suprathreshold compound spatial frequency gratings," *Vision Res.* **23** (1983) 1595-1606.

32. O. H. Schade, "Electro-optical characteristics of television systems. I. Characteristics of vision and visual systems," *RCA Review* **9** (1948) 5-37.

33. H. L. Snyder, M. E. Maddox, D. I. Shedivy, J. A. Turpin, J. J. Burke, and R. N. Strickland, "Digital image quality and interpretability: database and hardcopy studies," *Optical Engineering* **21** (1982) 14-22.

34. D. J. Tolhurst and L. P. Barfield, "Interactions between spatial frequency channels," *Vision Res.* **18** (1977) 951-958.

35. A. Watson, "Summation of grating patches indicates many types of detector at one retinal location," *Vision Res.* **22** (1982) 17-26.

36. A. Watson, "Detection and recognition of simple spatial forms," In Physical and Biological Processing of Images, ed. O. Braddick and A. Sleigh (Springer-Verlag, Berlin, 1983.)

37. A. Watson, "The cortex transform: rapid computation of simulated neural images," *Computer Vision, Graphics, and Image Processing* **39** (1987) 311-327.

38. G. Westheimer, "The eye as an optical instrument," in *Handbook of Perception and Human Performance*, ed. K. Boff, L. Kaufman, and J. Thomas (Wiley and Sons, New York, NY, 1986).

39. H. R. Wilson, "Psychophysical models of spatial vision and hyperacuity," in *Vision and Visual Dysfunction; Vol. 10: Spatial Vision.*, ed. D. Regan (CRC Press, Inc., Boston, MA, 1991).

40. H. R. Wilson and J. R. Bergen, "A four mechanism model for threshold spatial vision," *Vision Res.* **19** (1979) 19-32.

41. H. R. Wilson, D. K. McFarlane, and G. C. Phillips, "Spatial tuning of orientation selective units estimated by oblique masking," *Vision Res.* **23** (1983) 873-882.

42. H. R. Wilson and D. Regan, "Spatial-frequency adaptation and grating discrimination: predictions of a line element model," *J. Opt. Soc. Am. [A]* **1** (1984) 1091-1096.

TEMPLATE RECOGNITION BASED ON EXPANSION MATCHING WITH NEURAL LATTICE IMPLEMENTATION

JEZEKIEL BEN-ARIE and K. RAGHUNATH RAO
Department of Electrical and Computer Engineering,
Illinois Institute of Technology,
3301 S. Dearborn St., Chicago IL 60616 , USA

This chapter describes a novel method for template matching based on expanding the image with respect to basis functions that are shifted versions of the template. The coefficients of such a non-orthogonal expansion directly signify the presence of the template at the corresponding location in the image. This method, known as Expansion Matching (EXM), optimizes a new similarity measure called the Discriminative Signal-to-Noise Ratio (DSNR). The DSNR is a more practical criterion for matching tasks than the conventional SNR, since it penalizes all off-center responses, including off-center responses to the pattern itself. Thus, in comparison to the widely used correlation or matched filtering approach, EXM yields significantly better matching results with sharp peaks and minimal off-center response, even in conditions of noise, superposition and occlusion. EXM is shown to be equivalent to minimal squared error restoration via Wiener filtering, thus offering an efficient method for computing the expansion coefficients. EXM can also be implemented by a set of neural lattices. These parallel architectures are capable of multiple-scale Gaussian smoothing of multi-dimensional signals, and are used in an adaptive configuration to expand the image into template-similar basis functions. EXM is also extended for the simultaneous recognition of multiple templates using a single filter. Here, a single filter is designed to elicit user-defined responses from a given set of templates, while optimizing the DSNR criterion.

1. Introduction

Matching is a fundamental operation in any application that involves detection or recognition of patterns in multi-dimensional signals. Matching of pictorial templates is extensively used in many vision systems. Simply put, template matching is the process of comparing a given scene sub-image (could be a visual, infrared, radar or sonar image or any other representation of a target scene) and a known template (typically a stored model of the target) with the objective of detecting and locating the template in the input scene image. Model-based image understanding usually requires matching a database containing a set of models (represented here as templates) against a corresponding image pattern. Also, methods that employ primitive features, such as edges, corners, junctions, etc., employ template matching in the form of edge, corner and other feature detectors.

One can regard matching as assessing the similarity between two signals. Template recognition can then be performed by locating the peak in such a similarity measure. The problem is to develop a similarity measure which is robust in conditions such as additive noise, missing data (occlusion) etc. In this chapter, we introduce a novel matching method which maximizes a more practical similarity measure than the traditional approaches. This method is based on signal **expansion**. Unlike the traditional correlation approach, which is based on **signal projection**, the new similarity measure is based on **signal decomposition**. In other words, the new similarity measure signifies how much of the template signal is **contained** in the given signal.

1.1. Traditional Template Matching Methods

One simple method for template matching is called template subtraction[1,2]. Here, the absolute difference between the image and the template is used to detect the template. Since absolute control is required over the image intensity, such a method is useful only in stationary and perfect imaging conditions.

A far more popular method is matching-by-correlation, which is considered to be more robust to image degradations such as noise, illumination effects and minor distortions. Almost all the contemporary applications of template matching currently employ some sort of correlation matching technique (also known as matched filtering). The reason correlation matching is so popular is that for a given pattern, it provides the optimal filter which maximizes the Signal-to-Noise Ratio (SNR). As elaborated in Section 2, the approach of SNR optimization has a serious drawback since it maximizes the ratio between the filter's response to the signal at the pattern's center, with respect to the overall energy of the filter's response to the noise. This approach overlooks the filter's off-center response to the pattern which can be quite substantial. As demonstrated in Section 6, this approach results in filters that respond to their matched patterns with broad peaks which are quite hard to detect and to localize accurately. Correlation is also quite sensitive to partial occlusion, scale and orientation of the feature, and to the absolute gray level of the template. Normalizing the correlation[1] with respect to the template and local image variances, alleviates most of the gray level sensitivity of the matching at the cost of severe additional computation, but does not improve the sharpness of the matching peaks. Section 6 provides illustrative experiments that demonstrate this effect.

1.2. Discriminative Signal-to-Noise Ratio: A New Similarity Measure

To derive an optimal processing strategy, it is necessary to formulate a set of mathematical criteria and conditions that exactly represent the desired objective. In our case, the requirement is that the optimal linear processing should respond to the given template only at the center of the template, and have minimal off-center response. In addition, as in the case of the matched filter, the response to additive noise should be minimal all over the image. Once these requirements have been formulated, optimization of the criteria subject to the previously mentioned conditions will yield the optimal processing strategy.

In Section 3, we introduce a **new similarity measure** called Discriminative Signal-to-Noise Ratio (DSNR). The DSNR at a certain location of the image measures how much of the stored template is contained at that location of the image. Thus, the DSNR is also a measure of how similar the given image is to the stored template shifted to that location. Furthermore, optimizing the DSNR incorporates a competitive strategy since it involves decomposition of the signal into basis functions which compete in extracting energy from the image. Thus, the optimal matching output is sharp and impulse-like at the center of the template, with almost no response off the center. This optimal DSNR matching method is found to be exactly equivalent to the non-orthogonal expansion which is described in the following subsection.

1.3. Non-Orthogonal Expansion For Template Matching

Non-orthogonal Basis Functions (BFs) can be employed very effectively to represent signals. It is a well known fact that natural signals and images in particular, contain many redundancies, i.e. repeated patterns or highly correlated waveforms. Image compression techniques exploit these redundancies and often employ orthogonal representations such as Fourier, cosine or orthogonal wavelet transforms, primarily due to the ease of implementation. If the constraint on orthogonality is removed, the BFs are free to assume any shape and configuration (as long as they are independent and complete) and can be made to match the features in the signal. To obtain a direct relation between the expansion coefficients and the structural entities in signals (e.g. image features, speech patterns), it is reasonable to expand the signal with BFs that match the signal features. This requires a non-orthogonal representation, since the signal features are non-orthogonal in general.

Some specialized non-orthogonal expansions have been previously used for image compression and texture discrimination[3,4]. We have developed a generalized non-orthogonal expansion scheme, in which a complete BF set is formed using shifted/dilated versions of an arbitrary given signal[11,14,15,16]. This expansion can be implemented by a set of neural lattice architectures as described in Section 7. We use a special case of the generalized expansion scheme for template matching. The BFs suggested here are all spatially shifted versions (without dilation) of the template to be matched. Orthogonal expansions cannot be used here, since the shifted versions of the template are almost always non-orthogonal. If the signal is expanded in terms of this template-similar bases in the minimum squared error sense, **the magnitude of the coefficients of this expansion directly signify the presence of the template at the corresponding candidate locations**[5-7]. Expansion with this specially chosen template-similar basis set is shown to be exactly equivalent to optimizing the DSNR similarity measure[6].

1.4. Expansion Matching vs. Correlation Matching

Traditional correlation matching optimizes the SNR, which does not consider off-center response of the matched filter to the template itself. In contrast, the DSNR penalizes any filter response off the center of the template. Thus, the ideal response (in terms of DSNR) in the case of perfect matching is simply a delta function. As shown in Section 5, **the linear operation which maximizes the DSNR is expansion with BFs that are all similar to the pattern.** For this reason, Expansion Matching (EXM) generally provides better results in comparison to the traditional correlation matching (which maximizes the SNR). As demonstrated in Section 6, EXM outperforms correlation matching by a wide margin and yields results which are better by more than 25 dB. Furthermore, EXM alleviates the problems of localization, spurious responses and partial occlusion to a large extent. Results show that templates that are occluded more than 85% are successfully recognized with expansion and spurious responses are very much attenuated[5-7]. Localization is greatly enhanced with expansion and provides very sharp peaks even under severe occlusion (see Fig. 4).

It should be noted here that expansion is an operation which is fundamentally different from correlation. It is a **decomposition** operation while correlation is a **projection** operation. These operations are identical only when the basis set is orthogonal. Section 3.2 presents a simple two-vector example that illustrates this difference clearly. In effect, expansion diverts the signal energy into the nearest matching BF (shifted candidate template) and thus, neighboring BFs have low coefficients. The response is therefore sharp and well localized in the neighborhood if there is a match. On the other hand, if the template does not appear in the image, the signal energy is equally shared amongst all the neighboring BFs.

The decomposition capability of expansion matching also results in an improved performance in matching superimposed patterns. Such signals frequently occur in audio, sonar and radar signals. Since the signal patterns are substantially altered by superposition, correlation proves ineffective in such conditions, while expansion yields near-ideal results. An example of matching superimposed patterns is given in Section 6.

1.5. Expansion Matching Implemented by Image Restoration

Optimizing the DSNR and the template-similar non-orthogonal expansion have a strong relation to Minimum Squared Error (MSE) restoration using the Wiener filter[5-7]. If we regard the template as the blurring function, and 'restore' the image (although the image is assumed to be sharp and does not need any restoration), the **'restored' image corresponds to the set of non-orthogonal expansion coefficients described above**. This method is more elaborated in Section 6 and it is proved that the template-similar MSE image expansion is precisely implemented by MSE restoration (Wiener filtering). Employing restoration techniques provides efficient means to overcome the complexity of non-orthogonal image decomposition in the special case where the BFs are a template-similar dense set. Basically, the complexity of the expansion matching process implemented via MSE restoration is identical to that of correlation-matching, i.e. a linear shift-invariant filtering process.

1.6. Expansion Matching Implemented by Neural Lattices

Unlike the coefficients of orthogonal expansions which are determined simply by projecting the corresponding BF onto the signal, non-orthogonal expansion entails simultaneous solution of a set of equations Eq. (15). Since the number of equations required is proportional to the number of BFs, one might be required to deal with a very large set of equations which is computationally prohibitive. Two approaches for the solution of this problem are discussed in this chapter. The first approach is based upon the previously mentioned equivalence of expansion and restoration. This allows the usage of DFT techniques for the expansion, which greatly simplifies the solution. The second approach is a hardware implementation using a set of neural architectures that find the expansion coefficients with minimal squared error. This implementation transforms the set of equations for non-orthogonal expansion into a minimization problem which is solved by a gradient descent method.

The basic architectural component is the linear lattice (also called a web[11]) which generates a dense set of multiple-scale Gaussian smoothed versions of the input signal. Section 7.1 introduces the lattice structure which is composed of an array of linear summers (in our terminology, Processing Elements or PEs) that are arranged in consecutive layers. This lattice directly produces the scale-space description of the input signal that was originally obtained by Witkin[12]. The fundamental principle of operation of the lattice is based on the Central Limit Theorem (CLT)[13]. It is well known from the CLT that the cumulative convolution of many small kernels will result in a Gaussian convolution. The lattice structure performs such a repetitive convolution, and thus generates quite accurate Gaussian smoothing at any required scale (Gaussian standard deviation). Section 7.2 briefly describes the various forms of the lattice.

Section 7.3 describes the adaptive lattice which is used for signal expansion by arbitrary BFs[16]. The basic principle is that any arbitrary signal with compact support can be represented by a linear combination of Gaussian BFs (called a Gaussian Set or GS) with any desired accuracy. Furthermore, this arbitrary signal represented by a GS can itself be used to generate BFs to represent any given signal. In this case, the BFs used are Gaussian Set Wavelets (GSWs), which are translated and/or dilated versions of the original GS. Thus, the adaptive lattice offers a scheme for representing any given signal using translated/dilated versions of any arbitrary signal as a basis set.

In the implementation of expansion matching with the neural lattices, the stored template is represented by a GS, and a complete basis is formed by all translated versions of this GS (without any dilation). The adaptive lattice performs the gradient descent algorithm and yields the desired minimum squared error expansion coefficients.

1.7. Expansion Matching for Multiple Templates

In many applications, template recognition is required within a limited set of template classes. For example, a class of templates could be defined as the set of views or instances of an object thus providing invariant or generic recognition of this object respectively. In many cases, it is possible[18] to formulate a single filter or a small number of filters to perform a classification task. Compared to the paradigm of having to perform separate matching for every template, this approach is more attractive.

In Section 8, the DSNR similarity measure is extended to more than one template. The response to each individual template can be constrained to any desired value, and optimizing the DSNR criterion results in a generalized formulation of a single filter that can respond to multiple templates. For the special case of a single template this method reduces to expansion matching discussed previously. Special cases of the multiple-template EXM filter exactly correspond to previous formulations[17,18,19] depending on the assumed noise model.

2. The Traditional SNR and Correlation Matching

Correlation (also known as matched filtering)[1,2,13] is probably the most widely used method for template recognition in the field of computer vision. Correlation matching has a long history[21] and has been used extensively for character recognition, target recognition, stereo mapping, map-matching for navigation purposes, and change detection.

The problem of template matching can be formulated as follows: Given a $M \times M$ discrete image $s(x,y)$, it is desired to find a region which matches a two-dimensional template $\psi(x,y)$. Let the signal $s(x,y)$ contain the template at a certain location (x_0,y_0) and additive noise $\lambda(x,y)$. In correlation matching, a filter $h(x,y)$ is convolved with the signal to generate maximal response at the location (x_0,y_0). The filter response $z(x,y)$ is given by:

$$
\begin{aligned}
z(x,y) &= s(x,y) * h(x,y) \\
&= c_\psi \psi(x - x_0, y - y_0) * h(x,y) + \lambda(x,y) * h(x,y) \\
&= z_\psi(x,y) + z_\lambda(x,y)
\end{aligned}
\tag{1}
$$

where $*$ denotes discrete convolution and c_ψ is an amplitude scale factor.

The Signal-to-Noise Ratio (SNR) is defined[1,2,13] by the ratio between the energy of the response at the template center (x_0,y_0) and the energy of the overall noisy response:

$$
SNR = 10 \log \frac{\left[z_\psi(x_0,y_0)\right]^2}{\frac{1}{M^2} \sum_M \sum_M \left[z_\lambda(i,j)\right]^2} .
\tag{2}
$$

Optimization of this criterion[22] yields the optimal filter $h(x,y)$, which has a Fourier transform given by[1,2,13]

$$
H(u,v) = c_h \frac{\overline{\Psi}(u,v)}{S_{\lambda\lambda}(u,v)}
\tag{3}
$$

where $S(u,v)$ is the Fourier transform of $s(x,y)$, $S_{\lambda\lambda}(u,v)$ is the spectral density of the noise $\lambda(x,y)$, c_h is a constant and the bar symbol denotes complex conjugation. If the noise $\lambda(x,y)$ is wide sense stationary and white, $S_{\lambda\lambda}(u,v)$ is constant, and the optimal filter $h(x,y)$ is simply the mirror image of the template $\psi(x,y)$.

There is a **major drawback** in the matched filtering formulation. The response $z_\psi(x,y)$ at locations other than (x_0,y_0) is completely overlooked. For the purpose of template matching, these responses are **also unwanted and should also be considered as 'noise'**. Experimental results in Section 6 confirm that correlation can generate broad peaks and z_ψ is quite substantial in the neighborhood of (x_0,y_0) and should not be overlooked. In addition, correlation generates many spurious peaks that do not correspond to the correct feature, and interfere with the detection process. Moreover, the correct peaks are not sharp enough and their localization is often inaccurate. The peak response of correlation also depends on the magnitude of the sub-image (expressed here as c_ψ). In order to eliminate this effect and to somewhat enhance the sharpness of the peaks, it has been suggested to employ[1,2,11] the normalized correlation coefficient $\rho(x,y)$

$$
\rho(x,y) = \frac{s(x,y) * h(x,y)}{\left[\sum_{M_x} \sum_{M_y} h^2(i,j) \bullet \sum_{M_x} \sum_{M_y} s^2(x+i, y+j)\right]^{\frac{1}{2}}}
\tag{4}
$$

where M_x and M_y define the region of the template. The correlation coefficient is bounded by $-1 \le \rho \le 1$. Moreover, $|\rho| = 1$ iff $h(x,y) = c_\psi s(x,y)$ within the region of the template. As demonstrated in Section 6, even normalized correlation does not produce ideal results and is inferior to the recognition by expansion approach. Furthermore, normalized correlation requires a much larger amount of computation compared to unnormalized correlation.

3. DSNR and Why Expansion Matching Is Better

The conclusion of the previous section is that matched filtering (or the correlation approach) maximizes the ratio of signal to noise, where the noise does not include the off-center response of the filter to the template. According to this approach, a filter that provides a very broad peak is equivalent to a filter that provides a sharp peak with the same amplitude, the power of the noisy response being the same. Thus, a better SNR definition which provides a better measure of matching quality, **should define as 'noise', any response that is not located at the sub-image's center.** Accordingly, we introduce a new similarity measure called the Discriminative Signal-to-Noise Ratio (DSNR).

3.1. Definition of the DSNR Criterion

In the framework of the correlation matching defined in Section 2, we define the new *DSNR* for the correlation output as

$$DSNR_{cor} = 10\log \frac{\left[z(x_0,y_0)\right]^2}{\frac{1}{M^2-1}\sum_{(i,j)\ne(x_0,y_0)}\sum \left[z(i,j)\right]^2} \ . \tag{5}$$

Thus, the DSNR criterion penalizes any response off the center (x_0, y_0) and increases with larger on-center response. This is equivalent to defining any off-center response as unwanted 'noisy' response. The center of the template is assumed to be the origin, unless otherwise mentioned.

3.2. Expansion Matching vs. Correlation: An Illustrative Example

As a prelude to understanding the better performance of EXM over correlation, we present a simplified example using two multi-dimensional vectors, drawn as two-dimensional vectors in Fig. 1. The signal (or image) S is matched against the candidate templates Ψ_1 and Ψ_2 (which are normalized to a unit magnitude, i.e. $|\Psi_1| = |\Psi_2| = 1$), by two methods: correlation and EXM.

In Fig. 1a, which represents correlation matching, the projections of S onto Ψ_1 and Ψ_2 are the results of tentatively matching the signal with the candidate templates. In Fig. 1b, which represents EXM, the signal S is **decomposed into its components along the candidate template-vectors which are regarded as BFs.** The fundamental difference between correlation and EXM, is that correlation is basically a projection operation which does not divert the energy of the signal to the most similar template as does expansion. The projection of S onto Ψ_2 depends only on Ψ_2 and does not consider Ψ_1 at all.

On the other hand, in EXM, neighboring BFs compete for the signal energy, and the closest matching BF (candidate shifted template) wins the largest coefficient, while the other BFs (in this example, only one) share the residual energy. Thus, in contrast to correlation, EXM yields a sharp peak at the template center and minimal off-center response. The only case where correlation and EXM are equivalent is when all the BFs are mutually orthogonal. Such a case is impractical, since natural templates (like real images or speech waveforms) seldom form mutually orthogonal functions when subjected to translations.

Referring to Fig. 1, it is assumed without loss of generality, that the signal S is more similar to Ψ_1 than to Ψ_2. Since images have only positive values, the vectors S, Ψ_1 and Ψ_2, have only positive components (even in their multi-dimensional formulation). Hence, the inner products $<\Psi_1,S>$, $<\Psi_2,S>$ and $<\Psi_1,\Psi_2>$ are all positive and the expressions for Discriminative SNR can be simplified. In the case of correlation matching the DSNR is expressed as:

$$DSNR_{cor} = 10\log\left(\frac{<Y_1,S>}{<Y_2,S>}\right)^2 \tag{6}$$

whereas the DSNR in expansion matching is:

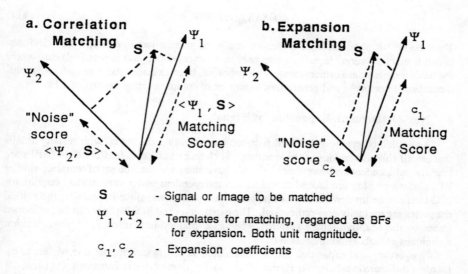

Figure 1. Expansion Matching versus Correlation: Two vector example.

$$DSNR_{exp} = 10\log\left(\frac{c_1}{c_2}\right)^2 . \tag{7}$$

From the geometry of the vectors in Fig. 1b, the coefficients c_1 and c_2 can be obtained from the equations:

$$c_1\Psi_1 = <\Psi_1,\mathbf{S}>\Psi_1 - c_2 R_{12}\Psi_1 \tag{8}$$

and

$$c_2\Psi_2 = <\Psi_2,\mathbf{S}>\Psi_2 - c_1 R_{12}\Psi_2; \text{ where } R_{12} = <\Psi_1,\Psi_2> \geq 0 . \tag{9}$$

Note that $|R_{12}| \leq 1$ always, since the BFs are assumed to be unit magnitude. By eliminating the vectors Ψ_1 and Ψ_2, and with a little manipulation[6] we can show that

$$\left(\frac{c_1}{c_2}\right)^2 = \left[\frac{<\Psi_1,\mathbf{S}> - R_{12}<\Psi_2,\mathbf{S}>}{<\Psi_2,\mathbf{S}> - R_{12}<\Psi_1,\mathbf{S}>}\right]^2 \geq \left[\frac{<\Psi_1,\mathbf{S}>}{<\Psi_2,\mathbf{S}>}\right]^2 \tag{10}$$

which implies that:

$$DSNR_{exp} \geq DSNR_{cor} \tag{11}$$

Thus the DSNR obtained from expansion is always greater than or equal to the DSNR obtained from correlation. Equality exists only in the exceptional (and impractical) case where the basis templates are orthonormal. This proof has been extended to more than two multi-dimensional vectors[5,7] and generalized to any set of complete template-similar BFs.

4. Non-Orthogonal Expansion of Signals

As explained previously, EXM is based on expanding the signal with respect to BFs that are all shifted versions of the template. Such an expansion is feasible if these BFs are linearly independent and complete[13,24]. We have shown[5,7] that the set of template-similar BFs that we employ are indeed complete and independent under very modest conditions. EXM cannot be implemented by orthogonal basis functions, since in practice, the shifted templates are mutually non-orthogonal. The expansion used in this paper can be performed either by the adaptive lattice system[11,14,15] as explained in Section 7, or by restoration techniques as elaborated in Section 6.

Non-orthogonal expansion can be formulated as follows: Suppose one wishes to estimate a d-dimensional discrete signal $s(x,y,...)$ by a set of basis functions $\{\psi_i(x,y,...)\}$ with the sum:

$$\hat{s}(x,y,...) = \sum_{i=1}^{m} c_i \psi_i(x,y,...); \quad (x,y,...) = 1...M \tag{12}$$

where $\{c_i\}$ are the coefficients of the expansion. The d-dimensional signal $s(x,y,...)$ is translated into a M^d-dimensional vector $\mathbf{S}$, the basis functions $\{\psi_i(x,y,...)\}$ are expressed by the basis vector set $\{\Psi_i\}$, and the approximation $\hat{s}$ by $\hat{\mathbf{S}}$. It is desired to obtain a representation with minimum squared error D given by the inner product:

$$D = < (\mathbf{S} - \hat{\mathbf{S}}), (\mathbf{S} - \hat{\mathbf{S}}) >= < (\mathbf{S} - \sum_{i=1}^{m} c_i \Psi_i), (\mathbf{S} - \sum_{i=1}^{m} c_i \Psi_i) > \quad . \tag{13}$$

From the orthogonality principle[2,13] we know that the approximation error $\mathbf{S} - \hat{\mathbf{S}}$ is orthogonal to the BFs. Alternatively, we can set $\partial D / \partial c_i = 0$ for $i = 1...m$. This yields the following set of m equations:

$$< (\mathbf{S} - \hat{\mathbf{S}}), \Psi_i >= 0; \; i = 1...m \quad . \tag{14}$$

This leads to a set of equations:

$$< \Psi_1, \Psi_1 > c_1 + < \Psi_1, \Psi_2 > c_2 + ... < \Psi_1, \Psi_m > c_m = < \mathbf{S}, \Psi_1 >$$
$$< \Psi_2, \Psi_1 > c_1 + < \Psi_2, \Psi_2 > c_2 + ... < \Psi_2, \Psi_m > c_m = < \mathbf{S}, \Psi_2 >$$
$$\cdots \quad \cdots \quad \cdots \cdots \quad \cdots \quad \cdots \quad \cdots \cdots \quad \cdots \quad \cdots ..=.. \quad \cdots$$
$$< \Psi_m, \Psi_1 > c_1 + < \Psi_m, \Psi_2 > c_2 + ... < \Psi_m, \Psi_m > c_m = < \mathbf{S}, \Psi_m > \quad . \tag{15}$$

As long as the set of BFs $\{\Psi_i\}$ is linearly independent, then the matrix $[\mathbf{R}_{\psi\psi}]_{ij} = [< \Psi_i, \Psi_j >]$ is positive definite and the above Eqs. (15) yield a unique solution for the coefficients c_i. Stability of the expansion is not a major consideration, since in practice, EXM is implemented via restoration techniques or the adaptive lattice architecture, both of which are regularized and stable solutions.

5. Expansion Matching

Let the given image $s(x,y)$ be expanded into a set of BFs that correspond to translated versions of the template, i.e. the template shifted to every candidate location. Then, the expansion coefficient obtained for a BF that corresponds to the template at a particular location, signifies the presence of the template at that location. Using the formulation in the previous section, the set $\{\Psi_i\}$ represents the translated templates. Ψ_i is a vector representation of $\psi(x - x_i, y - y_i)$, where (x_i, y_i) is the central location of the i-th translated template. In matrix notation, Eq. (15) is expressed as:

$$[\mathbf{R}_{\psi\psi}]\mathbf{C} \equiv [\Psi][\Psi]^T \mathbf{C} = [\Psi]\mathbf{S} \tag{16}$$

where the elements of the autocorrelation matrix are $[\mathbf{R}_{\psi\psi}]_{ij} = \langle \Psi_i, \Psi_j \rangle$, $\mathbf{C} = [c_1, c_2 \ldots c_{M^2}]^T$, $[\Psi] = [\Psi_1, \Psi_2 \ldots \Psi_{M^2}]^T$ and $\mathbf{S}$ is the M^2-dimensional vector formulation of the image $s(x,y)$.

The DSNR criterion with respect to the location (x_i, y_i) can be written for non-orthogonal expansion as

$$DSNR_{\exp} = 10 \log \left(\frac{c_i^2}{\frac{1}{M^2 - 1} \sum_{j \neq i}^{M^2} c_j^2} \right) \tag{17}$$

where the sub-image is considered as most similar to the basis function template Ψ_i and the remaining expansion coefficients are considered as 'noise'.

Given a template $\psi(x - x_l, y - y_l)$ to be recognized in the image, we seek the linear operator Θ that maximizes the DSNR. In matrix notation, the linear convolution is expressed as:

$$[\mathbf{S}]\Theta = \mathbf{C} \tag{18}$$

where $[\mathbf{S}]$ is a circulant matrix[5] derived by circulating the signal $\mathbf{S}^T$.

The DSNR optimization is detailed in reference[5] and the optimal DSNR linear filter Θ is found to be

$$\Theta = \tfrac{1}{k}\big[[\mathbf{S}]^T[\mathbf{S}]\big]^{-1}\mathbf{S}_l = \tfrac{1}{k}\big[\mathbf{R}_{SS}^T\big]^{-1}\mathbf{S}_l \tag{19}$$

where k is only a scaling factor (a scalar), $[\mathbf{R}_{ss}]$ is the autocorrelation matrix of the signal given by $[\mathbf{S}][\mathbf{S}]^T$, and $\mathbf{S}_l$ is the l-th column of $[\mathbf{S}]^T$.

The filter output is obtained from Eq. (18) as

$$\mathbf{C} = \tfrac{1}{k}\big[[\mathbf{S}]^T\big]^{-1}\mathbf{S}_l \ . \tag{20}$$

Also, if $\mathbf{S}_l$ is considered to be equal to the signal $\mathbf{S}$, Eq. (16) is reduced to

$$\mathbf{C} = \big[[\Psi]^T\big]^{-1}\mathbf{S}_l \ . \tag{21}$$

Thus, if $[\Psi] = k[\mathbf{S}]$, expansion by template-similar BFs as in Eq. (16) yields exactly the same results as optimal-DSNR filtering. This proves that maximal DSNR is obtained by expansion with BFs that are all similar to the template if the signal contains only the template. When the signal model has additive noise, the optimal filter is the Wiener filter described in Section 6 and the optimal expansion filter is slightly modified. Stability of the expansion is not a major consideration, since in practice, expansion matching is implemented via the Wiener filter, or by the adaptive lattice, both of which are regularized and stable solutions.

6. Restoration and the Equivalence to Expansion Matching

This section establishes the relationship between the restoration problem and the special case of non-orthogonal expansion that is suitable for matching. We deal with 1D functions for the sake of simplicity. However, the same formulation can easily be expanded to any number of dimensions.

Let a discrete function $s(x)$ be expanded by a set of self-similar basis functions $\{\psi_i(x)\}$

$$s(x) = \sum_{i=-\infty}^{\infty} c_i \psi_i(x) \ . \tag{22}$$

In our case, the BFs $\psi_i(x)$ are all shifted versions of the same template $\psi(x)$ i.e.,

$$\psi_i(x) = \psi(x) * \delta(x - i) = \psi(x - i); \ -\infty < i < \infty \ . \tag{23}$$

The function $s(x)$ can now be rewritten as a discrete convolution

$$s(x) = \sum_{i=-\infty}^{\infty} c_i \psi(x - i) = c(x) * \psi(x) \ . \tag{24}$$

The coefficients of expansion c_x are identical to the function $c(x)$, i.e. $c(x) = c_x$. Thus, for the case of template-similar dense BFs used in expansion matching, expansion and restoration are equivalent operations. Hence, in order to expand a signal $s(x)$ in terms of a dense set of self-similar BFs $\{\psi_i(x)\}$ as defined above, one has to simply 'restore' it with respect to the blurring kernel $\psi(x)$. This yields the 'restored' signal $c(x)$ which is identical to the expansion coefficients $\{c_x\}$. Of course, this equivalence is true only in the special case of dense self-similar BFs used in expansion matching. In other cases, such as if we were to recognize templates that are scaled as well as translated, non-orthogonal expansion is the more generalized scheme.

Suppose the signal $s(x)$ is composed of a linearly blurred signal with additive noise $\lambda(x)$

$$s(x) = \int c(\alpha) \psi(x - \alpha) d\alpha + \lambda(x) \ . \tag{25}$$

The Linear Least Square Estimate (LLSE) or Wiener filter[1,2,13] is the filter $\theta(x)$ which restores the signal $c(x)$ with the smallest squared error D. Assuming that the estimate $\hat{c}(x)$ is a linear function of the signal $s(x)$, i.e.

$$\hat{c}(x) = \int \theta(x - \alpha) s(\alpha) d\alpha \ , \tag{26}$$

the error is minimized as

$$D = E\left\{ \int [c(x) - \hat{c}(x)]^2 dx \right\} \rightarrow \min \tag{27}$$

with a filter $\theta(x)$ whose Fourier transform $\Theta(\omega)$ is

$$\Theta(\omega) = c_\theta S_{cs}(\omega) / S_{ss}(\omega) \tag{28}$$

where c_θ is a constant, $S_{ss}(\omega)$ is the spectral density of $s(x)$ and $S_{cs}(\omega)$ is the cross spectral density of $c(x)$ and $s(x)$. Assuming that $\lambda(x)$ is of zero mean and is uncorrelated with $c(x)$, we have

$$\Theta(\omega) = c_\theta \frac{\overline{\Psi}(\omega) S_{cc}(\omega)}{S_{cc}(\omega) |\Psi(\omega)|^2 + S_{\lambda\lambda}(\omega)} \tag{29}$$

where $S_c c(\omega)$ and $S_{\lambda\lambda}(\omega)$ are the spectral densities of $c(x)$ and $\lambda(x)$ respectively. Since the desired coefficients are ideally a delta function, $S_{cc}(\omega) = \sigma_c^2$ is assumed to be constant.

Suppose the signal $s(x)$ contains only the template $\psi(x)$ at x_0 and the noise $\lambda(x)$, i.e.,

$$s(x) = c_s \psi(x - x_0) + \lambda(x) \tag{30}$$

the ideal $c(x)$ would be

$$c(x) = \begin{cases} c_s & \text{for } x = x_0 \\ 0 & \text{elsewhere} \end{cases} \tag{31}$$

The Wiener filter approach will find the estimate $\hat{c}(x)$ which is closest to $c(x)$ in the least squared error sense, and thus maximizes the DSNR as defined in Eq. (5). The approach of matched filtering convolves the signal by a totally different filter:

$$H(\omega) = c_h \frac{\overline{\Psi}(\omega)}{S_{\lambda\lambda}(\omega)} , \tag{32}$$

c_h being a constant, and evidently arrives at an inferior DSNR. Since the Wiener filter is guaranteed to be optimal in a least squared error sense, any other approach including matched filtering, will have less DSNR and thus inferior performance. Intuitively, the Wiener filter has a high-pass characteristic compared to the matched filter, and thus yields a sharper matching peak. The EXM technique yields exactly the same result as the Wiener filter, since the expansion is also based on a minimization of squared error. Thus, EXM is always guaranteed[5-7] to have better DSNR than matched filtering.

It is important to note that EXM with the additive noise parameter does not lead to the inverse filter of the template. The inverse filter is unstable due to the possible presence of zeros in the Fourier transform of the template. In contrast, the Wiener filter is a regularized solution, adjustable to any level of noise, and is always stable. For any given noise level, the optimal DSNR expansion filter can be designed that will yield maximal DSNR for that noise level, and minimal off-center noisy response. In fact, we have shown[6] that in the limiting case of infinite noise, the optimal DSNR EXM filter approaches the matched filter exactly.

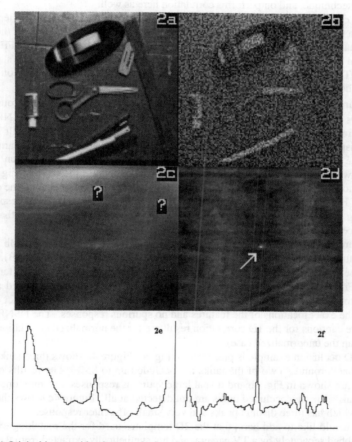

Figure 2. (a) Original image with scissors and other objects. (b) Noisy image (SNR = 2.9dB). (c) Results of correlation matching with the scissors template (DSNR = 1.6dB). Note the broad and spurious responses marked by question marks. (d) Result of expansion matching with scissors template (DSNR = 22.1dB). Note the sharp peak (marked by the arrow) and minimal off-center response. On previous page: (e) Profile (column 64) of correlation matching response. Note the broad and weak peak and large additional unwanted response. (f) Profile (column 64) of expansion matching response. Note the sharp peak and minimal off-center response.

6.1. Experimental Results

Experimental results comparing the traditional correlation (matched filtering) approach with our expansion method, show that the expansion approach has definite advantages over correlation especially in conditions of noise and severe occlusion. Natural images often contain occlusion, due to the interference of features and objects. In the case of audio or radar signals, such interference between features is in the form of superposition. Expansion matching is ideally suited to combat superposition, since it is a linear decomposition technique, and outperforms correlation here as well.

The expansion matching scheme is implemented as follows: First, the Wiener filter of the given template is computed from the Discrete Fourier Transform (DFT) of the template. The signal sizes are all chosen to allow the use of Fast Fourier Transforms (FFTs). Next, the given signal is convolved with the Wiener filter by multiplying their FFTs, and the inverse FFT yields the expansion matching coefficients. A similar implementation is used for the matched filtering approach as well.

Figure 2a is a 128×128 image of scissors with other objects in the background. Figure 2b shows the same image with strong additive Gaussian white noise with SNR = 2.9dB. Correlation matching of Fig. 2b with the scissors template yields the result in Fig. 2c, which displays substantial spurious response. Expansion matching with the same template yields the coefficients shown in Fig. 2d, with a sharp and distinct delta function The difference between correlation matching and EXM is easily seen in the plots of Fig. 2e and 2f which show profiles of Figs. 2c and 2d respectively. The matching peak in the correlation result of Fig. 2e is broad and weak, and there is strong off-center spurious response. The matching peak in the EXM result of Fig. 2f is sharp and well localized, and there is minimal off-center response.

Figure 3a shows a 1D feature extracted from the image in Fig. 2a. Fig. 3b shows two such features superimposed with additional Gaussian white noise (SNR=18dB). Figure 3c shows the result of normalized and unnormalized correlation matching of the template feature of Fig. 3a with the signal in Fig. 3b. The two features cannot resolved and only a single broad plateau is detected. The EXM results in Fig. 3d show two distinct delta functions at the exact locations of the features and no spurious responses. The DSNR quoted in the figure captions for the 1D correlation result are for the normalized correlation (which is better than the unnormalized case).

A 2D occlusion example is presented in Fig. 4. Figure 4a shows three tanks against a natural background. Two of the tanks are occluded up to 85%. The results of matched filtering are shown in Fig. 4b and reveal large spurious responses, and only one broad and weak peak. The two occluded tanks are not detected at all. Figure 4c shows the EXM response which has three distinct peaks and very small off-center response.

We would like to add here, that the 2D templates used for the matching experiments were grabbed separately by a TV camera, and not synthetically extracted from the test scene images, i.e. there are inherent rotation and size distortions as well as sensor noise in the templates that we use. The results show that the EXM scheme is quite tolerant to these perturbations. In fact, we have performed experiments that establish that expansion matching is quite robust in the presence of minor rotation and scale distortions[7].

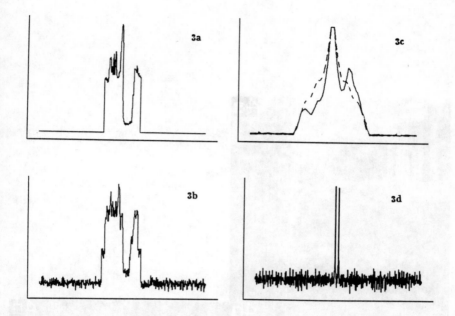

Figure 3. (a) Signal feature to be matched. (b) Supposition of two signal features with additive noise (SNR = 18dB). (c) Normalized (solid line) and unnormalized correlation (dashed line) coefficients (DSNR = 9.8dB). (d) Coefficients of expansion matching. Note the distinct and sharp peaks obtained (DSNR = 28.1dB).

7. Expansion Matching by Neural Lattice Architectures

This section describes a set of neural lattices that generate multiple-scale Gaussian smoothing of signals of any desired dimension. The operating principle of the lattice is based upon the Central Limit Theorem (CLT)[3]. The CLT proves to be very dominant and highly accurate Gaussian smoothing can be obtained with this simple and uniform architecture. The lattice can be used in two ways. The forward lattice accepts the input signal at its lowest layer and at each higher layer, generates increased smoothing of this signal. Thus, the forward lattice directly produces the scale-space description of the input signal that was originally obtained by Witkin[12]. The inverse lattice does the opposite: it takes coefficients of a Gaussian signal representation and reconstructs the signal. Both the forward and the inverse are especially useful in image processing and have been used for computing global

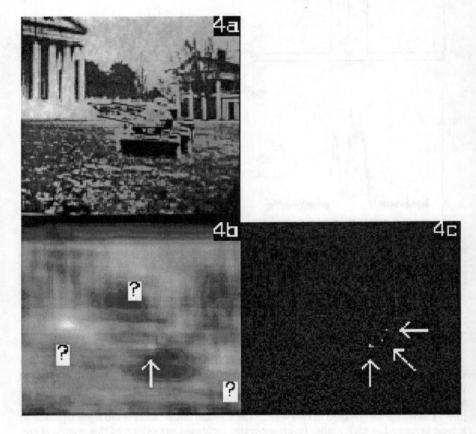

Figure 4. (a) Original image with three tanks against a natural background. The second and third tanks are occluded up to 85%. (b) Correlation matching results. Note the spurious responses and only one weak, blurred peak is detected (DSNR = 4.1dB). (c) Expansion matching results. The three distinct and sharp delta functions signify the locations of the centers of the tanks. No spurious responses elsewhere (DSNR = 29.2dB).

transforms (like the Fourier, Cosine, Sine transforms) of signal[14,15]. They are also used in the adaptive lattice system that is used for generalized signal representation by arbitrary basis functions (see Section 7.3).

7.1. The Lattice Architecture

From the central limit theorem[13] we know that a series of convolutions with small non-negative kernels tends to generate a cumulative Gaussian kernel. In this section, we implement this principle for discrete Gaussian smoothing of multi-dimensional arrays. The cumulative convolution is implemented by a lattice of analog summers (also called Processing Elements or PEs) which are arranged in layers. The general structure of the lattice is illustrated in Fig. 5. Each summer sums up a subset of PE outputs that belong to the layers beneath. In a 2D lattice, that can be used for Gaussian smoothing of 1D signals, the PE output $Q(\mu,x)$, at layer μ, and spatial location x, can be defined by the following equation:

$$Q(\mu,x) = \begin{cases} \sum_{i=1}^{N} q(\mu,\mu_i,i)Q(\mu_i,x_i+x) & ; \text{for } B_\mu < x < M - B_\mu \\ \sum_{i=1}^{N_x} q_x(\mu,\mu_i,i)Q(\mu_i,x_i(x)+x) & ; \text{for } M - B_\mu < x < M \text{ or } 1 < x < B_\mu \end{cases} \tag{33}$$

where μ_i is the layer of the i-th connection, x_i is the relative displacement of the connected PE, M is the size of the array (and also the lattice width), N is the number of connections to each PE (also called the order of the lattice), and B_μ is the size of the boundary region. The lattice is divided into a central region, and left and right boundary regions of width B_μ. According to Eq. (33), in the central region the configuration and the set of weights of every PE is identical for each PE in the same layer, whereas, the number of connections N_x, the weights q_x, and the relative displacements $x_i(x)$ are varied in accordance with the location x, in the boundary regions. It is important to note that the layer for $\mu = 0$ is the input data array and the input data points are marked by dark circles in Fig. 5. Outputs for different Standard Deviations (SDs) are obtained at the corresponding layers (PEs marked by white circles in Fig. 5).

By increasing the lattice's dimension, with the same general structure, we can generate multi-dimensional Gaussian smoothing. Hence, the general structure of the $d+1$-dimension lattice which could be used for smoothing of d-dimensional signals, can be expressed as

$$Q(\mu,\underline{x}) = \begin{cases} \sum_{i_1=1}^{N^1} \cdots \sum_{i_d=1}^{N^d} q(\mu,\mu_i,i)Q(\mu_i,\underline{x}_i+\underline{x}) & ; \text{for } \underline{B}_\mu < \underline{x} < \underline{M} - \underline{B}_\mu \\ \sum_{i_1=1}^{N_x^1} \cdots \sum_{i_d=1}^{N_x^d} q_{\underline{x}}(\mu,\mu_i,i)Q(\mu_i,\underline{x}_i(\underline{x})+\underline{x}) & ; \text{for } \underline{M} - \underline{B}_\mu < \underline{x} < \underline{M} \\ & \text{or } \underline{I} < \underline{x} < \underline{B}_\mu \end{cases} \tag{34}$$

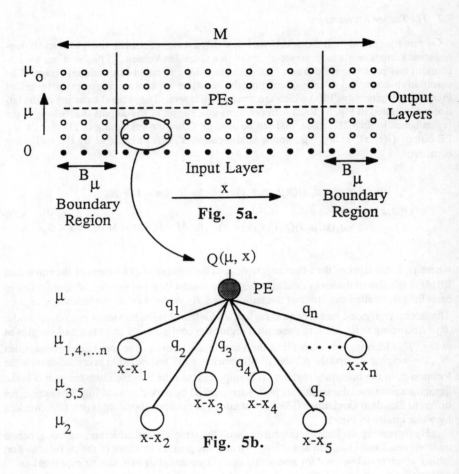

Figure 5. (a) General structure of the lattice architecture. White circles denote output layer PEs. Dark circles denote input layer PEs. (b) Illustration of connections and weights of one PE which is denoted in a shaded circle.

where all vectors are d-dimensional, $\underline{I} = [1,1,...,1]^T$ and $N_{\underline{x}}^m$ represents the number of connections in the mth dimension at location $\underline{x}$.

The special set of connections and weights for the boundary regions are incorporated to allow reduction of distortions of the generated Gaussian kernels in the boundaries of the signal's region of support (ROS). If the same set of weights are used through out a particular layer (including the boundary region), the Gaussian kernels generated at the boundaries will be distorted due to the missing contribution of lower PEs which lie outside the signal support. Two remedies are possible to overcome this problem: (1) Define a boundary region as in Eqs. (33) and (34) and design special connections and weights to minimize the distortion at each point. This involves an iterative approach for the desired weights, since we find that the analytical expressions are hard to solve. (2) Construct the lattice to be larger than the signal support and use the same weights throughout. This is equivalent to padding zeroes around the signal to increase the effective ROS and allowing the distorted boundary region of the lattice to fall outside the signal's actual ROS. The second method is much simpler, but involves more PEs than the first method.

7.2. Some Other Forms of the Lattice

There are a few special cases of the general form of the lattice in Eqs. (33) and (34). The simplest form of the lattice is the uniform lattice[14,15]. Here all the input weights are identical for every PE (any layer, any location) in the whole lattice. Higher order uniform lattices (each PE with inputs from a larger support) generate correspondingly higher amount of smoothing. However, this kind of lattice can generate only square-root progression of Gaussian smoothing with the number of layers in the lattice. Thus, for a practical amount of smoothing, a very large number of layers is required.

Since the CLT is so dominant, even if some of the PEs in the lattice are defective or missing, the Gaussian smoothing is still reasonably accurate. In fact, a statistical analysis[14,15] reveals that for a multiplicative noise with standard deviation as much as 20% of the weights, the lattice maintains an accuracy of 40dB SNR, which is very high in practice.

The geometric lattice overcomes the SD progression problem of the uniform lattice. Here, a special design procedure[14,15] is used and for each subsequent layer in the lattice, successively wider spread kernels (PE weight configurations) are used. Given the basic lattice dimensions (number of PEs and layers) and the desired SD at each layer, it is possible to compute the incremental smoothing required between consecutive layers which will generate all the desired Gaussian scales. Then, the weight configurations for each layer are simply a sampled Gaussian corresponding to the required incremental smoothing for that layer[14,15]. With such a design, the lattice can have substantially any desired progression of SD, though we find the geometric progression the most effective.

The above mentioned 'forward' lattices take an input signal and generate Gaussian smoothed versions of it at each layer. The inverse lattice is constructed by simply inverting the weight sets of the forward lattices, i.e. the bottom-most layer assumes the weight configuration of the top-most and so on. If the Gaussian representation of a signal is known, i.e. the signal is composed of a set of Gaussians with known locations, amplitudes and SDs, the signal can be easily reconstructed by simply injecting these coefficients at appropriate locations[14,15] in the inverse lattice. The output appearing at the top-most layer of the

304

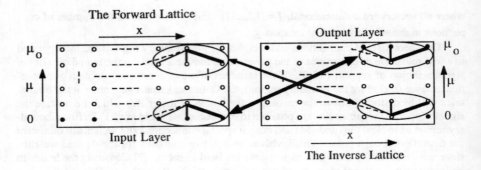

The Forward Lattice

Output Layer

Input Layer

The Inverse Lattice

Figure 6. The forward and inverse lattices and their relationship. The layers and weight configurations are inverted for the inverse lattice.

lattice will then be the reconstructed signal. Figure 6 illustrates the forward and inverse lattices and their inter-relationship.

All the different kinds of lattices discussed above have constant resolution at each layer. A pyramidal structure has also been developed called the Gradual Lattice Pyramid (GLP)[14,15] which significantly reduces the complexity (in number of PEs) of the lattice. The GLP is a piecewise multi-resolution structure composed of a number of stages. Each of these stages has an identical configuration as far as PE weights are concerned. However, each subsequent stage is decimated by half in resolution. Thus, the number of required PEs is less than twice the number of PEs in the lowest stage. In addition, as experiments reveal[14,15], high accuracy is still maintained. All the different kinds of lattices (uniform, geometric, inverse) can be incorporated in the GLP form in much the same manner.

7.3. The Adaptive Lattice for Expansion Matching

This section briefly describes a general method for non-orthogonal signal expansion using Gaussian Sets (GSs). The method outlined is an alternative expansion method to the restoration techniques suggested in Section 6. GSs are functions constructed from linear combinations of Gaussians, and are described in more detail in Ref. 15. It is proved in Ref. 15 that GSs can approximate $L^2(R)$ signals with any desired accuracy. Therefore, GSs can represent with arbitrarily small error, any compact BF with a finite number of Gaussians. In addition, GSs can be generated in real-time by the lattice architectures discussed above. The expansion system consists of three lattices and is described in Fig. 7. This system, called the adaptive lattice (AL), finds the expansion coefficients with minimal square error by gradient descent algorithm which is described in the following text.

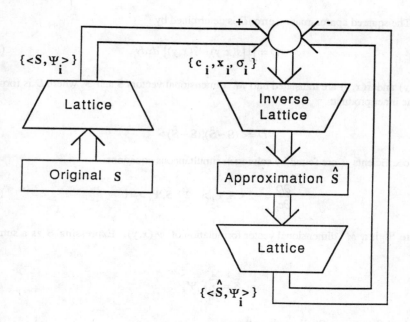

Figure 7. The adaptive lattice system

In the following equations we refer to 2D signals. However, a similar formulation can derived for any dimension. Consider a 2D image $s(x,y)$ that is to be decomposed into its basis function constituents. In this case, the template $\psi(x,y)$ is represented by a linear combination of n normalized Gaussians

$$\psi(x,y) = \sum_{j=1}^{n} \frac{a_j}{2\pi\sigma^2} \exp(-[(x-x_j)^2 + (y-y_j)^2]/2\sigma_j^2); \qquad (35)$$

$s(x,y)$ is approximated by m basis functions

$$\hat{s}(x,y) = \sum_{i=1}^{m} c_i \psi_i(x,y) \ . \qquad (36)$$

For EXM, the BFs are setup as $\psi_i(x-x_i) = \psi(x-x_i, y-y_i)$, where for a $M \times M$ discrete image, $m = M^2$ and $\{(x_i,y_i); i = 1...M^2\}$ spans the $M \times M$ spatial locations in the input image.

The squared approximation error D is determined by

$$D = \iint \left[s(x,y) - \hat{s}(x,y) \right]^2 dxdy \tag{37}$$

$s(x,y)$ and $\hat{s}(x,y)$ are translated into M^2 dimensional vectors $\mathbf{S}$ and $\hat{\mathbf{S}}$, where D is formed by the inner product:

$$D = <(\mathbf{S} - \hat{\mathbf{S}}),(\mathbf{S} - \hat{\mathbf{S}})> . \tag{38}$$

The coefficients c_i are found by solving m simultaneous equations:

$$\frac{\partial D}{\partial c_i} = -2 <\mathbf{S}, \Psi_i> +2 <\hat{\mathbf{S}}, \Psi_i> = 0 \tag{39}$$

where Ψ_i is a M^2 dimensional vector formulation of $\psi_i(x,y)$. Expressing $\hat{\mathbf{S}}$ as a sum of Ψ_i:

$$\hat{\mathbf{S}} = \sum_{j=i}^{m} c_j \Psi_j . \tag{40}$$

For $i = 1,2...m$, we finally arrive at:

$$\frac{\partial D}{\partial c_i} = -2 <\mathbf{S}, \Psi_i> +2 < (\sum_{j=1}^{m} c_j \Psi_j), \Psi_i> = 0 . \tag{41}$$

This result also conforms with the set of equations in Eq. (15). In general, it is extremely difficult to solve this enormous set of equations. It is therefore suggested to use an adaptive network that employs three lattices of the types discussed in reference[14,15]. The first lattice generates the set of terms $\{<\mathbf{S}, \Psi_i>\}$ which are the projections of the original image onto the basis functions Ψ_i. The second lattice is an inverse lattice which reconstructs the approximated image $\hat{\mathbf{S}}$ from the coefficient set $\{c_i\}$. The third lattice generates the set of projections $< (\sum_{j=1}^{m} c_j \Psi_j), \Psi_i >$. The adjustment rule for the coefficients is:

$$\Delta_{c_i} = -b \left[\frac{\partial D}{\partial c_i} \right] = \frac{b}{2} \left[<\mathbf{S}, \Psi_i> - <\hat{\mathbf{S}}, \Psi_i> \right] \tag{42}$$

where $b/2$ is the loop gain. All the coefficients are adjusted in parallel at iteration k by:

$$c_i^k = c_i^{k-1} + \Delta_{c_i}^{k-1}; \quad i = 1,2,...,m . \tag{43}$$

The entire system performs a gradient descent process on the error surface, and reaches the equilibrium state when the coefficients fulfill the original requirement:

$$\frac{\partial D}{\partial c_i} = 0; \quad i = 1,2,...,m; \quad = \quad D \to \text{min.} \tag{44}$$

Since D is quadratic in every c_i, only one global minimum exists. Therefore, convergence towards a unique solution is theoretically guaranteed.

In summation, to use the adaptive lattice to implement EXM, there are two stages. The first stage involves approximating the given template itself by using Gaussian BFs in Eq. (35). In other words, we need to find a_j, (x_j, y_j) and σ_j in Eq. (35) for a value of n that retains sufficient accuracy in approximating the given template. Once the Gaussian representation $\psi(x,y)$ of the template is computed, the shifted set of templates $\{\psi_i(x,y)\}$ are used as the BFs in the adaptive lattice to represent the input image $s(x,y)$. The resulting coefficients are the desired EXM coefficients $\{c_i\}$.

8. Generalized Expansion Matching for Multiple Templates

This section briefly describes the generalized EXM paradigm for simultaneously matching multiple templates using only a single filter. The formulation allows one to specify any desired output value for the matching peak of each template, and also maximizes the DSNR for matching each template. Such a filter can be used for generic recognition by demanding the same response for different instances of an object[20]. Scale and rotation invariant matching is also possible to an extent, by designing the filter to elicit the same response for different views of the template.

The problem is formulated in one-dimension using matrix-vector notation. The results can easily be generalized into two dimensions by using lexicographically ordered vectors and block-circulant matrices. Given a set of templates Ψ_i; $i = 1...L$, we expect a set of noisy input templates $S_i = \Psi_i + \Lambda$, where Λ is a random noise vector. We wish to design a filter Θ that yields as its expected peak correlation to each template S_i, a desired response u_i, i.e.,

$$E\{\Theta^T S_i\} = u_i; \quad i = 1...L . \tag{45}$$

The correlation coefficient vectors C_i (filter response) for the i-th template are obtained as $C_i = [S_i]^T \Theta$, where $[S_i]^T$ is a circulant correlation matrix obtained by circulating the noisy input template S_i. Note that in this formulation correlation, not convolution, is used to represent the linear filtering. This is merely for the sake of mathematical convenience. The correlation referred to in this section is the signal processing operation of correlating one signal with another, and should not be confused with correlation matching or matched filtering.

In addition to the constraints of Eq. (45), we also wish to maximize the DSNR criterion for the correlation response of the filter to each input template. The DSNR for matching the i-th template is

$$DSNR_i = 10 \log \frac{(M-1)(E\{\Theta^T S_i\})^2}{E\{C_i^T C_i\} - (E\{\Theta^T S_i\})^2} \quad . \tag{46}$$

Since all the $DSNR_i$ cannot be globally optimized[20], a weighted average of DSNR over all templates is maximized as

$$\sum_{i=1}^{L} \alpha_i DSNR_i \to \max; \quad \sum_{i=1}^{L} \alpha_i = 1 \tag{47}$$

where α_i are the weights, typically set to $1/L$. Note that maximizing $DSNR_i$ is equivalent to minimizing $E\{C_i^T C_i\}$ subject to the constraints of Eq. (45). Applying the method of Lagrange multipliers, the above constrained maximization problem can be reformulated as the unconstrained minimization of a single objective function

$$J(\mathbf{Q}) = E\left\{\sum_{i=1}^{N} \alpha_i C_i^T C_i\right\} + \sum_{i=1}^{L} \xi_i (E\{\mathbf{Q}^T S_i\} - u_i) \to \min \quad . \tag{48}$$

The solution of this minimization[20] yields Θ as

$$\Theta = \left[\sum_{i=1}^{L} \alpha_i [\mathbf{R}_{\psi\psi i}] + [\mathbf{R}_{\lambda\lambda}]\right]^{-1} \sum_{j=1}^{L} -\tfrac{1}{2}\xi_j \Psi_j = [\mathbf{R}]^{-1} \sum_{j=1}^{L} \xi_j \Psi_j \tag{49}$$

where $[\mathbf{R}_{\psi\psi i}]$ and $[\mathbf{R}_{\lambda\lambda}]$ are the autocorrelation matrices of the template Ψ_i and the noise Λ respectively. $\tilde{\Xi} = [\tilde{\xi}_1 \dots \tilde{\xi}_N]^T$ is found by enforcing the constraints of Eq. (45) on this solution for Θ to yield[20]

$$\tilde{\Xi} = [\mathbf{A}]^{-1}\mathbf{U}; \quad [\mathbf{A}]_{ij} = \Psi_i^T [\mathbf{R}]^{-1} \Psi_j \quad . \tag{50}$$

The matrix $[\mathbf{A}]$ is a non-singular (for distinct, non-zero Ψ_i), real symmetric $N \times N$ matrix and $\mathbf{U} = [u_1 \dots u_N]^T$ defines the constraints.

Since all the matrices in the formulation are circulant, they can be diagonalized by the DFT matrix[1,2] and an efficient implementation using the frequency domain is possible[20]. The filter Θ in the frequency domain is given by its Fourier transform

$$\Theta(\omega) = \frac{\sum_{j=1}^{L} \tilde{\xi}_j X_j(\omega)}{\sum_{i=1}^{L} \alpha_i S_{\psi\psi i}(\omega) + S_{\lambda\lambda}(\omega)} \tag{51}$$

where $X_i(\omega)$ represents the Fourier transform of the i-th template Ψ_i, $S_{\psi\psi i}(\omega) = X_i(\omega)\overline{X}_i(\omega)$ and $S_{\lambda\lambda}(\omega)$ is the power spectrum of the noise, the bar symbol representing complex conjugation. For the single template case, $L = 1$, and this is easily recognized as the Wiener filter. The matrix [A] can also be efficiently calculated in the frequency domain[20] by

$$[A]_{ij} = \sum_{\omega} \left(\frac{\overline{X}_i(\omega) X_j(\omega)}{\sum_{k=1}^{L} \alpha_k S_{\psi\psi k}(\omega) + S_{\lambda\lambda}(\omega)} \right) .$$ (52)

The above EXM formulation is quite generalized and special cases lead to previous approaches for multiple template matching. If the noise Λ is set to zero, the EXM formulation is identical to the Minimum Average Correlation Energy (MACE) filter[17]. As the noise power tends to infinity, the EXM filter approaches the Synthetic Discriminant Function (SDF)[18] if the noise is white, or the Minimum Variance SDF[19], if the noise is colored. Hence, it is found that EXM is the generalized solution that encapsulates other approaches, such as MACE, SDF and MVSDF, as only special noise parameter variations. Illustrative examples of applying multiple template EXM for generic recognition and occluded parts recognition can be found in reference 20.

Acknowledgments

The work described in this chapter was supported by the National Science Foundation under grant IRIS-9115280 and ARPA/ONR Grant No. N00014-93-1-1088.

References

1. A. Rosenfeld and A. Kak, *Digital Picture Processing* (Academic Press, New York, 1982).
2. A. Jain, *Fundamentals of Digital Image Processing* (Prentice Hall, Englewood Cliffs, NJ, 1989).
3. M. Rabbani and P. W. Jones, *Digital Image Compression Techniques.* (SPIE Optical Engineering Press, Bellingham, WA, 1991).
4. J. G. Daugman, "Complete discrete 2-D Gabor transform by neural networks for image analysis and compression" *IEEE Trans. on ASSP* **36(7)** (1988) 1169-1179.
5. J. Ben-Arie and K. R. Rao, "A novel approach for template matching by non-orthogonal image expansion," *IEEE Transactions on Circuits & Systems for Video Technology* **3(1)** (1993) 71-84.
6. J. Ben-Arie and K. R. Rao, "Optimal template matching by non-orthogonal image expansion using restoration," *International Journal of Machine Vision and Applications* **7** (1994) 69-81.
7. K. R. Rao and J. Ben-Arie, "Non-orthogonal image expansion related to optimal template matching in complex images," *Computer Vision, Graphics, and Image Processing: Graphical Models and Image Processing* **56(2)** (1994) 149-160.
8. R. J. Schalkoff, *Digital Image Processing and Computer Vision.* (John Wiley & Sons Inc., New York, 1989), pp. 77-209.
9. H. Wechsler, *Computational Vision.* (Academic Press, New York, 1990), pp. 267-291.

10. D. Casasent and D. Psaltis, "Position, rotation, and scale invariant optical correlation," *Applied Optics* **15(7)** (1976) 1795-1799.

11. J. Ben-Arie, "Multi-dimensional linear lattice for Fourier and Gabor transforms, multiple-scale Gaussian filtering, and edge detection," in *Neural Networks for Human and Machine Perception*, ed. H. Wechsler (Academic Press, New York, 1992), pp. 231-252.

12. A. P. Witkin, "Scale-space filtering: A new approach to multi-scale description," in *Image Understanding 1984*, eds. S. Ullman and W. Richards (Albex Publishing, Norwood, NJ, 1984), pp. 79-96.

13. A. Papoulis, *Probability, Random Variables, and Stochastic Processes* (McGraw-Hill, New York, 1989) pp. 480-532.

14. K. R. Rao and J. Ben-Arie, "Lattice architectures for multiple-scale Gaussian convolution, image processing, sinusoid-based transforms and Gabor filtering," *Analog Integrated Circuits and Signal Processing* **4(2)** (1993) 141-160.

15. J. Ben-Arie and K. R. Rao, "Lattice architectures for non-orthogonal representation of signals and generation of transforms using gaussian sets," *Report No. IIT ECE-TR-005-92 Department of Electrical and Computer Engineering* (Illinois Institute of Technology, Chicago, IL, 1992).

16. J. Ben-Arie and K. R. Rao, "Signal representation by generalized non-orthogonal Gaussian wavelet groups using lattice networks," in *IEEE International Joint Conference on Neural Networks* (IEEE Press, Singapore, 1991), pp. 968-973.

17. A. Mahalanobis, B. V. K. Vijaya Kumar and D. Casasent, "Minimum average correlation energy filters," *Applied Optics* **26(17)** (1987) 3633-3640.

18. D. Casasent, "Unified synthetic discriminant function computational formulation," *Applied Optics* **23F(10)** (1984) 1620-1627.

19. B. V. K. Vijaya Kumar, "Minimum variance synthetic discriminant functions," *J. Opt. Soc. of Am. [A]* **3** (1986) 1579-1590.

20. K. R. Rao and J. Ben-Arie, "Multiple template matching using expansion matching," *IEEE Transactions of Circuits and Systems on Video Technology* (1994, in press).

21. M. Horowitz, "Efficient use of a picture correlator," *J. Opt. Soc. of Am.* **47** (1957) 327-332.

22. J. L. Harris, "Resolving power and decision theory," *J. Opt. Soc. of Am.* **54** (1964) 606-611.

23. J. F. Andrus, C. W. Campbell, and R. R. Jayro, "Digital image registration using boundary maps," *IEEE Trans. Computers* **C-24** (1975) 935-940.

Peripheral Vision
and
Search

MODELING OFF-AXIS VISION I: THE OPTICAL EFFECTS OF DECENTERING VISUAL TARGETS OR THE EYE'S ENTRANCE PUPIL

ARTHUR BRADLEY and LARRY N. THIBOS

School of Optometry, Indiana University
Bloomington, IN   47405

Most of our knowledge about human visual performance describes foveal vision with a well centered pupil. However, these studies of "on-axis" vision do not provide much insight into the effects of moving the retinal image or the pupil off-axis. In this chapter we define the inherent optical and neural axes of the human eye, and we examine the optical and visual effects of decentering either the retinal image or the entrance pupil. The optical axis of the eye is usually well centered on the eye's neural axis, which provides best image quality at the fovea. Decentration of the eye's entrance pupil can occur when using any visually-coupled electro-optical device with a defined exit pupil. This decentration can lead to reduced light sensitivity, reduced spatial resolution, reduced contrast sensitivity, color distortions, unpredictable changes in refractive error, wavelength-specific distortions of visual direction and wavelength-specific errors in the judgment of apparent depth and size. We then examine associated problem of a centered pupil and an off-axis object and conclude with a simple computational model that accounts for the majority of the effects on contrast sensitivity and spatial resolution.

1. Introduction

Most of what we know about vision and the visual processes stems from experiments in which subjects fixate a target which is viewed through the eye's natural pupil. Although we implicitly consider this to be the typical visual environment, it represents a very specific set of viewing conditions in which the target and pupil are located on a particular axis called the *visual axis*. This chapter will examine the optical and visual consequences of displacing either the pupil or target from this axis. By examining the optical ramifications of off-axis vision, we reveal a more general model of human spatial vision that may be particularly pertinent to real world visual tasks performed with or without visually-coupled electro-optical systems.

In the human electro-optical imaging system, the quality of signal transmission is affected by the quality of the eye's optical system and the quality of the electrical (neural) image processing. Recent work in our laboratories [7, 50, 53, 55, 56, 67, 68, 71] has highlighted the substantial differences in both optical and neural image quality between on- and off-axis vision. Predictably, the quality of the optical image depends on the route taken by the light which forms the retinal image. The light path, and hence the optical image quality, varies with both target and pupil decentration. In addition to the off-axis decline in optical image quality, there are profound differences between on- and off-axis neural processing by the retina and brain and these are discussed in the following chapter (Modeling off-axis vision - II: the effect of spatial filtering and sampling by retinal neurons, by Thibos & Bradley).

The present chapter will define the optical axes of the human visual system and examine the optical properties and visual ramifications of off-axis vision. Since the neural processing of the eye's optical image exhibits an approximate radial symmetry about a high resolution fovea (see chapter by Thibos and Bradley), we can think of the fovea as defining a neural axis for the human eye. To begin the discussion, therefore, the location of the human eye's optical axes will be compared to that of the eye's inherent neural axis.

2. Establishing an Optical Axis for the Human Eye

Early optical studies of the human eye introduced the idea of an optical axis defined as the line which contains the centers of rotation of each of the optical elements of the eye. Aligning all of the optical elements within a multi-lens system is a typical optical strategy for optimizing image quality, and such a system will generally provide best image quality for targets placed along this axis. Because of the inhomogeneities in the quality of the neural processing (see chapter by Thibos and Bradley), optimal image quality at the fovea is visually most important. Therefore, early studies examined the location of the eye's optical axis relative to the eye's neural axis. That is, where does the eye's optical axis intersect the retina?

The eye's optical axis may be determined experimentally by identifying the location of a target which yields superposition of the reflected (catoptric) images, known as Purkinje images I through IV, from the four optical surfaces in the eye (front and back surface of the cornea, front and back surface of the lens, see Figure 1). If the optical axis of the human eye included the neural fovea, the Purkinje images would, to the experimenter, appear aligned with the fixation target. In general this alignment is only approximate for two reasons. First, it is rare that all four catoptric images perfectly superimpose for any target location,[37] which indicates that the different optical elements within the human eye are not perfectly aligned along a specific optical axis. Second, the axis that creates the best alignment generally does not intersect the fixation point, and therefore it does not intersect the neural fovea.[37] The horizontal angular separation (angle alpha) between the neural axis of the visual system (often referred to as the visual axis, see Figure 1) and the best approximation of an optical axis varies from +17 degrees temporal to -2 degrees nasal, and it appears to co-vary with refractive error.[37] Vertically, the visual and optical axes seem better aligned.[37] Although there are few contemporary studies of the eye's optical axis,[19] and the older data indicate significant inter-subject variability, many texts report that the optical axis is 5 degrees temporal to the visual axis. The visual and optical consequences of these naturally occurring misalignments have never been examined experimentally.

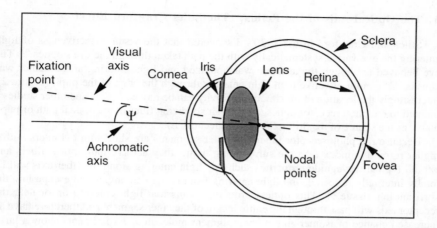

Figure 1 Schematic eye showing the principal optical surfaces, and the general anatomical structure of the eye. The optical axis (not shown) is defined as the line passing through or near the centers of rotation of the four optical surfaces of the eye. The achromatic axis follows the path of the chief nodal ray (passes through center of pupil and nodal points) and is the axis for which chromatic dispersion vanishes. The visual axis is defined as the axis connecting the fovea and the fixation target *via* the eye's nodal points.

A major limitation of this traditional formulation of the optical axis of the human eye is that it does not take into account the location of the eye's aperture formed by the iris. For this reason, Thibos *et al.* [55] suggested the path of the chief nodal ray as an alternative reference axis for the eye. They reasoned that, for a given pupil location, each object point in the visual field gives rise to a chief ray (i.e. a ray which passes through the center of the pupil). Of the infinite number of chief rays that are possible, only one is a nodal ray (i.e., enters through the eye's anterior nodal point and exits in a parallel direction from the posterior nodal point) and thus (by definition) avoids the effects of refraction. Since this unique chief ray is undeviated, it suffers no ray aberrations and thus the path of this ray assumes special significance for vision. In particular, rays traveling along this axis will be spared the effects of chromatic dispersion and for this reason the axis was dubbed the "achromatic axis" of the eye.[55] The magnitude of angle ψ between this achromatic axis and the visual axis (see Fig. 1) is of crucial importance for image quality of polychromatic targets[55] on the fovea and may also prove important for the analysis of off-axis, monochromatic aberrations. In a sample of 5 subjects we found that the pupil center was on average 0.14mm temporal to the visual axis, and therefore, angle ψ was only 2 degrees.[55] The close correspondence between the center of the natural pupil and the visual axis[46] indicates that the eye's pupil is located to provide best image quality in the fovea.

All of the reference axes defined above fail to incorporate the directional properties of the retina, which has its own inherent optical axis. This factor is considered in the next section.

3. The Optical Axis of the Retina: The Stiles Crawford Effect

Stiles and Crawford in the 1930's discovered that the visual effectiveness of light entering the eye varied systematically with the path taken through the eye's optics.[47] The eye behaved as though the aperture was apodized and light entering at the center was considerably more effective than light entering through the edge of the pupil (Figure 2). Interestingly the location of maximum sensitivity can be moved.[1] This and other studies[23] pointed to the photoreceptor optics, and not an apodizing filter in the optical path or pupil plane, as the source of the Stiles-Crawford effect (SCE).

Because the photoreceptor inner and outer segments are short thin cylinders with a higher refractive index than the surrounding tissue, they act as small optical fibers and exhibit typical waveguide properties such that light entering along the fiber axis will be totally internally reflected, and light entering from peripheral angles can escape into the surrounding tissue.[23] This optical property means that light entering on or near the receptor axis will pass through the entire length of the outer segment and therefore have an increased chance of isomerizing a photopigment molecule. Experiments show a large change in sensitivity to light entering the eye through different parts of the pupil. For example, rho values (Fig. 2) are typically around 0.05 mm^{-2}, which means that sensitivity for light entering the pupil 4mm from the peak of the SCE is about 16% of the peak sensitivity.[2] Although the source of the SCE is the angular selectivity of individual photoreceptors in the human retina, it has been modeled as an optical apodization function in the pupil plane.[38]

The SCE has important ramifications for optical image quality and light sensitivity. First, if the eye's pupil is decentered with respect to the receptor axes, light entering the eye will have less visual impact. It will be similar to viewing the world through a neutral density filter. Fortunately, in most subjects, the pupil location and the receptor axes appear very closely aligned. This is inferred from the extensive data showing that the peak of the SCE is centered near to the pupil center (typically less than 1mm nasal of center).[2, 21, 58] This close correspondence is not surprising because one study has shown that the peak of the SCE will track the location of the pupil similar to the way that plants follow the direction of light.[1] This movement of the SCE is interpreted as a phototropic response of the individual photoreceptors, which should ensure a close correspondence between receptor axis and pupil location in all eyes. Therefore, in the normal eye, the pupil's location approximately maximizes the visual response. This optimal arrangement can, of course, be disrupted if a small artificial entrance pupil is introduced. For example, if the observer is using an optical device that has a small exit pupil, and this exit pupil is decentered with respect to the eye's normal entrance pupil, the light will effectively be reduced in intensity. It is also important to realize that some people have a naturally decentered SCE.[1, 2]

The potential for inadvertant decentration of an artificial pupil or instrument exit pupil can be largest when the natural pupil is most dilated. Dilation occurs at low light levels and is greatest for young observers.[66] For example, at 9 cd/m^2 the pupil diameter of a 20-year old can be between 6 and 8 mm, and therefore light entering the eye at the pupil margin can be nearly an order of magnitude less effective than light entering through the pupil center.[2]

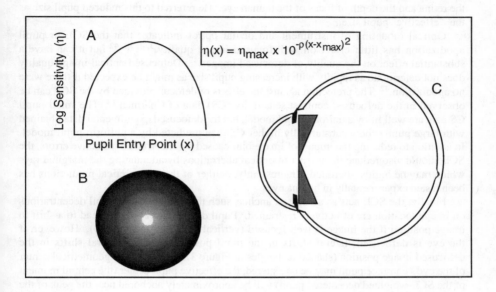

Figure 2 Schematic representation of the Stiles Crawford Effect (SCE). A: Visual sensitivity (η) is dependent upon the radial distance between the point (x) at which light passes through the eye's pupil and the peak of the SCE. In the equation relating sensitivity to pupil location ρ= rho determines the steepness of this function. B and C: Although the origin of the SCE is retinal, it can be modeled with an apodizing filter (B) which behaves as a radially symmetric neutral density wedge in the pupil plane (C).

The effect of pupil apodization on retinal image quality has been appreciated since some of the early work of Campbell who showed that the eye's depth of focus did not decrease with increasing pupil diameter by the amount predicted by geometrical optics.[8] Large pupils behaved as though they had a smaller diameter. Campbell was able to model the depth of focus data by substituting a uniform pupil with a radius of r_c for the natural apodized pupil according to the empirically determined formula

$$r_c = \sqrt{\frac{1 - e^{-0.105 r^2}}{0.105}} \tag{1}$$

where r_c is the radius of a uniform transmission pupil (no SCE) that would transmit the same amount of light as the larger (r) apodized pupil. In effect, Campbell showed that the apodization model of the retinal direction effect could predict the amount of light reaching the retina and the depth of focus of the human eye. He referred to this reduced pupil size as the "effective" pupil size.

Optical modeling of instrument and ocular optics indicates that the SCE or pupil apodization has little effect on well-focused image quality,[3, 4, 38, 42] but it can have a substantial effect on the quality of defocused images.[42] Defocused optical image quality does not deteriorate as rapidly with increasing pupil size as might be expected if there were no apodization.[42] The protection against the effects of defocus provided by the SCE can be observed in the defocused contrast sensitivity (CS) data of Charman.[14] The small-pupil CS data are well fit by a uniform pupil model, but the defocused experimental data obtained with large pupils show substantially higher CS than predicted by a uniform pupil model. In addition to reducing the impact of image blur caused by uncorrected refractive errors, the SCE should also reduce the impact of optical aberrations by attenuating the marginal rays which may be highly aberrated. Interestingly, neither of these theoretical predictions has been tested experimentally in humna eyes.

Finally, the SCE acts as an optical anchor, such that the effects of pupil decentrations on image location are effectively restrained. Pupil decentration will not lead to a shift in image position if the image is well focused (vertical dark bars in Figure 3). However, if the eye is defocused, lateral shifts in the pupil position produce lateral shifts in the defocused image position (shaded rectangles in Figure 3). Although the geometrical center of the eye's entrance pupil may be decentered, the effective pupil center (the central moment of the SCE-weighted decentered pupil) will be approximately anchored near the peak of the SCE (and hence near the center of the natural pupil). Therefore, problems of image misalignment that might be encountered in optical devices with exit pupils decentered from the eye's entrance pupil are partially ameliorated by the SCE. This interaction between decentered entrance pupil and the SCE and the impact on perceived visual direction has been modeled by Ye et al.,[68] and it is discussed in detail in the next section.

4. Optical Quality of On-axis Vision

In order to take full advantage of the functional capability of the high resolution area within the neural array, optical image quality must be high at the fovea. For example, typical adult humans can easily resolve up to 50 c/deg. [11] and some falcons and eagles can resolve more than 100 c/deg. with their foveae.[25, 45] In humans, 50 c/deg. corresponds to a grating period of about 6.5 microns on the retina. Numerous studies of retinal image quality in human eyes [5, 11-13, 16, 28, 29, 61] have shown that, in a well focused eye, with an intermediate pupil size, spatial frequencies up to about 50 c/deg can be imaged on the fovea with sufficient contrast to be visible.[11]

Three basic methods have been applied to the problem of measuring the optical quality of the human eye. First, the double-pass method examines the quality of an aerial image

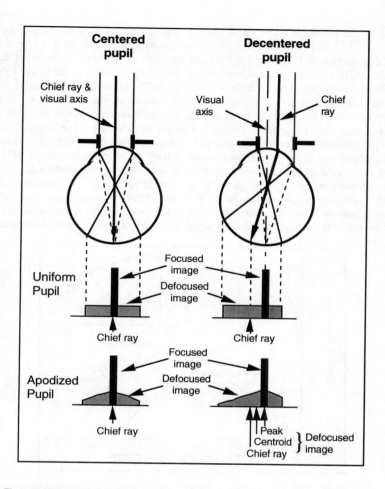

Figure 3 Schematic showing the anchoring effect of the SCE. The top section of this figure shows ray tracing for two model eyes, one with a pupil centered on the visual axis (left) and one with a pupil decentered to the right of the visual axis (right). The lower section of this figure shows schematic retinal illuminance profiles (black for focused and gray for defocused) for retinal images of a point source viewed through a uniform pupil (middle section) and through an apodized pupil (lower section). Although the chief ray (geometric center of the ray bundle, and hence center of the blur circle) for a defocused image shifts with pupil decentration, the peak and central moment of the SCE-weighted blur circle remain fairly centered. See Fig. 1 for definition of visual axis.

formed by the reflection back off of the retina of the image of a thin line or point of light.[12, 29, 43, 61] It is assumed that the retina acts as a plane diffuse reflector and that image degradation is the same for both passes. The single pass modulation transfer function (MTF) is taken as the square root of the modulus of the aerial image's Fourier Transform. In the second method, the eye's optical MTF is inferred by comparing contrast sensitivity measured under (1) normal viewing conditions in which contrast in the retinal image is attenuated by the eye's optics, and (2) interferometric conditions in which retinal image contrast is assumed to be unaffected by the eye's optics. The reduced contrast sensitivity observed with normal viewing is, therefore, attributed to optical attenuation, and the ratio of the two types of contrast sensitivity function is equivalent to the MTF.[11, 61] Both of these techniques produce similar results, but a recent comparison using the same subjects showed that the double-pass method tended to slightly underestimate optical quality,[62] probably due to an error in the first assumption (a plane cosine reflector). A third technique involving measurement of ray aberrations has been used to estimate the optical quality in the human eye. By measuring the monochromatic optical aberrations of

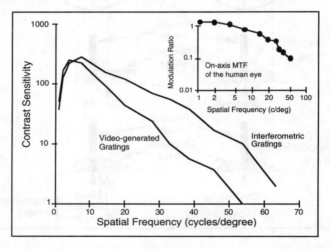

Figure 4 The average Contrast Sensitivity Functions of the two authors obtained using gratings generated on an oscilloscope and viewed through a 5mm pupil with those generated directly on the retina with an interferometer. Contrast sensitivity is the inverse of the minimum detectable contrast (contrast threshold). Although the retina can detect gratings with very high spatial frequencies (up to 120 c/deg),[64] optical attenuation limits normal foveal vision to about 50 cycles per degree. The ratio of these two contrast sensitivity functions is the optical MTF of the human eye (see inset).[11] At the foveal resolution limit for natural view, retinal image contrast is reduced by optical factors to about 10% (CS natural view =1, CS interferometry = 10, ratio = 0.1).

the eye, the MTF can be calculated. Subjective [31] and objective [59] versions of an ingenious device called an aberroscope were developed for this purpose. A comparison with the previous two methods [62] suggests that the aberroscope estimates of the MTF are better by about a factor of two than those estimated with the double-pass and CS methods. Because the aberrascope method only measures the lower order aberrations and does not evaluate the effects of higher order aberrations or scatter, it may overestimate retinal image quality.

Using the approach of Campbell and Green,[11] we have compared the authors' foveal contrast sensitivities obtained with interferometric and standard oscilloscope display technologies. Unlike the interferometrically generated gratings, retinal images of the oscilloscope gratings are degraded by the eye's optical aberrations and diffraction resulting in reduced contrast sensitivity (Figure 4). The ratio of the two contrast sensitivity functions provides a measure of the modulation transfer function of the human eye's optics (shown as an insert in Figure 4). This experiment was performed foveally with a well centered 5 mm natural pupil and well centered interference beams. The results show that, for example, at the normal high frequency cut-off (about 50 c/deg), the optics are transmitting about 10% of the object contrast to the retinal image. Similar results have been observed in earlier studies using this method.[11]

Simple sphero-cylindrical corrections can usually provide myopes, hyperopes, and/or astigmats with a retinal image of sufficient quality to achieve high spatial resolution approaching the neural limit at the human fovea.[63] In addition, many visually-coupled viewing instruments (e.g. Night Vision Goggles: NVG) incorporate an adjustable ocular lens to control the exit vergence in a way similar to that of a spectacle lens, but most of these only correct spherical and not astigmatic refractive errors. With a suitable refractive correction most subjects can be provided with a retinal image of sufficient quality to take full advantage of the high quality neural fovea.

However, in order for the retinal image quality to achieve these high levels, the optical path within the eye must be well centered. For example, failures in centration can lead to reduced light sensitivity, reduced spatial resolution, reduced contrast sensitivity, color distortions, unpredictable changes in refractive error, wavelength-specific distortions of visual direction and wavelength-specific errors in the judgment of apparent depth and size. The next section will consider the optical and visual consequences of decentering the optical path within the human eye.

Whenever we view the world through a visually coupled device that has an exit pupil, there is potential for optical path changes in the eye. Clearly, when viewing the world through a simple aperture or pupil, the location of the aperture determines the path taken by light in the eye. Also, when using a device that projects an exit pupil into the eye's pupil plane, any movement of the device with respect to the head will introduce displacements in this exit pupil with respect to the eye. If the instrument exit pupil does not completely cover the eye's natural pupil, these displacements will change the path of light in the eye that is used to form the retinal image. In active environments with significant changes in head position and acceleration (such as a fighter pilot in a combat environment), there will be significant changes in the relative location of the eye and the exit pupil of a visually coupled device (such as a NVG). Also, because the normal visual field extends about 160 degrees horizontally and about 120 degrees vertically, images of peripheral targets are created using quite different optical paths compared to the foveal images, and predictably their optical properties are quite different.

5. Decentration of the Eye's Entrance Pupil and its Effect on Vision

Optical theory predicts that decentration of the entrance pupil can introduce a variety of optical aberrations, e.g. transverse chromatic aberration, coma, and astigmatism. Over the last 30 years, each one of these has been blamed for the visual effects of pupil decentration. Of the few studies of the visual impact of pupil decentration, an early study by Green [26] is the most striking. He measured contrast sensitivity (CS) for sinusoidal gratings presented on an oscilloscope as a function of the location of a small (2mm) artificial pupil. He found that decentration of the pupil led to large decreases in visual acuity (VA) and an even larger decline in mid- and high-frequency contrast sensitivity (Figure 5). For example, when the small artificial pupil was decentered 3 mm, Green observed a 0.5 log unit reduction in VA and a 2 log unit reduction in CS at 15 c/deg. He noticed no such decline in CS when decentering the beams of a laser interferometer. Since CS for monochromatic interference fringes is unaffected by defocus or any other aperture dependent aberrations,[11] Green attributed the loss in CS observed in the normal incoherent

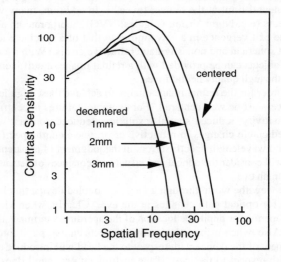

Figure 5 Data from Green [26] showing the effect of pupil decentration on foveal contrast sensitivity. These data were obtained by viewing a grating displayed on an oscilloscope with a P31 phosphor. Gratings were viewed through a small artificial pupil that was displaced from the point which provided best acuity. Note that the CS at 15 c/deg. has been reduced by about 2 log units.

experiment to coma caused by off-axis viewing in an eye with spherical aberration. Earlier studies of the refractive properties of the human eye had shown that the refraction of the marginal optics was generally different than the central optics [32] indicating that the human eye exhibits off-axis aberrations similar to spherical aberration, and more recently studies have indicated significant amounts of coma.[31, 59]

Subsequent to Green's study, van Meeteren and Dunnewold[57] and Thibos[53] both argued the ocular chromatic aberration and not spherical aberration or coma were responsible for the reduction in contrast sensitivity and visual acuity with pupil decentration. Recently, off-axis astigmatism was proposed as a significant contributing factor.[36] Finally, Campbell,[10] and Campbell and Gregory[9] argued that reduced visual acuity for decentered ray-bundles could be explained by the anatomical properties of the photoreceptors. The next section will examine these various hypotheses.

6. The Effect of Transverse Chromatic Aberration on Visual Performance with Decentered Pupils

The optical material of the human eye, like all refracting materials, exhibits chromatic dispersion. Obliquely incident rays will be spectrally dispersed, because short wavelengths are refracted more than long wavelengths. In an imaging system, this property can lead to

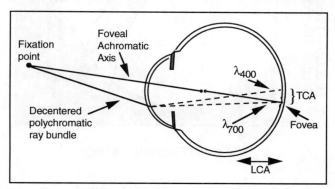

Figure 6 A schematic diagram showing the effect of beam decentration on foveal TCA and LCA. The magnitude of foveal transverse chromatic aberration (TCA) is directly proportional to the decentration of the entrance pupil from the visual axis (see Figure 1) and it is related to the LCA by a simple formula.[55] TCA (radians)= LCA (diopters) * Pupil Displacement (meters). The visual axis is defined theoretically as the axis that connects the fixation point, the eye's nodal points, and the fovea. Operationally, this axis can be identified by locating the ray path from the fixation point to the fovea that creates no foveal TCA.[55] For a simple model eye with a single refracting surface, the ray that passes through the nodal point strikes the optical surface orthogonally and therefore is the unique ray that is not refracted and hence experiences no chromatic dispersion.

324

wavelength dependent image planes (longitudinal or axial chromatic aberration), wavelength dependent image location within a given image plane (lateral or transverse chromatic aberration), and wavelength dependent image size,[50] all of which have been measured in the human eye.[30, 54, 71] Figure 6 shows a schematic representation of ocular longitudinal chromatic aberration (LCA) and transverse chromatic aberration (TCA).

Experimental studies of ocular TCA and pupil decentration show that the retinal location of the short and long wavelength images can differ by as much as 40 arc minutes for an artificial pupil decentered 4mm from the visual axis.[55] Therefore, when a polychromatic target is viewed through a decentered pupil, the visible spectrum is smeared across the retina in the same meridian as pupil decentration. The spectral smearing of polychromatic images created by ocular TCA demodulates contrast of polychromatic images by introducing wavelength-dependent phase-shifts into the image.[53, 57] The theoretical effects

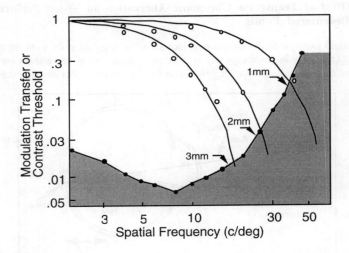

Figure 7 This Figure compares two optical models of the effect of pupil decentration on retinal image quality. The solid lines are from Thibos[53] and they are calculated using a single surface water eye, the open circles are the data from van Meeteren and Dunnewold,[57] who used a wave optics model of the eye. Both models predict the same reduction in polychromatic (P31 phosphor) MTF with increasing pupil decentration (1, 2, and 3 mm from top to bottom). Interestingly, Thibos's model only includes TCA. The filled circles are the retinal contrast thresholds from Campbell and Green,[11] and the arrows show the measured reduction in acuity observed by Green[26] with an artificial pupil decentered 1, 2, and 3 mm from the visual axis (see Fig. 5). The cross-over points between the model MTF and the retinal contrast threshold function predict the maximum acuity possible for decentered pupils. The predictions provide an accurate fit of the acuity data observed by Green (abscissa value for arrow tips).

of ocular TCA on retinal image contrast precisely predict the large decline in contrast sensitivity and visual acuity reported experimentally for polychromatic targets viewed through decentered pupils (Figure 7).[26, 53, 57, 70]

Using the contrast threshold function from Campbell and Green[11] and the predicted polychromatic MTFs for decentered pupils,[53] we can see that the highest detectable spatial frequencies imaged on the model eye retina for this polychromatic source correspond precisely with the measured fall-off in acuity seen in Green's data. The effectiveness of a TCA-based optical model to predict Green's data suggests that the reason Green observed no loss in contrast sensitivity for decentered interferometric gratings was not because they were created by interference on the retina, but because they were monochromatic. This conclusion is supported by results from our laboratories[6, 54] which show that interferometric monochromatic visual acuity is largely unaffected by beam decentration, but polychromatic interferometric acuity declines rapidly with increasing beam decentration (Figure 8). As predicted by the TCA models, the reduction in acuity and CS only occurs when the gratings were orthogonal to the axis of decentration (Figure 8).

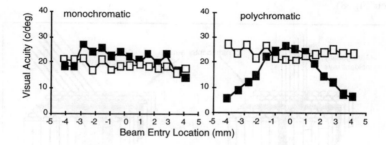

Figure 8 Data showing the effect of beam entry point on interferometric visual acuity. Filled and open symbols show data for vertical and horizontal gratings, respectively. The left and right panel show luminance matched data for monochromatic and polychromatic visual acuity. The polychromatic source was an incandescent bulb. Beams were decentered horizontally from the visual axis.

7. The Effect of Photoreceptor Structure on Visual Performance with Decentered Pupils

In addition to the effects of TCA, a component of the reduction in CS and VA is thought to originate in the retina. Due to the generally long axial length and narrow width of foveal photoreceptors, marginal rays in the pupil strike the retina obliquely and are thought to penetrate several photoreceptors as they pass through the retina (Figure 9). The "Retinal Direction Effect"[9, 10] proposed meridional smearing of the image across several receptors to account for some of the loss in VA that accompanied pupil decentration.

Interestingly, Campbell's model predicts a reduction in VA only for contours oriented orthogonal to the axis of pupil decentration, which is the same prediction made by TCA. In both cases (as shown schematically in Figure 9), a horizontally displaced pupil will lead to reduced contrast in the retinal images of vertical contours. However, this effect should be independent of spectral distribution of the light, and thus it probably accounts for the residual effects observed with monochromatic interferometric VA and CS.[17] Interestingly, Green[26] observed no effect on CS with his decentered monochromatic interferometer, and we only observed a small effect on VA (see Figure 8). Both of these studies suggest that the "retinal direction effect" is quite small, and virtually all of the visual problems associated with beam decentration are attributable to TCA.

Interestingly, the detailed study by Chen and Makous[17] points out the inadequacy of the simple model proposed by Campbell and described in Figure 9. Their results show that high spatial frequency interferometric contrast sensitivity is reduced by oblique retinal incidence for gratings oriented either orthogonal to or parallel to the axis of decentration. This result suggests that the light that escapes from each cone and continues on to be absorbed by a subsequent receptor is reflected in many directions before it leaves the cone (see their Fig. 8).[17]

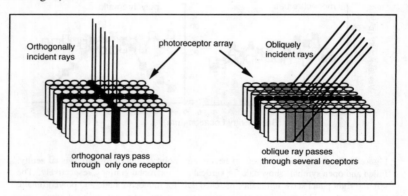

Figure 9   A schematic diagram showing that obliquely incident rays pass through multiple photoreceptors and produce a meridional smearing of the image for contours oriented orthogonal to the axis of pupil decentration. In this example, oblique rays are from a horizontally displaced pupil, and while the horizontal contour is unaffected, the image of the vertical contour has been smeared across several receptors. Campbell proposed this model to explain a reduction in VA that occurred with pupil decentration.

In summary, there are five clear hypotheses to explain the reduction in contrast sensitivity and visual resolution that accompanies decentered pupils: 1. Reduced retinal illuminance because of the SCE; 2. Coma and spherical aberrations (proposed by Green); 3. Oblique rays spreading to several photoreceptors because of the axial length of the receptors (Campbell and Gregory); 4. TCA creating a meridional spectral "smearing" of the retinal image (van Meeteren, Dunnewold, and Thibos); 5. Off-axis astigmatism due to the oblique incidence of the ray bundle.

Both the theoretical modeling and the experimental data point to TCA as the most important factor, but it is hard to explain the reduction in VA reported by Campbell and Gregory[9, 10] and Chen and Makous[17] for monochromatic stimuli without postulating a retinal direction effect. Coma and astigmatism perhaps contribute a small amount, but because of the large depth of focus afforded by the small pupils used by Green[26] and by Marcos,[36] these aberrations probably had a small effect. But in practice, with generally much larger pupils, the coma and astigmatism would be expected to play a more significant role.

Fortunately, recent studies[46, 54] have shown that the center of the eye's pupil is usually close to the visual axis and therefore, under normal viewing conditions, TCA is small near the fovea. However, TCA grows linearly with eccentricity from the achromatic axis and the rate of change in TCA across the retina is determined by the axial location of the pupil.[71] The pupil location the human eye appears to minimize foveal TCA and thus optimize polychromatic image quality at the fovea.

8. The Effect of Pupil Location of Perceived Direction and Depth

In addition to contrast demodulating effects observed with polychromatic stimuli, there are other very pronounced effects of TCA observed when viewing colored targets. For

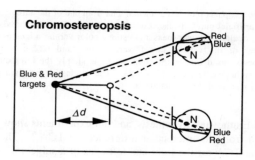

Figure 10 Schematic diagram showing how bi-temporal pupil decentrations can lead to an apparent difference in distance (Δd) between red and blue targets because of the interocular differences in monocular TCA. In this example, when viewing a red and a blue target at the same distance, the red will be imaged more temporally on the retina than the blue. Perceived visual direction and depth is found by back-projecting the red and blue retinal images into object space through the nodal points (N). In this example, it becomes clear that the red target will appear closer than blue, and the converse would be true for bi-nasal pupils. Most observers report seeing red slightly closer than blue and this probably reflects a bias in the population for the eye's pupil to be very slightly temporal relative to the visual axes.

example, it has been known for over 100 years that a simple optical model of TCA could account for the commonly observed color stereoscopy or chromostereopsis effect. When viewing equidistant, spatially adjacent objects of different colors (or wavelengths), most people report that the red objects appear closer than blue or green objects. Einthoven in 1885[22] realized that a horizontal interocular difference in monocular TCA created by unequal pupil decentrations (e.g., to the right in one eye and to the left in the other) would introduce a horizontal difference in the disparities of a long and a short wavelength target (Figure 10).

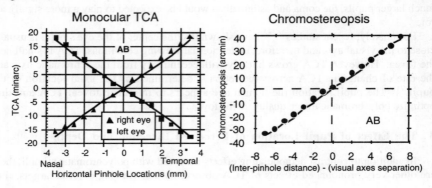

Figure 11 The left panel plots experimental data from one of the authors (AB) obtained with a small artificial pupil displaced nasally or temporally from the visual axis. For each location, ocular TCA was measured using a color vernier alignment procedure.[67] The two lines of the vernier target were 433nm and 622nm. The predicted chromostereopsis (solid line in the right panel) is simply the interocular difference between the right and left eye TCA data. The circles in the right panel are the experimentally measured chromostereopsis.

We have tested Einthoven's hypothesis, and our experiments show that the color depth effect are predicted from the interocular differences in TCA.[67] The data in Figure 11a show the monocular TCA for the right and left eyes of a subject as an artificial pupil is moved temporally or nasally. The interocular difference in horizontal TCA predicted for binocular viewing is simply the vertical separation between these two data sets. In Fig. 11b we show the calculated and experimentally measured chromostereopsis. It is clear that Einthoven's model precisely predicts the observed color depth "illusion". However, as described in Fig. 3, this geometrical optics explanation must be modified by the SCE anchoring effect,[58] which has an increasing effect with increasing pupil size.[68] The angular horizontal disparity (the ordinate in Fig. 11b) can be used to calculate the linear depth error introduced by TCA using the following approximate equation for small angles:

$$\theta = \frac{(-2a \times \Delta d)}{(D^2 + (D \times \Delta d))} \qquad (2)$$

where θ is the angular disparity, $2a$ is the interpupillary distance, D is the viewing distance, and Δd is the linear depth interval. It is important to emphasize that these predicted depth errors are not small, but extremely large. For example, ten arc minutes of disparity will create a 45 cm depth error when viewing a target at three meters. For spectrally pure stimuli viewed through small pupils, this sort of huge depth error can therefore be produced by an opposite lateral displacement of the right and left eye's entrance pupil by as little as 1mm (see Fig. 11b).

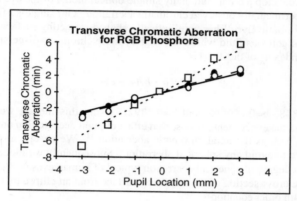

Figure 12 Transverse chromatic aberration of the human eye for targets displayed on a video monitor using either the red, blue, or green phosphors. TCA was measured as the amount of offset of two line segments required to make them appear collinear when viewed monocularly through a displaced, artificial pupil (zero displacement corresponds to alignment of the pupil on the visual axis). The two lines in this vernier alignment task were either red and green (filled circles), green and blue (open circles) or red and blue (open squares).

The color depth effect can be quite pronounced for broad spectrum stimuli.[65] For example, consider a red, green and blue phosphors on a typical TV monitor. Experimentally measured TCA for these stimuli are not as pronounced as observed between two monochromatic stimuli from the margins of the visible spectrum (e.g. Fig. 11), but large differences in apparent location of red and blue targets on a TV are produced when viewed through a displaced pupil (Fig. 12). This Figure provides an indication of the magnitude of the color misalignments that can be introduced with standard colored stimuli. As a worse-case example, the 6 arc minute of measured TCA produced between Red and Blue stimuli viewed through artificial pupils near the margins of the iris is approximately

100 times the typical vernier alignment threshold. This amount of TCA can introduce very significant errors into any alignment task that might involve two different colored targets. When viewed binocularly, this degree of asymmetric pupil decentration could introduce 12 arc minutes of horizontal disparity which, for an average person, corresponds to an error of about 2/3 meter in depth judgments at a 5 meter viewing distance.

9. Optical Model of Ocular TCA

The importance of ocular TCA for polychromatic image quality with decentered pupils, and its significant impact on the perceived location and depth of colored targets, has prompted us to develop a computationally simple optical model of the eye that accurately predicts the experimentally observed chromatic aberration. Our single-surface model eye, dubbed the Chromatic Eye,[51] has an elliptically shaped refracting surface separating air from an internal aqueous fluid which has slightly more chromatic dispersion than water. The refractive index n_λ of this fluid is

$$n_\lambda = a + b/(\lambda - c) \tag{3}$$

where a=1.31848, b=0.006662 and c=0.1292. Using this model, we were able to accurately model the experimentally observed effect of pupil decentration on foveal TCA in human eyes as well as the axial chromatic aberration.[51] We specifically employed an elliptical surface to avoid any spherical aberration. Subsequently we modified the model eye to include a degree of spherical aberration typical of human eyes.[52, 69] This was done by changing the cross-section of the refracting surface from an ellipse to a polynomial as defined by the 4th order equation

$$Y = 0.0899x^2 + 0.0006x^4 \tag{4}$$

This profile lies between a circle (which has too much spherical aberration) and an ellipse (which has too little spherical aberration). Refractive index was similar to the previous model,

$$n_\lambda = a + b/(\lambda - c) \tag{5}$$

where a=1.320535, b=0.004685 and c=0.214102. This model, called the Indiana Eye, accurately predicts both the eye's chromatic and spherical aberrations .

Application of the single-surface model to the problem of ocular chromatic aberration revealed the optical equivalence between displacing a target and displacing the pupil.[55] In both cases the target is being displaced from the achromatic axis of the eye, but in one case the target moves and in the other case the axis moves. To see this, imagine the result of moving a target in Fig. 1 off the achromatic axis. As a target is moved farther into the periphery, the angle of incidence of the chief ray departs more and more from the normal, resulting in chromatic dispersion. If, on the other hand, the target remains fixed and the entrance pupil is displaced, the achromatic axis of the optical system shifts because the achromatic axis, by definition, goes through the center of the pupil. Shifting the achromatic axis away from the target again increases the obliquity of the incident ray bundle, causing increased chromatic dispersion of a polychromatic chief ray. To quantify this equivalence relationship, Thibos et al ,[55] showed that the angle of incidence of the chief ray (and hence the amount of ocular TCA) was the same for eccentric targets and for decentered pupils when

$$H = NP \times \sin(\varepsilon) \tag{6}$$

where H is the decentration of the pupil and ε (in radians) is target eccentricity. The gain of this relationship is controlled by the axial separation NP between the entrance pupil and the nodal point.

10. Optical Effects of Target Eccentricity

The previous sections of this chapter have emphasized the impact of pupil decentration on foveal image quality. In this section we will examine the optical impact of off-axis targets. As noted above, many of the optical changes that accompany target decentration are equivalent, or at least qualitatively similar, to the optical effects of pupil decentration. In both cases the optical beam strikes the eye's optics with increasing obliquity and therefore the optical aberrations that accompany oblique rays (e.g. TCA, spherical aberration, coma, astigmatism) will affect retinal image quality. Despite this equivalence, the optical consequences of moving targets into the peripheral visual field are often dismissed as being unimportant since the spatial resolving power of the peripheral retina is so poor in comparison with foveal resolution. This dismissive attitude is changing, however, following the discovery of useful vision beyond the classical resolution limit in the periphery (see the chapter by Thibos & Bradley in this book) so it is worth reviewing the topic here.

There are few studies of the eye's optical system for peripheral targets, but early examination of peripheral refractive errors highlighted the significant differences between foveal and peripheral optics. For example, Ferree, Rand and Hardy[24] measured peripheral refractive error in 21 subjects out to 50 degrees in both the nasal and temporal fields. Their results, which have been replicated by others,[41] show that a very large amount of astigmatism develops in the far periphery (increasing to as much as 8 diopters at 50 degrees). As predicted by optical models,[20, 35, 60] most subjects had increasing peripheral astigmatism with increasing eccentricity with the tangential focus being myopic and the sagittal focus being hyperopic. In some subjects, both meridians were hyperopic, but again the sagittal meridian was more hyperopic. In general, real eyes tend to have much less peripheral astigmatism than spherical model eyes predict.[20, 35] This can be explained by the asphericity of the cornea and lens.[20] The location of the two foci (tangential and sagittal) will be influenced strongly by the shape of the eye-ball, which in turn is related to the spherical refractive error. This relationship was confirmed by Millodot,[39] who showed that, in more myopic eyes, both the tangential and sagittal meridians became more hyperopic than the fovea with increasing eccentricity. This reflects the lager reduction in peripheral posterior nodal distance in axially myopic eyes.

The oblique incidence of the rays forming retinal images of peripheral targets should lead to increased TCA[55] but experimental verification of this prediction has proved difficult. Experiments in our labs[18] have shown that the detection of peripheral polychromatic interference fringes varies with their orientation in a systematic fashion. Polychromatic fringes are easiest to detect when they are radially oriented (i.e. their orientation is parallel with a line connecting the fovea with the center of the target) and they are most difficult to detect when oriented tangentially. This behavior can be accounted for quantitatively using the Chromatic Eye model described above. However, using ordinary targets viewed through natural pupils, Ogboso and Bedell[44] failed to observe TCA consistent with any optical predictions. Also, Zhang et al[71], found only very small amounts of peripheral TCA. However, as predicted by a simple model,[72] the amount of peripheral TCA is amplified significantly if the natural pupil is substituted with an artificial pupil placed anterior to the eye (the typical location).[71] This should be a serious consideration in the design of any visually coupled instrument that creates an exit pupil.

Experimental measures of retinal image quality for peripheral targets have shown that image quality does deteriorate with increasing eccentricity.[33, 34, 43, 48] However, if peripheral refractive errors are corrected, image quality within the central 40 degrees (± 20 degrees) of the visual field remains uniformly high.[43, 48, 49]

Although peripheral aberrations can be very large, their impact on peripheral vision depends upon the visual task and whether known refractive errors are corrected with spectacles or contact lenses. As noted above, the detection of high-frequency, polychromatic fringes is optically limited and this holds as well for natural viewing of polychromatic gratings. However, this optically-imposed cutoff frequency for contrast *detection* is far beyond the Nyquist limit for spatial *resolution* imposed by the relatively coarse sampling density of neurons in peripheral retina.[56] Consequently, the optical quality of the well-focused human eye is not a limiting factor for peripheral resolution tasks such as reading letters or identifying the orientation of sinusoidal grating targets viewed eccentrically.[27, 40] On the other hand, if refractive errors are left uncorrected, they may be large enough to limit resolution, and the effect will likely vary with target orientation because of the large off-axis astigmatism present in human eyes.[24, 39, 41]

In addition to the increased off-axis optical aberrations that accompany target decentration, there are changes in retinal illuminance and distortions of the image. Fortunately, the combined effects of reduced pupil diameter and reduced posterior nodal distance with its decreased magnification (mm^2 per deg^2) may combine to provide almost constant retinal illuminance across all but the very far periphery,[15] but retinal illuminance will be lower in the very far periphery (>70 degrees).

11. Summary and Practical Considerations

The fortuitous alignment in most eyes of the visual axis, the pupil, and the SCE provides an approximate joint optical and neural axis for the human eye. Although some issues remain unresolved, it appears clear that deviations from this axis will lead to reduced optical quality of the retinal image, primarily due to transverse chromatic aberration and off-axis astigmatism. These aberrations will accompany both pupil and target decentration, but the visual ramifications of pupil decentration will generally be more pronounced because it will affect foveal vision.

In light of the above summary and the chapter on peripheral vision by Thibos and Bradley in this book, it becomes clear that optimal visual performance requires a well centered target and a well centered pupil. Target centration is usually well controlled by fixational eye movements that can maintain a small fixated target within the fovea and a large fixated target centered on the fovea. Also, when the eye's iris defines the entrance pupil for the eye, the entering optical beam will be well centered on the visual (foveal) axis. However, if an intervening visually coupled device employs a small exit pupil which is not centered on the visual axis, the optical problems summarized above would affect foveal image quality and hence foveal vision. Visually-coupled instruments that employ exit pupils larger than the natural pupil will be assured of a well centered optical path if the exit pupil completely covers the eye's entrance pupil. However, instrument decentration or relative movement between the head and instrument may lead to partial coverage, and hence the effective entrance pupil will be decentered. It is clear that any visually-coupled electro-optical device should employ an exit pupil large enough to ensure that it always covers the eye's entrance pupil.

Acknowledgments

The ideas presented in this paper have developed in parallel with the dissertation research of David Still, Xioaxioa Zhang and Ming Ye at Indiana University School of Optometry. Their work and ours has been supported by National Institutes of Health grants EY05109 and EY07638, and by a grant to the Indiana Institute for the Study of Human Capabilities provided by the USAFOSR.

References

1. R.A. Applegate and A.B. Bonds, (1981). Induced movement of receptor alignment toward a new pupillary aperture. *Invest. Ophthal. Vis. Sci.*, **21**, 869-873.
2. R.A. Applegate and V. Lakshminarayanan, (1993). Parametric representation of Stiles-Crawford functions: normal variation of peak location and directionality. *J. Opt. Soc. Am.-A*, **10**, 1611-1623.
3. P. Artal, (1989). Incorporation of directional effects on the retina into computations of optical transfer functions of human eyes. *JOSA-A*, **6**, 1941-1944.
4. D. Atchison, (1984). Visual Optics in man. *Aust. J. Optometry*, **67**, 141-150.

334

5. L.J. Bour, (1980). MTF of the defocused optical system of the human eye for incoherent monochromatic light. *J. Opt. Soc. Am.*, **70**, 321-328.
6. A. Bradley, L. Thibos and D. Still, (1990). Visual acuity measured with clinical Maxwellian-View systems: Effects of beam entry position. *Optom. Visual Sci.*, **67**, 811-817.
7. A. Bradley, X. Zhang and L.N. Thibos, (1991). Achromatizing the human eye. *Optom Vision Sc*, **68**, 608-616.
8. F. Campbell, (1957). Depth of Field of the Human Eye. *Optica Acta*, **4**, 157-164.
9. F. Campbell and A. Gregory, (1960). The spatial resolving power of the human retina with oblique incedence. *J. Opt. Soc. Am.*, **50**, 831.
10. F.W. Campbell, (1958). A retinal acuity direction effect. *J. Physiol.*, **144**, 25p-26p.
11. F.W. Campbell and D.G. Green, (1965). Optical and Retinal factors affecting visual resolution. *J Physiol (Lond)*, **181**, 576 - 593.
12. F.W. Campbell and R.W. Gubisch, (1966). Optical quality of the human eye. *J. Physiol.*, **186**, 558-578.
13. F.W. Campbell and R.W. Gubisch, (1967). The effect of chromatic aberration on visual acuity. *J. Physiol.*, **192**, 345-358.
14. W. Charman, (1979). Effect of refractive error on visual tests with sinusoidal gratings. *Brit. J. Physiol. Optics*, **33**, 34-39.
15. W. Charman, (1989). Light on the peripheral retina. *Ophthalmic Physiol. Opt.*, **9**, 91-92.
16. W.N. Charman, in *Progress in Retinal Research*, 1983), 1-50.
17. B. Chen and W. Makous, (1989). Light capture by human cones. *J. Physiol (Lond.)*, **414**, 89-109.
18. F. Cheney, *Detection acuity in the peripheral retina*, Masters Thesis (Indiana University, 1989)
19. C. Cui and M. Campbell, (1994). Two methods for measuring the tilt and decentration of the crystaline lens in Vivo. *Invest. Ophthalmol.*, **35**, 1258.
20. M. Dunne and D. Barnes, (1987). Schematic modelling of peripheral astigmatism in real eyes. *Ophthalmic Physiol Opt.*, **7**, 235-239.
21. C.J.W. Dunnewold, *On the Campbell and Stiles-Crawford effects and their clinical importance*, M.D. thesis Thesis (Rijksuniversiteit Utrecht, The Netherlands, 1964)
22. W. Einthoven, (1885). Stereokopiee durch Farbendifferenz. *Albert von Graefes Archiv. fur Ophthamologie*, **31**, 211-238.
23. J.M. Enoch and V. Lakshminarayanan, in *Vision Optics and Instrumentation*, ed. W.N. Charman (MacMillan Press, London, U.K., 1991), 280-308.
24. C. Ferree, G. Rand and C. Hardy, (1931). Refraction of the peripheral field of vision. *Arch. Ophthalmol.*, **5**, 717-731.
25. R. Fox, S. Lehmkuhle and D. Westendorf, (1976). Falcon Visual Acuity. *Science*, **192**, 263-265.
26. D. Green, (1967). Visual resolution when light enters the eye through different parts of the pupil. *J. Physiol. (Lond)*, **190**, 583-593.

27. D.G. Green, (1970). Regional variations in the visual acuity for interference fringes on the retina. *J. Physiol.*, **207**, 351-356.

28. D.G. Green and F.W. Campbell, (1965). Effects of focus on the visual response t a sinusoidally modulated spatial stimulus. *J. Opt. Soc. Am.*, **55**, 1154-1157.

29. R.W. Gubisch, (1967). Optical performance of the human eye. *J. Opt. Soc. Am.*, **57**, 407-415.

30. P.A. Howarth and A. Bradley, (1986). The longitudinal chromatic aberration of the human eye, and its correction. *Vision Res.*, **26**, 361-366.

31. H. Howland and B. Howland, (1977). A subjective method for the measurement of monochromatic aberrations of the eye. *J. Opt. Soc. Am.*, **67**, 1508-1518.

32. A. Ivanoff, (1956). About the spherical aberration of the eye. *J. Opt. Soc. Am.*, **46**, 901-903.

33. J. Jennings and W. Charman, (1978). Optical image quality in the peripheral retina. *Am. J Optom Physiol Optics*, **55**, 582-590.

34. J. Jennings and W. Charman, (1981). Off-axis image quality in the human eye. *Vision Res.*, **21**, 445-454.

35. Y. Le Grand, *Form and Space Perception,* ed. M. Millodot and G. Heath (Indiana University Press, Bloomington, 1967).

36. S. Marcos, P. Artal and D. Green, (1994). The effect of decentered small pupils on ocular modulation transfer and contrast sensitivity. *Invest. Ophthalmol.*, **35**, 1258.

37. F. Martin, (1942). The Importance and Measurement of Angle Alpha. *Brit. J. Physiol. Optics*, **3**, 27-45.

38. H. Metcalf, (1965). Stiles-Crawford Apodization. *J. Opt. Soc. Am.*, **55**, 72-74.

39. M. Millodot, (1981). Effect of ametropia on peripheral refraction. *Am J Optom Physiol Optics*, **58**, 691-695.

40. M. Millodot, A.L. Johnson, A. Lamont and H.W. Leibowitz, (1975). Effect of dioptrics on peripheral visual acuity. *Vision Res.*, **15**, 1357-1362.

41. M. Millodot and A. Lamont, (1974). Refraction of the periphery of the eye. *Opt. Soc. Am.*, **64**, 110-111.

42. M. Mino and Y. Okano, (1971). Improvement in the OTF of a Defocused Optical System Through the Use of Shaded Apertures. *Appl. Opt.*, **10**, 2219-2225.

43. R. Navarro, P. Artal and D. Williams, (1993). Modulation transfer of the human eye as a function of retinal eccentricity. *J. Opt. Soc. Am. A*, **10**, 201-212.

44. Y. Ogboso and H. Bedell, (1987). Magnitude of lateral chromatic aberration across the retina of the human eye. *J. Opt. Soc. Am. A*, **4**, 1666-1672.

45. L. Reymond, (1985). Spatial Visual Acuity of the Eagle Aquila Audax: A behavioural, optical, and anatomical investigation. *Vision Res.*, **25**, 1477-1491.

46. P. Simonet and M. Campbell, (1990). The transverse chromatic aberration on the fovea of the human eye. *Vis. Res*, **30**, 187-206.

47. W.S. Stiles and B.H. Crawford, (1933). The luminous efficiency of rays entering the eye pupil at different points. *Proc. Roy. Soc.*, **112**, 428-450.

48. D. Still, L. Thibos and A. Bradley, (1989). Peripheral image quality is almost as good as central image quality. *Invest. Ophthalmol Vis. Sci. (Suppl)*, **30**, 52.

49. D.L. Still, *Optical Limits to Contrast Sensitivity in Human Peripheral Vision*, Ph. D. Thesis (Indiana University, 1989)

50. L. Thibos N, A. Bradley and X. Zhang, (1991). Effect of ocular chromatic aberration on monocular visual performance. *Optom Visual Sc*, **68**, 599-607.

51. L. Thibos, M. Ye, X. Zhang and A. Bradley, (1992). The chromatic eye: a new reduced-eye model of ocular chromatic aberration in humans. *Applied Opt.*, **31**, 3594-3600.

52. L. Thibos, M. Ye, X. Zhang and A. Bradley, (1993). A new Optical Model of the Human Eye. *Optics and Photonics News*, **4**, 11.

53. L.N. Thibos, (1987). Calculation of the influence of lateral chromatic aberration on image quality across the visual field. *J Opt Soc Am A*, **4**, 1673-1680.

54. L.N. Thibos, A. Bradley and D. Still, (1991). Interferometric measurement of visual acuity and the effect of ocular chromatic aberration. *Appl Optics*, **In Press**,

55. L.N. Thibos, A. Bradley, D.L. Still, X. Zhang and P.A. Howarth, (1990). Theory and measurement of ocular chromatic aberration. *Vision Res.*, **30**, 33-49.

56. L.N. Thibos, D.J. Walsh and F.E. Cheney, (1987). Vision beyond the resolution limit: aliasing in the periphery. *Vision Res.*, **27**, 2193-2197.

57. A. van Meeteren and C.J.W. Dunnewold, (1983). Image Quality of the Human Eye for Eccentric Pupils. *Vision Res.*, **23**, 573-579.

58. J.J. Vos, (1960). Some new aspects of color stereoscopy. *J. Opt. Soc. Am.*, **50**, 785-790.

59. G. Walsh, W. Charman and H. Howland, (1984). Objective technique for the determination of monochromatic aberrations of the human eye. *J. Opt. Soc. Am. A*, **1**, 987-992.

60. G. Wang, O. Pomerantzeff and Pankratov, (1983). Astigmatism of oblique incidence in the human model eye. *Vis. Res.*, **23**, 1079-1085.

61. G. Westheimer and F.W. Campbell, (1962). Light distribution in the image formed by the living human eye. *J. Opt. Soc. Amer.*, **52**, 1040-1045.

62. D. Williams, D. Brainard, M. McMahon and R. Navarro, (1994). Double pass and interferometric measures of the optical quality of the eye. *J. Opt. Soc. Am. A*, **In Press**.

63. D.R. Williams, (1985). Aliasing in human foveal vision. *Vision Res.*, **25**, 195-205.

64. D.R. Williams, (1985). Visibility of interference fringes near the resolution limit. *J. Opt. Soc. Amer.*, **A2**, 1087-1093.

65. B. Winn, A. Bradley, N. Strang, P. McGraw and L. Thibos, (1994). Reversals of the color-depth illusion explained by ocular chromatic aberration. *Vision Res.*, **Submitted**.

66. B. Winn, D. Whitaker, D. Elliot and N. Philips, (1994). Factors Affecting Light-adapted Pupil Size. *Invest. Ophthalmol. Visual Sci.*, **35**, 1132-1137.

67. M. Ye, A. Bradley, L. Thibos and X. Zhang, (1991). Interocular differences in Transverse Chromatic Aberration Determine Chromostereopsis for Small Pupils. *Vision Res*, **31**, 1787-1796.

68. M. Ye, A. Bradley, L.N. Thibos and X.X. Zhang, (1992). The Effect of Pupil Size on Chromostereopsis and Chromatic Diplopia: Interaction between the Stiles-Crawford Effect and Chromatic Aberrations. *Vision Res.*, **32**, 2121-2128.

69. M. Ye, L. Thibos, X. Zhang and A. Bradley, (1993). A new single-surface model eye that accurately predicts chromatic and spherical aberrations of the human eye. *Invest. Ophthalmol. Vis. Sci.*, **34**, 777.

70. X. Zhang, A. Bradley and L. Thibos, (1991). Achromatizing the human eye: the problem of chromatic parallax. *Opt. Soc. Am. A*, **8**, 686-691.

71. X. Zhang, A. Bradley and L. Thibos, (1993). Experimental determination of the chromatic difference of magnification of the human eye and the location of the anterior nodal point. *J. Opt. Soc. Am. A.*, **10**, 213-220.

72. X. Zhang, L. Thibos and A. Bradley, (1991). Relationship between the chromatic difference of refraction and the chromatic difference of magnification of the human eye. *Optom. Vis. Sci.*, **68**, 456-458.

MODELING OFF-AXIS VISION II: THE EFFECT OF SPATIAL FILTERING AND SAMPLING BY RETINAL NEURONS

LARRY N. THIBOS and ARTHUR BRADLEY

School of Optometry, Indiana University
Bloomington, Indiana   47405

In Section 1 of this chapter we review the existing models of peripheral vision, most of which are based on the appealing conception that peripheral vision is just a spatially scaled version of central vision. We argue against scaling models, however, on the grounds that they cannot account for the primary factor which limits resolving power in the periphery: neural undersampling of the optical image formed on the retina. In order to account for sampling effects, we adopt an engineering perspective to develop in Section 2 a simple model of optical and neural processing of the retinal image. In Section 3, we apply our neuro-optical model to human eyes in order to discover the relative importance of the optical and neural limits to pattern detection and resolution. The results show that, although the optical system of the eye is the dominant factor limiting central vision, spatial undersampling by the optic nerve cells of the retina limits resolution in the periphery. Neural undersampling of the retinal image leads to perceptual aliasing and spurious detection of patterns up to an order of magnitude finer than the Nyquist limit. Aliasing is curtailed at very high frequencies by a combination of optical filtering and spatial summation over the finite aperture of cone photoreceptors. We conclude with some comments on practical applications of the model.

1. Spatial Vision in the Peripheral Field

1.1. Differences between Central and Peripheral Vision

Most of what is known about human vision is the result of experimental investigations of the central few degrees of the visual field. This emphasis is understandable since central vision is critical for everyday living and the loss of central vision to disease or aging is a severe physical handicap. Nevertheless, it is ironic to note that probably 99% of all research on the human visual system has been devoted to the central 1% of our visual field. As a result, the performance characteristics and mechanisms of peripheral vision are poorly understood by comparison to those of central vision.

Spatial resolving power is the most important difference between central and peripheral vision. In a classic study published in 1857 by Aubert and Förster[4] and summarized in Helmholtz's authoritative *Treatise on Physiological Optics*[83] (see p. 39), two fundamental facts were established. First, the minimum dimensions of letters and numerals that can be resolved in the peripheral field varies in direct proportion to the eccentricity of the letters from the fixation point. Second, the iso-acuity contours in peripheral vision for two-point resolution are slightly elliptical with the major axis oriented horizontally. Numerous subsequent studies have confirmed these findings (see Genter *et al.*[26] for a review), the most thorough of which was by Wertheim.[102] Using gratings as a test target, Wertheim performed an exhaustive series of measurements which documented the acuity of his own left eye throughout the visual field, an heroic feat which has only recently been repeated.[105] His results showed that the ability of the human eye to resolve the individual bars of a grating pattern varies by nearly two orders of magnitude over the visual field, falling from about 50 cyc/deg in central vision to less than 1 cyc/deg in the far periphery. Although Wertheim and many subsequent authors describe acuity as falling inversely with target eccentricity, this description simply reflects the convention of using spatial frequency, rather than its inverse, as a measure of acuity.[26]

Accounting for the huge loss of spatial resolving power in peripheral vision is a major challenge to visual scientists and to the models of spatial vision which they invent. Such models are important not only for summarizing our understanding of the physical factors which limit visual resolution, but also for solving applied problems and for yielding sensible answers to practical questions such as: "What are the functional consequences of a 6 deg foveal scotoma?", "Is a central scotoma equivalent to low-pass filtering the image?", "Is scotopic vision just photopic vision with more low-pass filtering?", "Does contrast threshold for patterned targets scale with eccentricity?", "Over what range of stimulus parameters is detection equivalent to recognition, and does the answer vary with retinal eccentricity?"

Variation of resolving power across the visual field is, in a broader context, an example of the common biological strategy of distributing individual sensory transducers non-uniformly in order to selectively emphasize some regions of the environment at the expense of others. In the sense of touch, for example, there are many more tactile sensors in the finger tips and lips than along the arm or leg. As a result, spatial resolution of tactile stimuli is much higher for our fingers and lips and there is a far greater portion of our brains devoted to the representation and analysis of these areas by comparison to other parts of the body.[55] Similarly, many animals (including mammals) which live in an open habitat dominated visually by the horizon have retinas which contain a specialized region called the *visual streak*,[33, 85] a pronounced band of tightly packed retinal receptors that supports especially high visual acuity over a horizontal region of visual space.

The evolution of a visual streak in insects and other arthropods is just one of many examples of biological adaptation that Wehner calls "matched filtering".[97] According to this general principle, the fundamental spatial aspects of crucial sensory problems are incorporated into the spatial design of the sensory surface itself. By this simple trick, sensory systems avoid the need for complex neural circuitry to solve difficult problems such as navigation by honey bees or desert ants using the celestial pattern of polarization to steer the course, or long-distance navigation by migratory birds and homing pigeons. A similar problem described by Wehner is illustrated in Fig. 1. During forward locomotion

340

(or during the approach of a predator) the retinal image of an off-axis object grows larger as it gets closer. In order to avoid misinterpreting this enlargement of the retinal image as physical growth of the object, the visual system must take into account the fact that the image is also moving into the periphery as it grows. It is conceivable that a neural circuit could be built to achieve the desired "neural size constancy" by extracting the correlation between image size and retinal eccentricity and using the result to calculate object size from image size. However, there is a much simpler solution which takes advantage of the geometry of Fig. 1. If the spatial grain of the retina increases in direct proportion to eccentricity, as is true in man (and sand crabs!), then the retinal image of an approaching object will stimulate the same number of neural elements regardless of viewing distance. One consequence of this arrangement is that if a visual object of size x is just resolvable in peripheral vision at one viewing distance, then it will be just resolvable at all viewing distances. From Wehner's perspective, then, the dramatic variation of resolving power of the human eye across the visual field is just one more example of biological evolution of matched filtering to simplify sensory coding of the visual environment through the technique of spatial distortion of the retinal array.

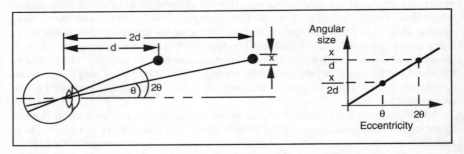

Figure 1. Non-uniform resolving power of the eye as a mechanism for achieving neural size-constancy. An object of constant absolute size located a fixed distance from the visual axis doubles in angular size and its eccentricity doubles when the viewing distance is halved. For the neural image of the object to be the same size in either case, the minimum resolvable angle of the visual system should vary in direct proportion to eccentricity. The weight of experimental evidence in humans is consistent with this model.[26]

The aim and scope of this chapter is to review the salient features of spatial vision in the peripheral field for the purpose of developing a useful model. In our view, the variation of spatial resolution across the visual field so prominent in man is due entirely to just two ocular factors: variation of optical image quality and changes in the architecture of the neural retina. The latter of these two factors is the topic of this chapter, whereas the former is dealt with in detail in the chapter by Bradley and Thibos (1995) in this book.

1.2. Filtering Models of Peripheral Vision

Perhaps the simplest approach to modeling spatial vision in the periphery is to adapt existing models of central vision by adjusting the parameters of the model. Current models of central vision emphasize two fundamental, physical factors which limit performance: filtering and noise. For example, in the "Static Performance Model" of the USAF Night Vision Laboratory[59] the human visual system is represented by a concatenation of two linear filters (one optical and the other a spatio-temporal filter of a neural contrast detector) and performance is quantified statistically to account for the effects of noise.[40] Such filtering-limited and noise-limited models have a firm scientific basis which is well documented in the literature on human foveal vision[20] and many applied models follow a similar approach,[50] including ACQUIRE,[40] VIDEM,[1] ORACLE,[51] and PHIND.[84]

To adapt foveal models for peripheral vision, the usual approach is to broaden the filter's impulse response function (or, equivalently, reduce the low-pass cutoff frequency) sufficiently to account for the reduced resolving power in the peripheral field. A conceptually simple way to broaden a spatial filter is to rescale the spatial dimension and so it has become popular to conceive of peripheral vision as just a spatially-scaled version of central vision. This rescaling approach gained considerable momentum from early experiments by Rovamo and Virsu[62] and others [35, 36] which demonstrated that if visual targets were magnified in the periphery in order to compensate for the reduced representation of the peripheral field in the visual cortex, and if the size of targets were expressed in cortical dimensions rather than visual space dimensions, then visual performance is invariant across the visual field. This idea fit in neatly with the well-known anatomical fact that the cortical representation of the visual world is highly distorted in favor of the central field of view.[19] It is also consistent with emerging evidence that the "cortical magnification factor", defined as the number of mm on the surface of the cortex representing 1 deg of visual field, is correlated with peripheral visual acuity.[14, 92]

The basic concept of the Rovamo-Virsu rescaling model in its current form[108] is illustrated schematically in Fig. 2. The foveal contrast sensitivity function (CSF) in Fig. 2A indicates the minimum contrast required by human observers to detect a small patch of sinusoidal grating as a function of the grating's spatial frequency. Since all points in the graph below the CSF represent grating contrasts which exceed psychophysical threshold, the CSF may be regarded as the upper boundary of a region of visibility. The lower boundary of this region of visibility is set by the horizontal line representing 100% contrast, which is the maximum physical contrast possible for sinusoidal gratings. The spatial frequency for which contrast sensitivity falls to unity thus represents the highest detectable spatial frequency and this cutoff spatial frequency is a universally accepted definition of visual acuity, i.e. the resolving power of central vision. By comparison, the CSF for the same small patch of grating displayed in peripheral vision was displaced increasingly downwards and to the left as the visual stimulus moved progressively further into the periphery (Fig. 2B). Rovamo and Virsu argued that contrast sensitivity and resolving power falls dramatically when the target is imaged on peripheral retina because the amount of visual cortex stimulated by the visual target is much smaller. In support of this interpretation, they found that if the peripheral target was enlarged to compensate for the difference in cortical representation, then contrast sensitivity increased to the levels measured for central vision. By scaling the targets in this way, the CSFs for central and peripheral retina were found to be indistinguishable when spatial frequency was expressed as a fraction of the cutoff frequency, as shown in Fig. 2C. Thus, on the basis of their experimental data, Rovamo and Virsu proposed the unifying concept of a universal CSF which, when properly scaled by a "cortical magnification factor", applies anywhere in the visual field.

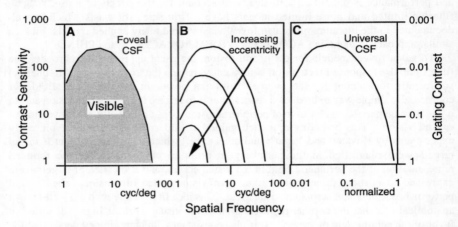

Figure 2. The Rovamo-Virsu filtering model of contrast detection across the visual field. Ordinate may be specified either as the contrast of a just detectable grating (right) or as contrast sensitivity (i.e. the inverse of threshold contrast, left). Abscissa is object spatial frequency specified either in absolute angular dimensions (A, B) or normalized by the cutoff spatial frequency for each curve (C). A: foveal vision. B: peripheral vision for targets of fixed angular size. C: a universal CSF which applies for all parts of the visual field, provided that the stimulus size is scaled according to cutoff spatial frequency.

1.3. Evidence of Sampling Limitations to Peripheral Vision

Our objection to the rescaling model as described above is that it contains a hidden assumption which is not valid for peripheral vision. To expose this hidden assumption we return to our earlier interpretation of the cutoff spatial frequency, which was offered as a definition of the resolving power of the eye. In so doing, no distinction was made between the ability of observers to *detect* the presence of a luminance pattern and the ability to *resolve* the spatial structure of the pattern. Although this may sound like a minor distinction, it is in fact fundamental to the problem of modeling peripheral vision. In psychophysical experiments designed to measure contrast detection, observers are asked to distinguish the grating from a uniform patch of the same mean luminance. The rationale of this paradigm is that, in a properly controlled experiment, the presence of spatial contrast is the only feature of the grating required by subjects to successfully perform the task. To measure resolution on the other hand, the experimenter must force the observer to demonstrate some evidence that the features of the detected pattern are correctly perceived. The most common way to gather such evidence experimentally is to ask the subject to identify the orientation of the grating (e.g. is it vertical or horizontal?).

When these two different psychophysical tasks of detection and resolution are performed using central vision, they give essentially identical results. Consequently, there is normally no need to distinguish between visual acuity for detection and visual acuity for resolution when viewing targets foveally. However, in peripheral vision there can be as much as an order of magnitude difference in these two measures of visual acuity when high-contrast interference-fringes are used to stimulate the retina,[82] thereby avoiding many of the optical limitations of the eye.[78] The difference between the cutoff frequency for resolution and detection tasks is not as great when the retinal image is formed by the eye's optics in natural view, but substantial differences remain provided the retinal image is clearly focused. For example, at 20 deg in the nasal field *detection acuity* for gratings displayed on an oscilloscope is four times greater than *resolution acuity* as demonstrated by the psychometric performance curves of Fig. 3A. The open symbols in this graph show that performance for the resolution task was flawless below 5 cyc/deg but then falls to 75% correct at about 6 cyc/deg and is no better than chance beyond about 7 cyc/deg. Nevertheless, just beyond this resolution limit the pattern is still detected without error (solid symbols) and detection performance does not fall to the 75% correct level until the spatial frequency goes beyond about 24 cyc/deg. Thus there is a large range of spatial frequencies, shown by the shaded area, for which gratings can be detected but not resolved. For reasons that we discuss next, this area is labeled the *aliasing zone*.

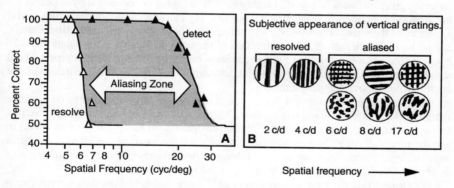

Figure 3. A: Comparison of performance for resolution and detection tasks. B: Drawings of subjective appearance of gratings. Eccentricity = 20 deg, horizontal nasal visual-field.

To gain some insight into the reason for the large difference in performance for the detection and resolution tasks in peripheral vision, we asked the observer in this experiment to sketch the subjective appearance of the stimulus. One observer's drawings of a 1.5 deg circular patch of vertical grating set to several different values of spatial frequency are shown in Fig. 3B. These sketches reveal that when the grating frequency was less than the resolution cutoff (i.e. < 6 cyc/deg), the subjective appearance was veridical. That is, the pattern appeared to contain the correct number of cycles and its orientation was correctly perceived. However, for frequencies beyond the resolution cutoff the subjective appearance was erroneous in several different ways. The pattern often did not look like a grating at all, but was fragmented and splotchy and it always appeared much coarser than when the stimulus was viewed foveally. On those occasions when the pattern did look like a grating, it frequently had the wrong orientation and always had too few cycles (for example, a 1.5 deg patch of 8 cyc/deg grating contains 12 cycles, but the drawing has only 5 cycles). Such percepts were highly unstable and changed significantly from moment to moment, as may be seen in the pairs of sketches drawn for the same test frequency. Despite this instability, the presence of spatial contrast was reliably observed across the full range of frequencies from the resolution limit to the detection limit.

Our interpretation of the non-veridical drawings in Fig. 3B is that subjects were experiencing the effects of neural undersampling of the retinal image. In other words, we believe the observer perceived an *alias* of the stimulus rather than the stimulus itself. Our reasoning is as follows. Because the continuous retinal image is sampled by the mosaic of retinal neurons, the fidelity of the discrete *neural image* will be constrained by Shannon's sampling theorem of communication theory.[67] Consequently, if the spatial frequency of the retinal image exceeds the Nyquist limit set by the density of retinal neurons, then the pattern will be misrepresented by the neural array. This erroneous pattern of neural activity is indistinguishable from the pattern of neural activity that would have been produced by a different, and much coarser, visual stimulus which is below the Nyquist limit. Thus, undersampling produces an essential ambiguity which cannot be reconciled by appeal to the information contained in the neural signals leaving the eye. Consequently, the neural apparatus of the visual cortex (which may interpolate the neural image onto a finer scale[6]), has no basis for attempting a reconstruction of the original stimulus rather than the sub-Nyquist alias. In other words, the observer's brain has no option but to misinterpret retinal signals generated by a relatively fine, undersampled pattern as being generated by a relatively coarse, oversampled stimulus.

The sketches of Fig. 3 reveal that although the aliased percept is always on a coarse spatial scale, it is not always grating-like. This is probably because the array of retinal neurons is not completely regular.[52, 109] For this reason, in biology it is more useful to use the term "aliasing" in a more general sense than the usual moiré effect familiar in engineering. Accordingy, *we define aliasing as the misperception of spatial features of objects caused by neural undersampling of the retinal image.*

We suspect that the temporal instability of aliasing is due to random eye movements which cause the stimulus to land on a slightly different part of the retina at different instants. Such eye movements have little consequence for gratings below the Nyquist limit of the neural array, but for gratings beyond the Nyquist limit small displacements of the target can induce large changes in orientation, spatial frequency, phase, and spatial structure of the neural image. It is perhaps surprising that the brain does not take advantage of eye movements to increase the effective sampling density of the retinal mosaic through temporal integration of a sequence of neural "snap-shots", each with a slightly different position of the retina relative to the image. This seems like a reasonable strategy to avoid the misperception of aliasing, but experimental evidence of such interpolation is lacking.

A growing body of evidence supports the interpretation that neural undersampling, rather than spatial filtering, is the primary factor which limits pattern resolution in the periphery. Although the original observations of aliasing in peripheral vision were for interference fringes,[82] Smith & Cass[68] and Still[73] have independently reported observations of aliasing for naturally-viewed gratings in the peripheral field. In addition to errors in the perceived structure of visual patterns, the undersampling hypothesis also predicts that drifting gratings should appear to move in the wrong direction. Experimental observations confirming this prediction of motion reversal have been reported independently by several groups.[3, 13, 88] Finally, if filtering were the limiting factor for resolution in the periphery, then the contrast of the visual target would need to be 100% in order to achieve the resolution limit. However, Still[73] has shown that stimulus contrast as low as 10% is sufficient to achieve maximum resolution acuity at an eccentricity of 30 deg.

If the resolving power of peripheral vision is sampling-limited, how are we to interpret the earlier evidence that resolution is filtering limited? One possible explanation is that the contrast sensitivity functions measured by Rovamo & Virsu were attenuated by optical filtering caused by uncorrected refractive errors, uncompensated changes in viewing distance of the stimulus, and off-axis optical aberrations of the eye (see the chapter by Bradley & Thibos in this book). To investigate this possibility, Still avoided the filtering effects of the eye's optical system by measuring subjects' ability to detect a small patch of high-contrast interference-fringes formed directly on the peripheral retina.[73] His measurements of contrast sensitivity were much higher than those reported by Rovamo & Virsu,[62] which suggests that optical factors may have been responsible for the very low values of contrast sensitivity which motivated the original rescaling model. This seems a plausible explanation since optical filtering by the eye is also responsible for the lack of sensitivity in central vision for high-frequency gratings beyond the neural resolution limit.[106] The implication of this line of reasoning (which we will revisit in Section 3.2) is that the optical system of the eye provides an effective anti-aliasing filter for central vision but not necessarily for peripheral vision. If the peripheral optics are well focused, then patterns beyond the neural Nyquist limit are imaged on the retina and perceptual aliasing becomes possible. However, if the retinal image is sufficiently blurred by defocus or aberrations, even peripheral vision may be protected by the anti-aliasing effects of low-pass, optical filtering in the eye.

In summary, there is now good evidence that a fundamental, qualitative difference exists between central and peripheral vision which cannot be accounted for by spatial rescaling of filters. When modeling foveal vision it is often permissible to ignore the sampling effects of converting a continuous retinal image into a discrete neural image because the eye's optical system is an effective anti-aliasing filter which prevents spatial frequency components beyond the Nyquist limit from being imaged on the retina. However, the Nyquist sampling limit drops rapidly in the peripheral retina and therefore optical anti-aliasing filtering does not necessarily occur for peripheral targets. Consequently, the ultimate factor limiting target resolution in the periphery is not filtering but retinal undersampling. This explains why filter models adapted from the fovea are inadequate for the periphery and suggests that to improve applied models of spatial vision one must take sampling effects into account. This is the goal of the next section.

2. Sampling Theory of Retinal Function

In this section we develop a mathematical model for the initial stages of image processing by the eye. Linear filter theory is used to describe the cascading effects of spatial filtering by the optical system of the eye and by neural receptive fields in the retina. The conditions necessary to prevent aliasing in the sampled neural image are then formulated in terms of optical filtering and the amount of spatial overlap of retinal samplers.

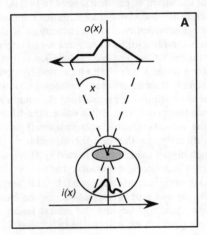 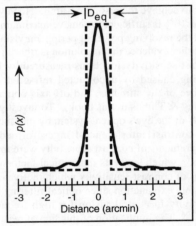

Figure 4. A: Coordinate reference frame for vision. The angular light distribution $o(x)$ of the object is imaged on the retina as $i(x)$. B: Point spread function $p(x)$ for a diffraction-limited optical system (solid curve) and it's equivalent width D_{eq}.

2.1. Optical Filtering

Vision begins with the formation of a light image upon the retina by the optical system of the eye, as illustrated in Fig. 4A. In order to develop optical models of the eye which are independent of viewing distance, it is common practice to specify object and image dimensions in angular units of visual direction (x). Optical imperfections of the eye and diffraction at the pupil inevitably reduce image contrast in a way that may be described as low-pass spatial-filtering. The highest quality retinal image (i.e. least amount of filtering) occurs for a well-focused eye with a pupil diameter of about 2.5 mm.[9] For smaller pupils, diffraction at the margin of the iris is the major limiting factor whereas for larger pupils, ocular aberrations dominate.[11] Given an optimum pupil diameter, the modulation transfer function of the human eye is slightly less than that of an ideal, diffraction-limited optical system.[9, 10] The corresponding statement of image quality expressed in the spatial domain is that the smallest point-spread function of the eye is somewhat larger than that of a diffraction-limited system with 2.5 mm pupil. To quantify this lower bound on the width of the point-spread function, it is convenient to apply Bracewell's[8] concept of the *equivalent width* of a function, which is defined as the width of the rectangular function with the same height and area as the given function. As illustrated in Fig. 4B, the equivalent width of the ideal system (2.5 mm pupil, 550 nm light; see Goodman,[27] Eq. (6-31)) is 0.87 arcmin and so an approximate value of about 1 arcmin would be a reasonable figure-of-merit for the equivalent width of the eye's point-spread function under optimal conditions.

Psychophysical experiments[73, 74] and physical measurements[49] have shown that optical image quality at 30 degrees of eccentricity can be nearly as good as in central vision, provided refractive errors and off-axis astigmatism are corrected with appropriate spectacle lenses. Nevertheless, systematic changes in the refractive power, magnification, and off-axis aberrations are well documented,[11] which means that a single optical transfer function is usually inadequate for describing image quality over the entire visual field. Despite this global non-uniformity, it is not unreasonable to assume that the optical system of the human eye is characterized on a local scale by a linear, shift-invariant system. Under this assumption, we may calculate the retinal image $i(x)$ by convolution ($*$) of the optical point spread function $p(x)$ of the eye with the intensity distribution of the object $o(x)$. Thus the first stage of the visual system will be characterized by the equation

$$i(x) = o(x) * p(x) \tag{1}$$

where the visual direction x applies interchangeably to angular distances in object space or image space.

2.2. Retinal Architecture and the Receptive Fields

Neural processing of the retinal image begins with the transduction of light energy into corresponding changes of membrane potential of individual light-sensitive neurons called photoreceptor cells. Photoreceptors are laid out as a thin sheet which varies systematically in composition across the retina. At the very center of the foveal region, which corresponds to our central field of view, the photoreceptors are exclusively cones but just outside the fovea rods appear and in the peripheral retina rods are far more numerous than cones.[58] Each photoreceptor is thought to integrate the light flux entering the cell through its own tiny aperture which, for foveal cones, is about 2.5 μ in diameter or 0.5 arcmin of visual angle.[17, 48] Since this entrance aperture is wholly within the body of each photoreceptor, apertures from neighboring receptors will not physically overlap on the retinal surface. Given this arrangement of the photoreceptor mosaic, we may characterize the first neural stage of the visual system as a sampling process by which a continuous optical image on the retina is transduced by an array of non-overlapping samplers into a discrete array of neural signals which we call a *neural image*.

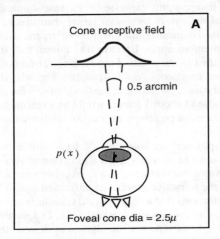 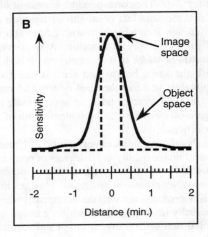

Figure 5. Receptive fields of cone photoreceptors in the fovea. A: Cone apertures on retina are blurred by eye's optical system when projected into object space. B: Spatial sensitivity profile of foveal cone in object space (solid curve) is broader than in image space (dashed curve).

Often it is useful to think of the cone aperture as being projected back into object space where it can be compared with the dimensions of visual targets, as illustrated schematically in Fig. 5A. This back-projection can be accomplished mathematically by convolving $p(x)$, the optical point-spread function of the eye, with the uniformly-weighted aperture function of the cone. (In taking this approach we are ignoring the effects of diffraction at the cone aperture, which would increase the cone aperture still further.) The result is a spatial weighting function called the *receptive field* of the cone. Before examining this receptive field in detail, we may draw two important qualitative conclusions. First, since foveal cones are tightly packed on the retinal surface, and since the effect of the eye's optical system is to broaden and blur the acceptance aperture of cones, the receptive fields of cones in object space must overlap to some degree. Second, the convolution result will be dominated by $p(x)$ since the equivalent width of the optical point spread function is about double that of the cone aperture. To substantiate these inferences quantitatively, we convolved the optical point-spread function of Fig. 4B with the uniformly weighted aperture function of a cone (0.5 arcmin diameter, circular shape). The 1-dimensional profile of the result is shown by the solid curve in Fig. 5B. As expected, this profile is very similar to the point-spread function of the optics alone and it has a calculated equivalent width of 0.93 arcmin. Since this figure is about twice that of the cone aperture on the retina, we conclude that receptive fields of neighboring cones will overlap significantly. The functional implications of this overlap are discussed below in Section 2.6.

The neural image encoded by the cone mosaic is transmitted from eye to brain over an optic nerve which, in man, contains roughly one million individual fibers. Each fiber is an outgrowth of a third order retinal neuron called a ganglion cell. It is a general feature of the vertebrate retina that ganglion cells are functionally connected to many rods and cones by means of intermediate, second order neurons called bipolar cells as illustrated schematically in Fig. 6A. As a result, a given ganglion cell typically responds to light falling over a relatively large region of the retina with the middle of the receptive field weighted most heavily. Neighboring ganglion cells may receive input from the same receptor, which implies that ganglion cell receptive fields may overlap. Thus in general the mapping from photoreceptors to optic nerve fibers is both many-to-one and one-to-many. The net result, however, is a significant degree of image compression since the human eye contains about 5 times more cones than optic nerve fibers and about 100 times more rods.[16, 17]

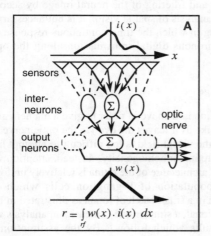 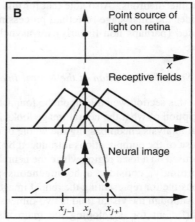

Figure 6. A: Formation of a neural response to the retinal image. Signals transduced by rods and cones are relayed by bipolar inter-neurons to ganglion cell output neurons for transmission along the optic nerve. B: Neural image for a point source of light on the retina is found by sampling the reflected receptive field at each visual direction represented by the array of output neurons.

A full account of spatial image processing by the retinal network would involve a description of the propagation of the neural image through each stage, taking account of neural pooling and sub-sampling of a fine mosaic by a coarse mosaic at multiple levels. Unfortunately, such a detailed model is beyond our present grasp despite the availability of a conceptual framework and mathematical tools.[25, 44] The reason is that although we understand retinal connectivity well enough to draw a rough schematic diagram for the mammalian eye,[43] detailed understanding of the complex retinal circuitry which connects input photoreceptors to output ganglion cells is lacking. Fortunately, such detailed knowledge is not necessary to achieve the more modest goal of describing the end result of retinal processing as revealed by the output neural image.

Ganglion cells come in many varieties, but one particular class called P-cells dominates throughout the primate retina.[60] Physiological experiments in monkey and cat indicate that a P-ganglion cell (or analogous X-cell in cat) responds to a linear combination of light falling on its receptive field.[34] Accordingly, the response r of an individual P-cell to the intensity distribution $i(x)$ would be found by integrating the product of the input $i(x)$ with the weighting function $w(x)$ over the receptive field (rf) of the neuron. That is,

$$r = \int_{rf} w(x) \cdot i(x) \, dx \ . \tag{2}$$

Notice that the weighting function $w(x)$ for the output neurons of the retina subsume the spatial weighting effects of the two previous stages of neural processing, namely, integration over the photoreceptor aperture and filtering of the neural image by second-order inter-neurons. Also note that for this analysis of spatial vision it is not necessary to consider the final stage of retinal processing in which the time-continuous response r is encoded (perhaps non-linearly) for asynchronous digital transmission along the optic nerve.

2.3. Spatial Description of the Neural Image

In this section we build upon the foundation laid above in order to give a mathematical description of what the neural image looks like as it leaves the eye *via* the optic nerve. A global analysis encompassing the whole of the visual field is too difficult to attempt here because of the complications introduced by retinal inhomogeneity. Instead, attention will be focused on a local region where the neural architecture of the retina is relatively uniform. Accordingly, consider a homogeneous population of P-ganglion cells which are responsible for representing the retinal image in a small patch of retina as illustrated in Fig. 6B. Although the visual field is two-dimensional, a simpler one-dimensional analysis will be sufficient for developing the main results which follow. By the assumption of homogeneity, the weighting function of each receptive field has the same form but is centered on different x values for different output neurons. The cells need not be equally spaced for the following general results to hold.

If we let x_j be the location of the receptive field center of the jth neuron in the array, then the weighting function for that particular cell will be

$$w_j = w(x - x_j) \tag{3}$$

and the corresponding response r_j is found by combining Eq. (2) and (3) to give

$$r_j = \int_{rf} w(x - x_j) \cdot i(x) \ dx. \tag{4}$$

It is important to emphasize at this point that although the neural image and light image are distinctly different entities, they share a common domain and similar language can be used to describe optical and neural images. For example, both kinds of image are functions of x, the visual direction, and a natural correspondence exists such that when the jth output neuron responds at level r_j it is sending a message to the brain that a certain amount of light (weighted by the receptive field) has been received from visual direction x_j. The variation of these neural responses across the array indicates the presence of contrast in the neural image just as the variation of light intensities across the retina signifies the presence of spatial contrast in the optical image. On the other hand, because of the regional specialization of the retina, the difference between visual directions of neighboring cells is small in the fovea and large in the periphery. Consequently, on a global level the neural image is spatially distorted causing the fovea to be highly magnified in comparison with the periphery.[20] This complication will be avoided in the present analysis by assuming local uniformity of scale over small regions.

The result embodied in Eq. (4) can be placed on more familiar ground by temporarily ignoring the fact that the neural image is discrete. That is, consider substituting for x_j the continuous spatial variable u. Then Eq. (4) may be re-written as

$$r(u) = \int_{rf} w(x - u) \cdot i(x) \ dx \tag{5}$$

which is recognized as a cross correlation integral.[8] In other words, the discrete neural image is *interpolated* by the cross-correlation of the input with the receptive weighting function of the neuron. We may therefore retrieve the neural image by evaluating the cross-correlation result at those specific locations x_j which are represented by the neural array. Using standard pentagram ($\star$) notation for cross correlation, the result is

$$r(x_j) = w(x) \star i(x), \quad x_j = x_1, x_2, \dots \ . \tag{6}$$

Replacing the awkward cross correlation operation with convolution yields

$$r(x_j) = w(-x) * i(x), \quad x_j = x_1, x_2, \dots \ . \tag{7}$$

In other words, *the discrete neural image is interpolated by the result of convolving the retinal image with the reflected weighting function of the neural receptive field.*

2.4. Neural Point-Spread Function

By analogy with the optical point-spread function, it is useful to define the neural point-spread function $n(x_j)$ as the neural image for a point source of stimulation on the retina. An expression for the neural point-spread function is obtained by letting $i(x)$ be the impulse function $\delta(x)$ in Eq. (7) and then applying the sifting property[8] of the impulse function

$$n(x_j) = w(-x) \ast \delta(x) = w(-x), \quad x_j = x_1, x_2, \ldots \tag{8}$$

where $n(x_j)$ denotes the response of the neuron at location x_j to the point source. This fundamental relationship between the neural point-spread function and the receptive field is summarized by the following theorem, which is illustrated graphically in Fig. 6B: *The neural image formed by a homogeneous array of linear neurons in response to a point of light on the retina is equal to their common receptive field weighting function, reflected about the origin, and evaluated for those visual directions represented by the array. This neural image is called the neural point-spread function.* In what follows, the discrete neural point-spread function will be designated $n(x_j)$ while its continuous interpolation will be designated $n(x)$.

The concept of a neural point-spread function is useful for specifying the output neural image for an arbitrary visual stimulus. Combining Eqs. (1), (7) and (8) we obtain

$$r(x_j) = o(x) \ast p(x) \ast n(x), \quad x_j = x_1, x_2, \ldots . \tag{9}$$

For the same reasons mentioned above in relation to Fig. 5, it is sometimes useful to interpret the term $p(x)*n(x)$ as the neural image projected optically back into object space where it is convolved with the stimulus. To put these results in a form which emphasizes the role of neural sampling, we multiply the right-hand side of (9) by a continuous "array function" $a(x)$, which is defined to be unity at each visual direction x_j represented by the neural array but is zero for all the in-between directions. By this maneuver the result of Eq. (9) takes on its final form

$$r(x) = a(x) \cdot [o(x) \ast p(x) \ast n(x)],$$
$$\ldots \text{where} \quad a(x) = \begin{cases} 1, & x = x_1, x_2, \ldots \\ 0, & \text{otherwise.} \end{cases} \tag{10}$$

It may be helpful to think of this result as the neurophysiological counterpart to the well-known "array of arrays rule" in the engineering study of antennas.[8] According to this rule, the field pattern of a set of identical antennas is the product of the pattern of a single antenna and an "array factor", which is the pattern that would be obtained if the set of antennas were replaced by a set of point sources.

Equation (10), which is illustrated graphically in Fig. 7, exposes the conceptual simplicity of signal processing by the common P-class of optic nerve fibers of the human eye. The final neural image is seen to be the result of three sequential stages of processing. First the object is optically filtered (by convolution with the optical point-spread function) to produce a retinal image. Next the retinal image is neurally filtered (by convolution with the neural point-spread function) to form a hypothetical, continuous neural image. Finally, the continuous neural image is point-sampled by the array of ganglion cells to produce a discrete neural image ready for transmission along the optic nerve to the brain. Notice the change of viewpoint embodied in Eq. (10). Initially the output stage of the retina was portrayed as an array of finite, overlapping receptive fields which simultaneously sample and filter the retinal image. Now this dual function is split into two distinct stages: neuro-optical filtering by the receptive field followed by sampling with an array of point samplers. Thus we see that neural filtering by non-point samplers is functionally equivalent to more traditional forms of filtering, such as that provided by optical blurring, which occur prior to the sampling operation.

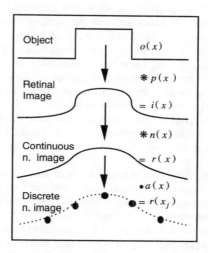

Figure 7. Sequential model of neural image formation by the eye. Objects are first filtered by the optical system of the eye and then sampled by the retinal array of neurons. Conceptually a retinal array of non-point samplers is equivalent to a filter followed by point sampling.

2.5. Frequency Description of the Neural Image

A spectral description of the neural image may be obtained by either of two methods. One approach is to compute the Fourier transform of $r(x)$, the hypothetical, continuous interpolation of the neural image specified in Eq. (10). One disadvantage of this method is that it invites the potential conceptual error of supposing that the spatial frequency spectrum of the neural image may contain frequency components beyond those which can actually be supported by the discrete neural array. An alternative approach is to determine the discrete Fourier transform of Eq. (9). This is straightforward when the sample points of the neural array are evenly spaced but is significantly more complex for an irregular, two-dimensional sampling mosaic.[110] In either case, aliasing in the neural image will occur unless the combined filtering action of the optics and receptive fields eliminates all frequency content beyond the Nyquist limit. This issue is the topic of the following section.

2.6. Aliasing in the Neural Image

An important design criterion for man-made digital communications systems is to avoid the prospect of aliasing caused by undersampling of analog signals. Often it is preferable to discard high-frequency information by pre-filtering the signal rather than to allow corruption of the remaining low-frequencies by aliasing. The design of the human eye seems to follow this good engineering practice to protect foveal vision from aliasing since the optical cutoff frequency is about equal to the Nyquist limit of the mosaic of cone photoreceptors.[9] On the other hand, the penalty of optical anti-alias filtering is an unavoidable loss of image contrast for all spatial frequencies. It is not obvious that the benefits gained by avoiding aliasing are worth the cost of contrast attenuation in biological vision systems. To the contrary, the fact that the optical cutoff frequency exceeds the neural sampling limit over most of the visual field in humans and other animals suggests that the cost of an optical solution is prohibitively high.[69, 76] From a different viewpoint, it may actually be advantageous to allow undersampling since this will reduce the statistical correlation between the outputs of neighboring ganglion cells, reduce redundancy in the neural image, and hence make more efficient use of the available channel capacity of the optic nerve.[42]

A strategy which the visual system might adopt in order to avoid conspicuous moiré effects when undersampling periodic patterns is to introduce irregularity into the sampling mosaic.[109] This view is supported by anatomical evidence of a degree of irregularity in the mosaic of retinal ganglion cells,[96] although the array is surprisingly regular in humans even in the peripheral retina.[18] Perceptually the subjective appearance of aliasing often lacks distinct periodicity (see Fig. 3B), an observation which lends further support to the irregularity hypothesis. However, it is not uncommon for the alias to look very much like a grating which suggests that the degree of irregularity is not so great as to completely eliminate moiré effects altogether. Perhaps regularity persists even in peripheral retina because the penalties of irregular sampling outweigh the benefits. Irregular sampling causes a deterioration of the quality of the neural image because of image demodulation and distortion[23, 29] which has serious consequences for spatial resolution[30] and for feature localization.[7]

The processing cascade depicted in Fig. 7 suggests that the eye's optical system in combination with neural receptive fields could act as a low-pass, anti-aliasing filter. If low-pass filtering by visual neurons is to be an effective anti-aliasing filter, then neural receptive fields must be relatively large compared to the spacing of the array. We can develop this idea quantitatively without detailed knowledge of the shape of the receptive field weighting function by employing Bracewell's equivalent bandwidth theorem.[8] This theorem states that the product of equivalent width and equivalent bandwidth of a filter is unity. In the present context, the equivalent width of the neuro-optical filter equals the equivalent diameter (d_E) of the receptive fields of retinal ganglion cells as measured in object space. The equivalent bandwidth of this filter is the bandwidth of the ideal, low-pass filter which has the same height and area as the Fourier transform of the receptive field. If we adopt the equivalent bandwidth as a measure of the highest frequency passed to any significant extent by the filter, then by applying Bracewell's theorem we find that the cutoff frequency is $1/d_E$. (This is a conservative criterion. In Bracewell's terminology, the bandwidth of an ideal low-pass filter is twice the cutoff frequency. Here we are effectively assuming that the tail of the neural low-pass filter is insignificant beyond twice the cutoff frequency of the equivalent, ideal filter.) To avoid aliasing, the cutoff frequency of the filter must be less than the Nyquist frequency (0.5/S) as set by the characteristic spacing S of the array. Thus aliasing will be avoided when $d_E > 2S$, that is, when the equivalent radius of the receptive field exceeds the spacing between fields.

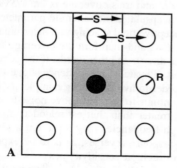 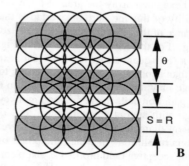

Figure 8. Coverage of visual field by square array of circular receptive fields. Left (A): visual field is subdivided into nearest-neighbor regions. S = spacing between fields, R = radius of field. Right (B): critical case where cutoff spatial frequency for individual receptive fields just matches the Nyquist frequency of the array. θ = period of grating at the Nyquist frequency for the array.

A similar line of reasoning can be developed for two-dimensional receptive fields. In Fig. 8 the visual field is tessellated by an array of square tiles, with each tile containing the circular receptive field of a visual neuron. Assuming radial symmetry of the fields, the generalization of Bracewell's theorem to two dimensions states that the product of equivalent width and equivalent bandwidth is $4/\pi$ and so (by the above conservative criterion) the cutoff frequency for individual neurons will be $4/(\pi d_E)$. The Nyquist frequency of the array will vary slightly with grating orientation,[57] but 0.5/S remains a useful lower bound. Thus the anti-aliasing requirement is that $d_E > 8S/\pi$. In other words, aliasing will be avoided if the equivalent radius of the receptive field exceeds $4/\pi$ times the spacing between fields. To within the level of approximation assumed by this analysis, $4/\pi$ is the same as unity and so the one-dimensional and the two-dimensional requirements for avoiding aliasing are essentially the same. Thus, we conclude from these arguments that effective anti-alias filtering requires that the radius of receptive fields be greater than the spacing between fields (i.e., $R > S$). The critical case ($R = S$) is depicted in Fig. 8B, along with that grating stimulus which is simultaneously at the Nyquist frequency for the array and at the cutoff frequency of the neuro-optical filter.

Neuroscientists are well aware of the importance of aliasing as a limit to the fidelity of the visual system and so have devised a simple measure called the *coverage factor* to assess whether a given retinal architecture will permit aliasing.[21, 33, 52] Conceptually, the coverage factor of a neural array measures how much the receptive fields overlap. To calculate this overlap we tessellate the visual field into nearest-neighbor regions (also called Voronoi or Dirichlet regions) as illustrated for a square array in Fig. 8A and then define

$$\text{Coverage} = \frac{\text{Area of receptive field}}{\text{Area of tile}} = \frac{\pi R^2}{S^2} \tag{11}$$

(For a hexagonal array the area of a tile is $0.5S^2/\sqrt{3}$ and thus coverage is $2\pi(R/S)^2/\sqrt{3}$.) The utility of this measure of overlap is that it encapsulates into a single parameter the importance of the ratio of receptive field size to receptive field spacing as a determinant of aliasing. For the critical case shown in Fig. 8B, $R=S$ and therefore the coverage factor equals π (for square array) or $2\pi/\sqrt{3}$ (for hexagonal array). In other words, if the coverage is less than about 3 we can expect aliasing to result. Physiological evidence suggests that coverage may have to be as high as 4.5 to 6 in order to avoid aliasing completely since retinal ganglion cells in cat[12, 52] and monkey [15] continue to respond above noise levels to gratings with spatial frequency 1.5 to 2 times greater than that estimated from their equivalent diameter. Such responses to very high frequencies may represent a kind of "spurious resolution" in which the phase of the response reverses, as is to be expected when the receptive field profile has sharp corners or multiple sensitivity peaks.[72, 81]

Analysis of the X-cells in cat[32, 33] and P-cells in monkey retina [15, 56, 90] suggests that the total population of these classes of ganglion cells has sufficient coverage to avoid aliasing, although this is not the case for other, more sparsely populated classes of ganglion cells. These conclusions were based upon physiological assessments of receptive field sizes in object space, which are much larger than corresponding dendritic fields in monkey peripheral retina.[15, 56] Consequently, if calculations are based on anatomical measurements of dendritic field size, then coverage is much less.[15, 56, 90] Furthermore, it has been argued that coverage should be assessed separately for the various sub-types of ganglion cells.[94] For example, X-cells in cat are split equally into two independent populations of opposite polarity ("ON-center" and "OFF-center") which, when considered separately, have insufficient coverage to avoid aliasing.[33, 52] This debate over whether it is more appropriate to consider the combined population of heterogeneous neurons, or the separate sub-populations of homogenous neurons, is compounded in monkey where P-cells are further subdivided into color-coded sub-populations (e.g., receptive field centers connected exclusively to either red-sensitive or green-sensitive cone receptors, with either ON- or OFF- polarity). The available evidence indicates that if each of these sub-populations is separately considered, then none would have sufficient coverage to avoid aliasing.[90]

Recent studies on human retina[16-18, 61] and other primates[93] have provided valuable new data on the cell-to-cell spacing of cones and of retinal ganglion cells at various locations across the visual field. Human data for the horizontal meridian of the visual field are shown by the solid curves in Fig. 9A,B. A prominent feature of the human retina revealed by these data is that cells are more widely spaced in the nasal field (i.e. temporal retina) than they are at equivalent eccentricities in the temporal visual field. To be useful here in estimating coverage of the visual field, these anatomical dimensions must be projected into object space as described above in Section 2.2. To do this for cones, we first estimated the mean anatomical diameter of cone inner segments (believed to be the entrance apertures of cones[48]) from published photomicrographs at various retinal locations (Figs. 2,3 of Curcio et al.[17]). Assuming a circular cone aperture, we next convolved a two-dimensional cylinder function with the optical point-spread function for a diffraction-limited optical system (shown above in Section 2.1 to be the lower-bound estimate of the optimal point-spread function of the human eye for central and mid-peripheral vision). The result is the cone receptive field in object space, from which we calculated the equivalent radius (an example of this calculation for foveal cones was described above in Section 2.2). In Fig. 9A we compare the results (indicated by symbols) with cone spacing (solid curves, taken from Fig. 7 of Curcio et al.[17]).

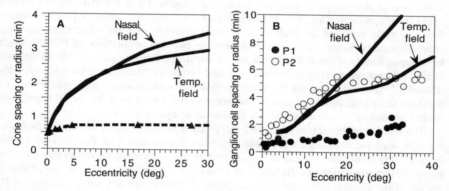

Figure 9. Coverage of visual field by cone receptors (A) and by retinal P-ganglion cells (B) in human retina. Solid curves show average linear spacing between cells and symbols show equivalent receptive field radius in object space. Data are from Curcio et al. and from Kolb et al. (see text).

The comparisons drawn in Fig. 9A reveal that, over most of the visual field, the receptive-field radius of cones is much smaller than their spacing. This implies that aliasing of peripheral targets by the cone array is inevitable when the eye's optics are well focused. In the fovea, however, the situation is quite different. As mentioned earlier (see Section 2.2), minimum cone radius in object space and cone spacing are both about 0.5 arcmin even though the physical radius of the cone aperture on the retinal surface is about half this value. This is precisely the critical situation depicted earlier in Fig. 8B (except that cones are typically packed in a more efficient hexagonal array). In effect, the eye's optics broaden the functional receptive fields of the foveal cones, thereby increasing their coverage factor to achieve the critical value needed to avoid aliasing. Thus we conclude that the neuro-optical filtering of the cone receptors is sufficient to provide effective anti-alias filtering for foveal vision but not for peripheral vision. It is interesting to note that cone undersampling appears to be widespread in the animal kingdom and so the foveal case, which has spawned a well-entrenched view that the photoreceptor mosaic should "match" the optical image quality of the eye, is more the exception than it is the rule.[69]

A similar analysis of coverage of the visual field by the retinal ganglion cell array in humans is depicted in Fig. 9B. The solid curves show the anatomical spacing between human P-ganglion cells as derived from the anatomical study of Curcio & Allen.[16] assuming that 80% of all ganglion cells are P-cells.[56] and that 1 mm on the retina corresponds to 3.3 deg of visual angle. Notice that the curves do not extend to zero eccentricity since retinal ganglion cells which are functionally connected to foveal cones are anatomically displaced into the parafoveal region. Physiological receptive field sizes of retinal ganglion cells in humans are unknown and so we must rely upon indirect estimates based on anatomical size of dendritic fields. It is generally accepted that the dendritic field of a ganglion cell provides the anatomical support for the central component of the cell's functional receptive field and so the size of dendritic fields is a good, lower-bound estimate of the size of physiological receptive fields.[53] Anatomical data are available for human retina from several studies,[18, 39, 61] and in Fig. 9B we show the radius of P-cell dendritic fields recently reported by Kolb et al.[39] (their Fig. 19). Unlike other contemporary neuroanatomists, Kolb et al. distinguish between two sub-populations of P-cells which have significantly different dimensions of dendritic fields. In Fig. 9B these two populations are separately represented by closed symbols (P1-cells) and by open symbols (P2-cells). (Note that, unlike the previous analysis with cones, it wasn't necessary to convolve these relatively large, anatomical receptive fields with the point-spread function of the eye in order to achieve an acceptable level of accuracy).

The relative proportion of P1 and P2 cell types in human retina is presently unknown. Nevertheless, the comparison drawn in Fig. 9B suggests that if all P-cells were of the larger (P2) type then receptive field radius matches cell-to-cell spacing and so the coverage factor for this population of cells (about 3) would be sufficient to avoid most, but probably not all, of the aliasing effects of undersampling. It follows that any sub-population of P-cells will render an even greater degree of aliasing since coverage is necessarily lower in a sparser array. For example, if a significant number of P-cells are of the smaller (P1) type described by Kolb et al., then the coverage factor for the remaining P2 cells will be that much less than the critical value needed to suppress aliasing. Similarly, P1-cells must generate a significant degree of aliasing since they have such small receptive fields. As may be deduced from Fig. 9B, even if every P-cell were a P1-type, their coverage factor would still be less than 1, which is far below the critical value needed to avoid aliasing.

The most direct examination of coverage factor in human retina is from an elegant series of recent experiments by Dacey.[18] By visualizing and staining individual neurons in fresh human tissue, Dacey was able to identify and study all of the P-ganglion cells in a small patch of retina. His observations revealed a large variation in the size of dendritic fields which did not fall neatly into P1 and P2 subclasses. However, he did confirm that P-cells form two independent mosaics (the "ON-" and "OFF-" systems described in greater detail in Section 3.1 below) just as they do in other species.[94] When these two mosaics were examined separately, Dacey found that adjacent dendritic trees apposed one another but did not overlap. Instead they fit together like pieces of a jigsaw puzzle, tiling the retinal surface with interlocking, irregularly shaped areas. This intriguing arrangement was observed first in cat[94] and it is supposed that a highly specific mechanism must be at work during development of the fetal retina that allows the growing dendritic trees of cells in the same mosaic to expand to fill their space, yet not overlap, just as prescribed by a Dirichlet tessellation scheme.[95] The relevant point here is that, since the ON and OFF sub-mosaics each have coverage no greater than 1, the total population of P-cells will have coverage no greater than 2, which is too small to avoid aliasing.

In summary, if all P-cells participate in a unified sampling mosaic then their coverage of the peripheral visual field would be sufficient to avoid most aliasing effects even when the retinal image is well focused. However, if P-cells are subdivided into known, functional sub-populations, all of the anatomical studies to date indicate that coverage would be too low to prevent aliasing in the peripheral field for a well-focused human eye. In the next Section we explore the quantitative implications of this conclusion.

3. Filtering and Sampling Limits in Human Vision

3.1. Comparison of Anatomical and Visual Nyquist Limits

In the preceding sections we have argued that neural sampling of the retinal image presents a fundamental limitation to visual resolution. We have also shown how each stage of neural processing in the retina can be conceptually and computationally projected back into object space and therefore be conceived as a sampling mosaic impressed upon the visual world. Given that the visual system consists of a series of anatomically distinct stages (e.g., photoreceptors, bipolars, ganglion cells), we may ask which of these arrays of neurons sets the ultimate limit for peripheral acuity? Since the beginning of this century the textbook answer to this question has been stated in the negative: the cone array cannot be responsible since peripheral acuity declines much more rapidly with increasing eccentricity than does cone spacing.[111] Each subsequent generation of vision scientists, with its refined measurements of anatomical dimensions and visual performance, has reaffirmed that cones are too tightly packed to limit resolution in peripheral retina and pointed instead to post-receptoral neural circuitry as the determining factor.[3, 28, 75, 80, 104]

It stands to reason that the sampling limit of the visual system will be set by the coarsest array of the visual pathway. A comparison of Figs. 9A,B reveals that over most of the retina (excluding the very central area) photoreceptors greatly outnumber ganglion cells, which implies that peripheral ganglion cells sub-sample the photoreceptor array. Wässle *et al.* have shown in monkey retina that out to 30 deg of eccentricity the number of cones matches the number of interneurons (midget bipolar cells) connecting cones to P-ganglion cells.[91] This implies that the cone array and the array of bipolar interneurons have the same Nyquist limit, which means the neural image carried by the cone mosaic is effectively transferred to the input stage of ganglion cells without loss of spatial resolution. Consequently, if retinal undersampling is the limiting factor for pattern resolution, then human resolution acuity should be well correlated with the Nyquist frequency of the ganglion cell array rather than the cone or bipolar arrays. This basic premise that ganglion cell spacing is the limiting factor for visual resolution has a long history in vision science, having been reaffirmed many times [33, 75, 80, 93, 104]

The comparison between anatomical predictions and human visual performance is drawn in Fig. 10. The symbols in this figure show how resolution acuity for interference fringes varies across the retina.[80, 82] In these experiments resolution acuity was defined as the highest spatial frequency which did not elicit perceptual aliasing (see Section 1.3). Given this criterion, we interpret these resolution data as a direct, non-invasive measurement of the sampling density of the underlying neural array. These estimates are compared with recent anatomical estimates of the Nyquist sampling rate of the population of P-type (i.e. midget) ganglion cells in humans,[16] and cone photoreceptors in human.[17] For a given density D of neurons, the highest Nyquist frequency occurs when the sampling points are arranged in an hexagonal array.[57] In this case the center-to-center spacing S of the sample points is given by the formula $S^2 = 2/(D\sqrt{3})$ and the Nyquist frequency which applies to gratings of all orientations is $1/(S\sqrt{3})$.[71] Using these two formulas, we computed the Nyquist frequency of neural arrays from anatomical estimates of cell density measured along the horizontal meridian of the human retina.[16, 17] The results for the mosaic of cone photoreceptors are shown by the dashed curve in Fig. 10. We estimated the Nyquist frequency of the sub-population of P-type ganglion cells from measurements of total ganglion cell density by assuming that 80% of all human ganglion cells are P-cells, just as in the monkey.[56] To plot these anatomical data in visual coordinates, the nonlinear projection of the retinal image (which has the effect of reducing the Nyquist rate at larger eccentricities) was computed according to the wide-angle model of Drasdo and Fowler.[70]

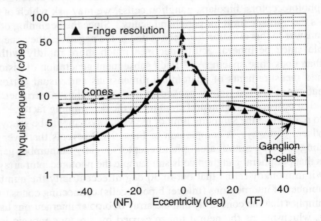

Figure 10. Comparison of human resolution acuity (symbols, from Thibos *et al.* 1987) with anatomical predictions based on the sampling density of retinal neurons (dashed = human cones (Curcio *et al.*, 1990), solid = human ganglion cells (Curcio & Allen, 1990)). NF=nasal field, TF=temporal field.

Inspection of Fig. 10 reveals that the cone Nyquist frequency falls rapidly over the first few degrees of eccentricity before leveling off to a much shallower slope in the peripheral retina. It is difficult to measure the density of ganglion cells in central retina because, although they are functionally connected to central cones, their cell bodies are physically displaced from the fovea into surrounding retina. (This accounts for the break in the solid curve near 0 deg. The other break, between 10-15 deg in nasal retina, corresponds to the optic nerve head.) Despite this uncertainty, it is clear that beyond about 10 deg of eccentricity the sampling density of P-ganglion cells is significantly lower than that of cones. Comparing these two curves with the psychophysical measurements of resolution acuity for interference fringes shows that, beyond about 10-15 deg of eccentricity, human resolution acuity is much lower than that predicted by the sampling density of cones but closely match the predictions based on ganglion cell density. These predictions are different for nasal and temporal visual fields (because of the well-known nasal/temporal asymmetry of the human and primate retinas[60]) and the psychophysical data reflect these differences. In fact, the onset of aliasing is so sensitive to small changes in neural sampling density that this psychophysical technique can reveal subtle variations across the visual field associated with the human visual streak (see Section 1.1).[2]

Similar experiments have been conducted on macaque monkeys trained to fixate a small spot of light while making resolution judgments about visual targets placed in the peripheral visual field.[46] While it is far easier to train humans to do the same task, the reward for pursuing this arduous experiment in monkey is that it provides invaluable behavioral data to compare with the substantial literature on the physiology and anatomy of the macaque visual system. The results indicated a decline in resolution acuity with eccentricity that followed the density of P-cells in a manner that is very similar to that shown for humans in Fig. 10.

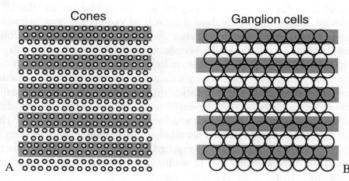

Figure 11. Illustration of the spatial scale of neural arrays in human nasal retina, 30 deg from fovea. A: cone photoreceptors (rods fill the space between cones but are too small to show here). B: P-ganglion cells (receptive fields are shown at half their true diameter to avoid the confusion of overlapping fields). Anatomical dimensions are taken from Fig. 9. Grating patch is 1 deg square and has spatial frequency (5.3 cyc/deg) equal to the psychophysical resolution limit.

To help gain an intuitive appreciation of these results, it may be helpful for the reader to inspect a scale drawing of the various neural arrays in the eye overlaid upon the visual stimulus. For example, in Fig. 11A we show a 1deg × 1deg patch of grating which is just at the resolution limit (5.3 cyc/deg, from Fig. 10) when placed 30 deg from the fovea in the temporal visual field. This target is imaged on nasal retina where cone diameter is about 1.5 arcmin and cone spacing is about 3.0 arcmin (from Fig. 9). Cones are depicted by circles arranged in an hexagonal array, but of course in reality the array is not perfectly regular. The space between the cones is filled by numerous rod photoreceptors which are about 0.5 arcmin in diameter . Rods are too small to illustrate here but notice that the space available between neighboring cones is large enough to accommodate about 3 rods side-by-side. For comparison with the cone array we show in Fig. 11B the array of P-ganglion cells in the same retinal location. Spacing and receptive field radius are both about 5.2 arcmin for the P2-ganglion cells (Fig. 9) chosen for illustration. From this comparison it is clear that the cone array significantly oversamples the grating target but the ganglion cell array is just adequate to meet the Nyquist requirement of two samples per period of the grating. One misleading feature of Fig. 11 is the apparent lack of overlap. The receptive fields of ganglion cells in Fig. 11 are drawn at half their true diameter because if drawn at full size their overlap would make it difficult to appreciate their spacing. When drawn to scale, the P2-ganglion cell picture looks very much like Fig. 8B.

On the basis of the close correlations evident between anatomical predictions and human performance, *we conclude that undersampling by retinal ganglion cells is the primary limiting factor for pattern resolution in human peripheral vision beyond about 10 deg of eccentricity (provided the retinal image is well focused).* However, in the parafoveal region (less than 10 deg of eccentricity) the cone mosaic determines the neural sampling limit[107] since ganglion cells outnumber cones over this region of retina.[16, 93] The same conclusion was drawn for the macaque monkey by Merigan and Katz.[46]

An important issue still to be resolved is the role of various sub-populations of P-cells in determining visual resolution performance. There is a large body of anatomical and physiological evidence from numerous vertebrate species demonstrating a fundamental dichotomy in the polarity of neural responses to light. Some cells are visually excited when the receptive field center receives more light than the surrounding areas, and conversely, are inhibited when the central region is darker than the surround. These are called "ON-cells" and are to be contrasted with "OFF-cells" which behave in just the opposite manner (i.e. are excited when the center is dark and inhibited when the center is light). This separation of visual signals into parallel neural channels signaling "brighter than ambient" and "darker than ambient" begins at the very first synapse in the visual system (between photoreceptors and bipolar cells) and is maintained by separate anatomical structures throughout the initial stages of the visual pathway.[90]

Since nature seems to have gone to great lengths to separate the neural image into complementary ON- and OFF- neural channels, it might be thought that the two arrays should be considered separately when estimating the sampling density of retinal ganglion cells. On the other hand, it is also conceivable that at some stage the ON- and OFF-channels are recombined with the overall sampling density determined by the combined array. The rationale for this view is that the ON array provides good dynamic range for signaling the bright bars of a grating and OFF cells provide good, but complementary, dynamic range for the dark bars. Thus ON/OFF parallel pathways in vision bear a striking resemblance to the positive and negative circuits in the classic, push-pull design of electronic amplifiers. Given the very close correlation evident in Fig. 10 between psychophysical resolution and anatomical predictions based on the combined (ON + OFF) populations of ganglion cells, it is tempting to reject the hypothesis that psychophysical performance is limited by sampling density of either sub-array alone. However, this would be pushing the data further than is warranted. Curcio and Allen[16] reported a large degree of inter-subject variability in the density of human ganglion cells, especially in the periphery. For the six retinas in their study, up to threefold differences in ganglion cell density were found at corresponding points in peripheral retina, which implies a $\sqrt{3}$-fold difference in Nyquist frequencies. Given such large variability between individuals, the psychophysical experiments of Fig. 10 cannot reveal the relatively small, $\sqrt{2}$-fold difference in Nyquist frequencies that distinguishes the combined (ON + OFF) hypothesis from the separate (ON or OFF) hypothesis. For the same reason it is not yet possible to decide whether there is any substantive disagreement between the approach of Thibos *et al.*[80] who compared resolution to the total P-cell population and that of Merigan & Katz[46] who compared monkey resolution to the sub-population of ON (or OFF) P-cells.

3.2 The Aliasing Spectrum of Human Vision

Results of our own systematic exploration of the limits to aliasing in human vision are summarized in Fig. 12. A series of experiments were conducted in which cutoff spatial frequency was measured for two different tasks (contrast detection, pattern resolution), for two different types of visual targets (interference fringes, sinusoidal gratings displayed on a computer monitor with the eye's refractive error corrected by spectacle lenses), at various locations along the horizontal nasal meridian of the visual field.[74, 80, 82]

Inspection of Fig. 12 reveals that, for the resolution task, cutoff spatial frequency was the same regardless of whether the visual stimulus was imaged on the retina by the eye's optical system (natural view; open triangles) or produced directly on the retina as high-contrast, interference fringes (closed triangles). This is consistent with our earlier conclusion that, for a well-focused eye, pattern resolution is limited by the ambiguity of aliasing caused by undersampling, rather than by contrast attenuation due to optical or neural filtering. Aliasing first occurs for frequencies just above the resolution limit, so the triangles in Fig. 12 also mark the lower limit to the aliasing portion of the spatial frequency spectrum. Recall that this lower boundary of the aliasing zone is accurately predicted by the Nyquist limit calculated for human P- ganglion cells (data from Fig. 10 replotted in Fig. 12 as a dotted curve).

The upper limit to the aliasing zone is determined by performance on the detection task. Detection acuity is significantly lower for natural viewing (open squares) than for interferometric viewing (filled squares) at all eccentricities. Consequently, the spectrum of frequencies for which aliasing occurs is narrower for natural viewing (shaded region) than for interference fringes (shaded + cross-hatched regions). This difference is directly attributable to imperfections of the eye's optical system [9] since all else is equal (in both cases the neural apparatus is faced with identical tasks (contrast detection) of the same stimulus (sinusoidal gratings)). Notice that for natural viewing the aliasing zone narrows with decreasing eccentricity and vanishes completely at the fovea, where contrast sensitivity for detection and for resolution of gratings is nearly identical. Thus under normal viewing conditions, the fovea is protected from aliasing because of optical low-pass filtering whereas in the periphery the optical quality of the human eye remains quite good (assuming refractive errors are corrected) and so the eye's optics are ineffective as an anti-aliasing filter for the coarse sampling of the peripheral retina.

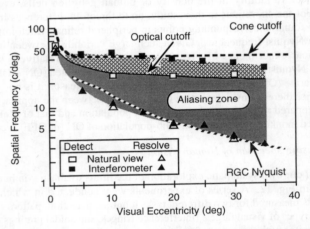

Figure 12. Summary of optical and neural limits to pattern detection and pattern resolution across the visual field in humans. Symbols show psychophysical performance (mean of 3 subjects from Thibos *et al.*, 1987) for grating detection (squares) and resolution (triangles) tasks under normal viewing conditions (open symbols) or when viewing interference fringes (closed symbols). The aliasing zone extends from the resolution to the detection limits. Solid curve drawn through open squares indicates the optical cutoff of the eye and marks the upper limit to the aliasing zone for natural viewing (shaded). The expanded aliasing zone observed with interference fringes (cross-hatched area) extends beyond the optical cutoff to a higher value set by neural factors. Dashed curve shows computed detection limit of individual cones (from Curcio *et al.*, 1990) and dotted curve shows computed Nyquist limit of retinal ganglion cells (RGC; from Curcio & Allen, 1990).

The neuro-optical model discussed in Section 2 above suggests that the optical limits to pattern detection revealed in Fig. 12 may be described in two ways, corresponding to image-space and object-space viewpoints. For an image space analysis, we conceive of the eye as a concatenated series of image processing stages as in Fig. 7. From this viewpoint the eye's optical system plays the role of a low-pass filter which attenuates the contrast of the retinal image, thus lowering the maximum detectable spatial frequency. Alternatively, if we imagine the projection of neural receptive fields into object space as in Fig. 5, then the effect of the eye's optical imperfections is to blur the neural receptive fields, creating a greater degree of overlap and thus lowering the cutoff frequency for contrast-detection by the neural array. From both of these viewpoints emerges the same question: which neural receptive fields limit pattern detection? Evidently the fields in question are extremely small since the cutoff spatial frequency for detecting interference fringes is over 30 cyc/deg even in the far periphery beyond 30 deg of eccentricity. This implies (if we assume, to first approximation, that cutoff spatial frequency is equal to the inverse of receptive field diameter) that the limiting field diameter must be less than 2 minutes of arc in visual angle, which corresponds to less than 10 microns on the retinal surface. The only visual neurons with such small receptive fields are the cone photoreceptors.

To pursue the idea that human detection of interference fringes throughout the visual field is limited by the size of cone apertures, we estimated the cutoff spatial frequency of cones (assuming cutoff = inverse of aperture diameter) from the data of Curcio *et al.*[17] and compare this result with the upper boundary of the aliasing zone determined psychophysically.[80] As may be seen from Fig. 12, the calculated cutoff for cones (dashed curve) closely matches the psychophysical detection limit, thereby lending quantitative support to the suggestion that aliasing is curtailed by spatial averaging over the entrance aperture of individual cone photoreceptors. Although this argument is widely accepted for foveal vision[48, 70, 71, 106] it was surprising to find evidence in favor of this hypothesis also for peripheral vision since receptive fields of even the smallest primate retinal ganglion cells were thought to pool many cone receptive fields in peripheral retina.[5, 61] However, recent anatomical experiments add considerable weight to the idea that some human ganglion cells (the P1 class identified by Kolb *et al.*[39]) have receptive field centers consisting of a single cone in peripheral vision, just as Polyak first described for foveal vision.[58]

In his classic description of the architecture of the human fovea,[58] Polyak coined the term "monosynaptic pathway" to stand for the exclusive, 1-to-1 pathway from single cones to single ganglion cells *via* single bipolar cells. Although Polyak believed the monosynaptic pathways were restricted to the foveal region, a growing body of evidence suggests the existence of a monosynaptic pathway also in human peripheral retina. It has been known for 25 years that an individual midget bipolar cell of the primate retina makes exclusive synaptic contact with only one cone photoreceptor,[37] but only recently has it been reported that the output of some individual midget bipolars is directed to single midget ganglion cells (the P1 sub-class).[38, 39] Although there are enough midget bipolar cells to act as interneurons in such a monosynaptic pathway,[91] there aren't enough ganglion cells available to provide a 1-to-1 pathway for every cone. Nevertheless, the anatomical evidence clearly shows that <u>some</u> P-ganglion cells exist in the periphery which are functionally connected to single bipolar cells, which in turn are connected to single cones. Corroborating physiological evidence of extremely small receptive fields has been reported by Crook *et al.*[15] who found that about 20% of cells recorded in peripheral monkey retina responded to gratings well above the Nyquist limit.

Although the anatomical and physiological evidence reviewed above is consistent with the psychophysical measurements of detection acuity, a 1-to-1 connection from cones to ganglion cells is not strictly required by the psychophysical evidence. A small degree of convergence of cone signals onto ganglion cells could be present and not markedly limit detection acuity because, unlike the foveal region, the peripheral cones are not tightly packed (numerous, smaller rods fill the space between cones). Given a grating with a half-period smaller than cone spacing yet larger than the cone radius, individual cones will act as functional subunits that sample the sinusoidal stimulus at random locations. If the number of these subunits per ganglion cell is small, a significant degree of neural contrast may persist across an array of such neurons. However, if the number of randomly located subunits is large, then their effects will tend to cancel and the contrast in the neural image will vanish, thus precluding the possibility of psychophysical detection.

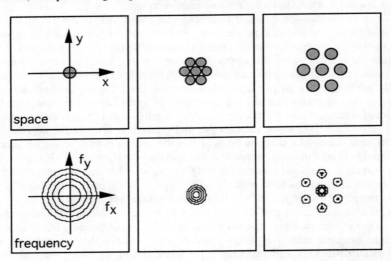

Figure 13. Frequency response characteristics of hypothetical P-ganglion cells. Top row shows receptive field maps of 3 examples (left: one cone/ganglion cell; middle: seven closely-packed cones per ganglion cell; right: seven widely-spaced cones per ganglion cell for which $R/S=0.3$). Bottom row shows contour plot of the magnitude portion of the 2-dimensional Fourier transform of the corresponding receptive field.

To quantify these arguments, we computed the Fourier transforms of three hypothetical receptive fields illustrated in the top row of Fig. 13. At the left is a small receptive field the size of a single cone, in the center is a medium-sized field formed by summing the outputs of 7 closely-packed cones, and on the right is a large field formed by summing the outputs of 7 widely spaced cones. To make the latter case representative of the mid-peripheral retina (30 deg eccentricity; see Fig. 9), cone radius R was set to 30% of the spacing S between cones. Directly below each receptive field map is shown a contour plot of the corresponding two-dimensional frequency spectrum of the receptive field. As expected from the equivalent width theorem, since the medium field is three times larger than the small field, it has one-third the bandwidth. However, for a peripheral ganglion cell connected to widely spaced cones, the equivalent width theorem is not a useful guide to understanding the more complicated filtering characteristics of the neuron. As may be seen in the bottom, right panel of Fig. 13, the overall bandwidth is similar to that of a single cone, but there are gaps in the spectrum at intermediate frequencies for which the cell is less sensitive. Evidence of such gaps in the spectrum has not been reported in perceptual aliasing experiments, but this is not surprising since it is very unlikely that all ganglion cells in a given region of the retina would be connected in precisely the same fashion. Instead, the anatomical evidence of large variance in dendritic field diameters indicates that neighboring ganglion cells are probably connected to a small but variable number of cones.[18] As a population, this would have the effect of filling in any gaps in the frequency spectrum and yet allow the array to signal the presence of patterns which are much finer than the Nyquist limit of the array and so produce the aliasing phenomenon of peripheral vision.

3.3. Practical Applications

For many real-world tasks there is considerable pressure to increase the amount of information presented to a human operator through a visually-coupled interface. However, this demand inevitably leads to central vision overload and so new strategies must be considered for alleviating some of the workload. One idea is to improve the information-handling capacity of central vision by avoiding the optical limitations normally present in the eye. Another idea is to shift some of the information from the overcrowded central portion of the visual field into the vastly larger peripheral field. This latter strategy is also an option for many forms of visual dysfunction in which central vision is reduced or lost completely due to disease, injury, or the normal aging process. In this section we critically examine these two approaches in the context of the neuro-optical model of human visual performance presented above. In that model, low-pass filtering by the optical system of the eye, followed by image sampling by the mosaic of retinal neurons, set absolute limits to the transmission of visual information to the human operator. These limits are different for central and peripheral vision and thus have implications for both of the design strategies just mentioned. We conclude with a discussion of biological visual systems as a model for space-variant image processing by machine vision systems.

Design idea #1: Bypass optical limitations of central vision

Developing methods to by-pass the optical limitations of central vision is an attractive goal of current research in visual and ophthalmic optics. The optical system of the human eye acts as a low-pass spatial-filter which significantly reduces the contrast of the retinal image.[11] For small pupils the major limiting optical factor is diffraction at the pupil margin. Theory predicts that for a diffraction-limited optical system, the optical cutoff spatial frequency for a 2 mm pupil is in the range 60-100 cyc/deg for the visible spectrum. Although the diffraction cutoff is proportionally higher for larger pupils, these potential values are never realized in normal vision since optical aberrations of the eye limit image quality for larger pupils. On the other hand, it is conceivable that future optical designs of contact lenses, spectacles, or visual stimulation devices will correct the eye's aberrations and thus greatly increase the quality of the retinal image, approaching the very much higher limits set by diffraction. In fact, even the contrast attenuation due to diffraction can be circumvented to some extent by employing a Maxwellian-view design. By this method light is concentrated within the pupil in the form of the Fourier transform of the object.[103] Consequently diffraction is avoided for all frequencies low enough to pass through the pupil, although optical aberrations of the eye are not necessarily avoided.[77, 79, 103].

Given these potential technologies for significantly improving retinal image quality, it is important to ask the following question. *What would be the consequences of avoiding normal optical limitations on retinal image quality?* As shown in Fig. 12, the optical cutoff for central vision closely matches the Nyquist limit imposed by the sampling mosaic of foveal cones, which implies that low-pass optical filtering in the naked eye protects central vision from aliasing due to undersampling. Consequently, very fine spatial details are normally filtered out by the eye's optical system before they can be undersampled by the retina. However, when these limitations are avoided experimentally by using Maxwellian-view interferometric stimulation, perceptual aliasing can occur when viewing patterns too fine to be resolved in the fovea.[106] Thus, in the attempt to avoid optical imperfections and improve image quality, the fovea becomes exposed to the effects of undersampling and the result is likely to be misperception of both stationary [82, 106] and moving [3, 13] spatial patterns. On the other hand, Snyder and colleagues have argued convincingly that the penalty of aliasing would be significantly offset by the greater contrast of sub-Nyquist image components resulting from improved image quality.[69]

Design idea #2: Shift information from central to peripheral vision

Our understanding of the performance limits of peripheral vision have expanded greatly over the past few years through basic research into the anatomy, physiology, and psychophysics of the primate/human visual system. We now know that the quality of the eye's optical system is nearly as good in the periphery as it is for foveal vision provided that focusing errors are corrected with spectacle lenses. However, the functional sampling density of the retinal mosaic of neurons is much lower in the periphery than it is in the fovea. Consequently, the peripheral retinal image is subject to retinal undersampling, which will cause perceptual aliasing of spatial frequencies greater than the classical resolution limit. The bandwidth of the aliasing spectrum can be very large in the peripheral field since the lower limit (e.g. about 3 cyc/deg at 30 deg of eccentricity) is set by the sampling density of a very sparse array of retinal ganglion cells while the upper limit (about 30 cyc/deg) is set either by the optical system or ultimately by spatial averaging over the entrance aperture of individual cone photoreceptors. These findings imply that the aliasing spectrum of normal peripheral vision may extend up to an order of magnitude beyond the classical resolution limit as shown in Fig. 12.

In orthodox engineering circles, aliasing is generally held to be an undesirable consequence of undersampling which is to be avoided by anti-alias, low-pass filtering. In a biological system, on the other hand, anti-alias filtering may have a greater cost than benefit. For example, optical low-pass filters attenuate not only the high frequencies to be rejected, but they also attenuate the low frequencies to be passed. Evidently the design trade-off nature has made in the human visual system is to tolerate the possibility of erroneous perception caused by aliasing in exchange for improved retinal contrast. As pointed out by Snyder *et al.*,[69] retinal image contrast is greatly increased by avoiding the substantial amount of low-pass filtering which is required to avoid aliasing altogether. What is needed in future research is an assessment of the benefits and/or costs of various strategies for filtering the aliasing spectrum. Depending upon the specific visual task or application, such filtering may or may not be desirable. At this early stage of research we only know that the spectrum of spatial frequencies subject to aliasing is potentially much larger than the resolvable spectrum in the peripheral field.

Although laboratory experiments have demonstrated aliasing phenomena for simple grating patterns, the impact of aliasing on real-world stimuli with rich frequency spectra is largely unknown. Initial experiments in this area have used edges or compound gratings containing just a few harmonic components. Early results indicate that different grating components can interact with each other, with one masking the appearance of the other. That is, although aliased components can still be seen in the presence of sub-Nyquist components[86] their visibility is reduced[89] or completely eliminated.[24] Conversely, the visibility of sub-Nyquist gratings is reduced in the presence of supra-Nyquist gratings.[87] Given these interactions, it is perhaps not surprising that aliasing in peripheral vision was not even discovered until only recently, and that neural undersampling may not be a significant handicap in everyday vision.

The foregoing discussion raises another question relevant to the design of visually-coupled systems: what kind of information is appropriate for peripheral display? Although central vision is commonly regarded as greatly superior to peripheral vision, in many regards just the opposite is true. Night vision is an obvious example for which the central scotoma is attributed to the lack of rods in the retinal fovea. Another broad area in which peripheral vision excels is in the sensing and control of body movement. For example, the visual control of posture, locomotion, head, and eye movements are largely under the control of motor mechanisms sensitive to peripheral stimulation.[31, 45] Many of these functions of peripheral vision are thought of as reflex-like actions which, although they can be placed under voluntary control, largely work in an "automatic-pilot" mode with minimal demands for conscious attention. This suggests that information regarding body attitude, self-motion through the environment, and moving objects are ideally suited for peripheral display since such a strategy matches the information to be displayed with the natural ability of the peripheral visual system to extract such information. However, retinal undersampling in the periphery can lead to erroneous perception of motion direction.[3, 13]

Design idea #3: Use space-variant imaging in machine-vision systems

In the beginning of this chapter we used the language of the vision scientist to motivate our investigation of peripheral vision by asking the question: what is the physiological and anatomical basis of the variation of acuity across the visual field? From the viewpoint of the design engineer, however, it is more interesting to ask what advantages accrue from the particular implementation of space-variant imaging found in the human visual system? We mentioned in Section 1.1 that one advantage of having the spatial grain of the retina increase in direct proportion to eccentricity is that it provides an anatomical substrate for neural size constancy. In an elegant series of papers, Schwartz and colleagues have shown that this simple idea has deep mathematical roots and profound implications for how the topographic mapping of retinal space onto the visual cortex is organized and its functional implications.[22, 41, 64-66] Schwartz found that the distortion of the visual field revealed by anatomical and physiological mapping experiments in animals could be accounted for by a simple, logarithmic mapping function from retinal coordinates to cortical coordinates. That is, if the retinal image is referenced to a polar (r, ϕ) coordinate frame, and the neural image representation on the surface of the lateral geniculate nucleus (LGN) or visual cortex is referenced to a rectangular coordinate frame (u, v) then the transformation from one coordinate frame to the other is given by the pair of equations

$$u = \log r$$
$$v = \phi.$$

(12)

This "log-polar" mapping function can be placed in more compact form by using complex-valued coordinates and is recognized as a complex logarithmic conformal map.[65]

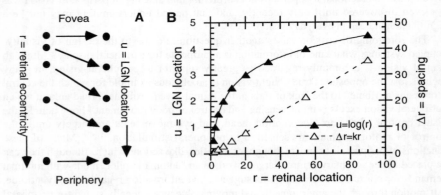

Figure 14. Retinotopic mapping from a non-uniform retina to a uniform lateral geniculate nucleus (LGN) distorts the brain's representation of the visual field. A: Schematic diagram of topographic map illustrates why the mapping magnifies the central field and compresses the periphery. B: In Schwartz's logarithmic conformal model the mapping function $x = log(r)$ transforms a set of retinal neruons for which local spacing (open symbols, right ordinate) is proportional to eccentricity into a series of equally spaced locations in the LGN (filled symbols, left ordinate). The magnification du/dr of this transformation process varies as $1/r$.

How might the log-polar transformation be implemented in the anatomical wiring of the visual pathway? Perhaps the simplest model is that the output ends of the optic nerve fibers spread uniformly over the surface of the LGN, the next stage of the primary visual pathway, and this basic organization transferred more or less intact to the visual cortex. A simplified schematic of the basic idea is shown in Fig. 14A. Although ganglion cells are tightly packed in the central regions of the retina and more widely spaced in the periphery, subsequent stages of the visual pathway are just the opposite: the LGN and visual cortex are conspicuously homogeneous. Consequently, if the optic nerve fibers of the eye fan out to cover the LGN surface uniformly, the result will be a distortion of the neural image yielding a disproportionately large representation of the foveal region of the visual field.

Quantitative support for this model emerges from its predictions about ganglion cell spacing. As illustrated in Fig. 14B, the spacing of a radial sequence of retinal cells must be directly proportional to their eccentricity if the logarithmic function is to be used to map their axons onto evenly spaced target-cells in the LGN. To see why this is true, let the local (linear) magnification of the topographic map be given by $\Delta u/\Delta r$, the ratio of spacing of nearest neighbors in the LGN to the spacing of corresponding nearest neighbors in the retina. This LGN magnification factor is given, in the limit, by the derivative of u with respect to r

$$\text{magnification} = \frac{du}{dr} = \frac{d(\log r)}{dr} \propto \frac{1}{r} . \tag{13}$$

Since the spacing Δu of the LGN cells is assumed constant, the implication is that retinal spacing of neighboring cells must be proportional to eccentricity,

$$\frac{\Delta u}{\Delta r} \propto \frac{1}{r} \Rightarrow \Delta r \propto r \tag{14}$$

which is precisely the result inferred from psychophysical studies of visual acuity (see Section 1.1). Thus Schwartz's logarithmic model of cortical magnification, created initially to describe anatomical and physiological measurements of topographic mapping, also accounts for the variation of visual resolution across the visual field determined psychophysically. Furthermore, the model provides a mathematical and conceptual framework for understanding the intriguing finding that visual acuity is directly proportional to cortical magnification.[14] Since cortical magnification and the Nyquist limit are both proportional to ganglion cell density[92] they must be proportional to each other.

We cannot hope to give justice here to the many and varied functional implications of the logarithmic conformal model of topographic mapping in biological or machine vision systems.[22, 41, 64-66, 98-101] Instead, we close with a brief description of just two of the more obvious features of the images transformed by this scheme.[65] We have already mentioned the idea of size constancy in the context of "matched filtering" (see Section 1). It is now possible to appreciate the full, two-dimensional nature of this idea and relate it to the concept of cortical magnification as illustrated in the top of Fig. 15. Suppose an object viewed from afar occupies the area of the visual field marked by the shaded area (left panel). When the viewing distance is reduced, the object grows larger and more eccentric as shown by the cross-hatched area (middle panel). However, in the transformed neural space of the brain, the neural image remains the same size and is merely translated to a new location (right panel). Thus the cortical image remains a fixed neural size for a looming object of fixed physical size despite the fact that the retinal image is growing in proportion to its eccentricity from the fovea (see geometry of Fig. 1). Furthermore, the visibility of the object remains roughly constant as it moves into the peripheral field since contrast sensitivity in the periphery depends on the ratio of eccentricity to retinal image size[54] (see the chapter by Peli in this book), which is constant in this scenario.

A different kind of invariance is illustrated in the bottom half of Fig. 15. Here the object (or the eye) rotates around the visual axis, maintaining constant eccentricity. Once again the cortical image is translated, but this time in the orthogonal direction to that for zoom. Such a neural mapping scheme would seem ideally suited for detecting and correcting rotational misalignment of the two eyes about their individual visual axes, an important prerequisite for binocular fusion and depth perception.

Size Constancy of Neural Image for Zoom (looming objects)

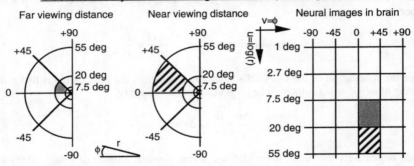

Orientation Constancy of Neural Image for Rotation

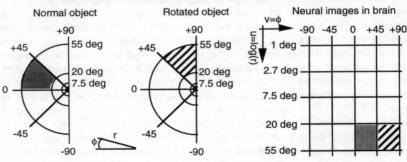

Figure 15. Top: Perceptual size constancy is facilitated by the logarithmic conformal mapping scheme for image transformation. If retinal image size is proportional to eccentricity, cortical image size of a looming object is constant. Bottom: The logarithmic mapping scheme converts the rays and exponentially-spaced rings of a polar coordinate reference frame into an evenly spaced, orthogonal grid of a rectangular reference frame. As a result, rotation of the field about the visual axis (r=0) causes translation of the cortical neural image.

Sensors which mimic the design of the human retina, alternatively known as log spiral, conformal logarithmic, and polar exponential grid (PEG) arrays, have found applications in a variety of machine vision systems. These include robot vision,[47, 63] spacecraft docking,[99] and video compression for remote driving.[100] The advantages of log-polar mapping for machine vision would seem to be the same as for biological vision. For example, PEG arrays permit a wide field of view with high central resolution and progressively decreasing resolution for peripheral objects, which greatly reduces memory requirements and processing loads on image processing computers.[99] Rotation and zoom operations, which require matrix multiplication in rectangular coordinates, are more simply computed as addition of log-polar coordinates. Exponential sensor arrays also ease the burden of computing target range from perspective changes, time-to-collision from optic flow velocity, and stereographic depth from binocular images.[98]

Perhaps no other aspect of vision science has resulted in such mutual benefit for engineers and biologists. The discovery of log-polar image processing by neurobiologists has been exploited by engineers to improve the design of man-made vision systems. In return, design engineers are revealing the practical advantages of such a system which previously had been mere biological speculation. Together, they have provided fresh ideas about how the eye evolved into such a marvelous instrument for extracting useful information from our visible world.

Acknowledgment.

The ideas presented in this paper have developed in parallel with the dissertation research of D. Walsh, F. Cheney, D. Still, M. Wilkinson, R. Anderson, and Y. Wang. This research was supported by National Institutes of Health grant EY05109.

References

1. A. Akerman and R.E. Kinzly (1979) "Predicting aircraft detectability", *Human Fact.* **21**, 277-291.
2. R.A. Anderson, M.O. Wilkinson and L.N. Thibos (1992) "Psychophysical localization of the human visual streak", *Optom. Vis. Sci.* **69**, 171-174.
3. S.J. Anderson and R.F. Hess (1990) "Post-receptoral undersampling in normal human peripheral vision.", *Vision Res.* **30**, 1507-1515.
4. H. Aubert and R. Förster (1857) "Beiträge zur Kenntniss des indirekte Sehens (I) Untersuchungen über den Raumsinn der Retina", *Arch. f. Ophth.* **3**, 1-37.
5. M.S. Banks, A.B. Sekuler and S.J. Anderson (1991) "Peripheral spatial vision: limits imposed by optics, photoreceptors, and receptor pooling", *J. Opt. Soc. Am. A* **8**, 1775-1787.
6. H.B. Barlow (1981) "Critical limiting factors in the design of the eye and visual cortex", *Proc. Roy. Soc. (Lond.) B* **212**, 1-34.
7. T.R.J. Bossomaier, A.W. Snyder and A. Hughes (1986) "Irregularity and aliasing: solution?", *Vision Res.* **25**, 145-147.

8. R.N. Bracewell, *The Fourier Transform and Its Applications,* (McGraw-Hill, New York, 1978).

9. F.W. Campbell and D.G. Green (1965) "Optical and retinal factors affecting visual resolution", *J. Physiol.* **181**, 576-593.

10. F.W. Campbell and R.W. Gubisch (1966) "Optical quality of the human eye", *J. Physiol.* **186**, 558-578.

11. W.N. Charman, in *Prog. Retinal Res.,* ed. N.N. Osborne and G.J. Chader (Pergamon Press, Oxford, 1983), 1-50.

12. B.G. Cleland, T. Harding and U. Tulunay-Keesey (1979) "Visual resolution and receptive field size: examination of two kinds of cat retinal ganglion cell", *Science* **205**, 1015-1017.

13. N.J. Coletta, D.R. Williams and C.L.M. Tiana (1990) "Consequences of spatial sampling for human motion perception", *Vision Res.* **30**, 1631-1648.

14. A. Cowey and E.T. Rolls (1974) "Human cortical magnification factor and its relation to visual acuity", *Exp. Brain Res.* **21**, 447-454.

15. J.M. Crook, B. Lange-Malecki, B.B. Lee and A. Valberg (1988) "Visual resolution of macque retinal ganglion cells", *J. Physiol.* **396**, 205-224.

16. C.A. Curcio and K.A. Allen (1990) "Topography of ganglion cells in human retina", *J. Comp. Neurol.* **300**, 5-25.

17. C.A. Curcio, K.R. Sloan, R.E. Kalina and A.E. Hendrickson (1990) "Human photoreceptor topography", *J. Comp. Neurol.* **292**, 497-523.

18. D.M. Dacey (1993) "The mosaic of midget ganglion cells in the human retina", *J. Neurosci.* **13**, 5334-5355.

19. P.M. Daniel and D. Whitteridge (1961) "The representation of the visual field on the cerebral cortex in monkey", *J. Physiol.* **159**, 203-221.

20. R.L. De Valois and K.K. De Valois, *Spatial Vision,* (Oxford University Press, New York, 1988).

21. B. Fischer (1973) "Overlap of receptive field centers and representation of the visual field in the cat's optic tract", *Vision Res.* **13**, 2113-2120.

22. C. Frederick and E.L. Schwartz (1990) "Conformal image warping", *IEEE Comp. Graph. & Appl.* **10/2**, 54-61.

23. A.S. French, A.W. Snyder and D.G. Stavenga (1977) "Image degradation by an irregular retinal mosaic", *Biol. Cyber.* **27**, 229-233.

24. S.J. Galvin and D.R. Williams (1992) "No aliasing at edges in normal viewing", *Vision Res.* **32**,

25. W.S. Geisler and D.B. Hamilton (1986) "Sampling-theory analysis of spatial vision", *J. Opt. Soc. Am. A.* **3**, 62-70.

26. C.R. Genter, G.L. Kandel and H.E. Bedell (1981) "The minimum angle of resolution vs angle of regard function as measured with different targets", *Ophthal. Physiol. Opt.* **1**, 3-13.

27. J.W. Goodman, *Introduction to Fourier Optics,* (McGraw-Hill, New York, 1968).

28. D.G. Green (1970) "Regional variations in the visual acuity for interference fringes on the retina", *J. Physiol.* **207**, 351-356.

29. J. Hirsch and R. Hylton (1984) "Quality of the primate photoreceptor lattice and the limits of spatial vision", *Vision Res.* **24**, 347-355.

30. J. Hirsch and W.H. Miller (1987) "Does cone positional disorder limit resolution?", *J. Opt. Soc. Am. A* **4**, 1481-1492.

31. I. Howard, in *Handbook of Perception and Human Performance*, ed. K.R. Boff, L. Kaufman and J.P. Thomas (John Wiley & Sons, New York, 1986), Ch. 18.

32. A. Hughes (1981) "Cat retina and the sampling theorem: the relation of transient and sustained brisk-unit cut-off frequency to alpha and beta-mode cell density", *Exp. Brain Res.* **42**, 196-202.

33. A. Hughes, in *Progress in Retinal Research*, ed. N.N. Osborne and G.J. Chader (Pergamon Press, Oxford, 1985), 243-313.

34. E. Kaplan, B.B. Lee and R.M. Shapley, in *Progress in Retinal Research*, ed. N. Osborne and G. Chader (Pergamon Press, Oxford, 1990), 273-336.

35. D.H. Kelly (1984) "Retinal inhomogeneity. I. Spatiotemporal contrast sensitivity", *J. Opt. Soc. Am. A* **1**, 107-113.

36. J.J. Koenderink, M.A. Bouman, A.E. Bueno de Mesquita and S. Slappendel (1978) "Perimetry of contrast detection thresholds of moving spatial sine wave patterns", *J. Opt. Soc. Am.* **68**, 845-865.

37. H. Kolb (1970) "Organization of the outer plexiform layer of the primate retina: electron microscopy of Golgi-impregnated cells.", *Phil. Trans. R. Soc.* **B 258**, 261-283.

38. H. Kolb and L. Dekorver (1991) "Midget ganglion cells of the parafovea of the human retina: a study by electron microscopy and serial section reconstructions", *J. Comp. Neurol.* **303**, 617-636.

39. H. Kolb, K.A. Linberg and S. Fisher (1992) "Neurons of the human retina: a Golgi study", *J. Comp. Neurol.* **318**, 147-187.

40. G.H. Kornfeld and W.R. Lawson (1971) "Visual-perception models", *J. Opt. Soc. Am.* **61**, 811-820.

41. P. Landau and E.L. Schwartz (1992) "Computer simulation of cortical polymaps: a proto-column algorithm", *Neur. Net.* **5**, 187-206.

42. S.B. Laughlin, in *Progress in Retinal and Eye Research*, ed. N.N. Osborne and G.J. Chader (Pergamon Press, Oxford, 1994), 165-196.

43. W.R. Levick and L.N. Thibos, in *Prog. Retinal Res.*, ed. N.N. Osborne and G.J. Chader (Pergamon Press, Oxford, 1983), 267-319.

44. B. Levitan and G. Buchsbaum (1993) "Signal sampling and propagation through multiple cell layers in the retina: modeling and analysis with multirate filtering", *J. Opt. Soc. Am. A* **10**, 1463-1480.

45. L. Matin, in *Handbook of Perception and Human Performance*, ed. K.R. Boff, L. Kaufman and J.P. Thomas (John Wiley & Sons, New York, 1986), Ch. 20.

46. W.H. Merigan and L.M. Katz (1990) "Spatial resolution across the macaque retina", *Vision Res.* **30**, 985-991.

47. R.A. Messner and H.H. Szu (1986) "An image processing architecture for real time generation of scale and rotation invariant patterns", *Computer Vision, Graphics & Image Processing* **31**, 50-66.

48. W.H. Miller and G.D. Bernard (1983) "Averaging over the foveal receptor aperture curtails aliasing", *Vision Res.* **23**, 1365-1369.

49. R. Navarro, P. Artal and D.R. Williams (1993) "Modulation transfer of the human eye as a function of retinal eccentricity", *J. Opt. Soc. Am. A* **10**, 201-212.

50. L.A. Olzak and J.P. Thomas, in *Handbook of Perception and Human Performance,* ed. K. Boff, L. Kaufman and J.P. Thomas (J. Wiley & Sons, New York, 1986), 7.1-7.56.

51. I. Overington (1982) "Towards a complete model of photopic visual threshold performance", *Opt. Engin.* **21**, 2-13.

52. L. Peichl and H. Wassle (1979) "Size, scatter and coverage of ganglion cell receptive field centres in the cat retina. ", *J. Physiol.* **291**, 117-141.

53. L. Peichl and H. Wassle (1983) "The structural correlate of the receptive field centre of alpha ganglion cells in the cat retina", *J. Physiol.* **341**, 309-324.

54. E. Peli, J. Yang and R.B. Goldstein (1991) "Image invariance with changes in size: the role of peripheral contrast thresholds", *J. Opt. Soc. Am. A* **8**, 1762-1774.

55. W. Penfield and T. Rasmussen, *The Cerebral Cortex of Man,* (Macmillan, New York, 1950).

56. V.H. Perry, R. Oehler and A. Cowey (1984) "Retinal ganglion cells that project to the dorsal lateral geniculate in the macaque monkey", *Neuroscience* **12**, 1101-1123.

57. D.P. Petersen and D. Middleton (1962) "Sampling and reconstruction of wave-number-limited functions in N-dimensional Euclidean spaces", *Inf. Control* **5**, 279-323.

58. S.L. Polyak, *The Retina,* (Univ. Chicago Press, Chicago, 1941).

59. J.A. Ratches (1976) "Static performance model for thermal imaging systems", *Opt. Engin.* **15**, 525-529.

60. R.W. Rodieck (1988) "The primate retina.", **4**, 203-278.

61. R.W. Rodieck, K.F. Binmoeller and J. Dineen (1985) "Parasol and midget ganglion cells of the human retina.", *J. Comp. Neurol.* **233**, 115-132.

62. J. Rovamo and V. Virsu (1979) "An estimation and application of the human cortical magnification factor", *Exp. Brain Res.* **37**, 495-510.

63. P.S. Schenker, E.G. Cande, K.M. Wong and W.R. Patterson, (1981). New sensor geometries for image processing: computer vision in the polar exponential grid. *Proc. IEEE Int'l. Conf. Acoustics, Speech, and Signal Processing*, 1144-1148.

64. E. Schwartz (1985) "On the mathematical structure of the retinotopic mapping of primate striate cortex", *Science* **277**, 1066-.

65. E.L. Schwartz (1977) "Spatial mapping in the primate sensory projection: Analytic structure and relevance to perception", *Biol. Cyber.* **25**, 181-194.

66. E.L. Schwartz (1980) "Computational anatomy and functional architecture of striate cortex: a spatial mapping approach to perceptual coding", *Vision Res.* **20**, 645-669.

67. C.E. Shannon (1949) "Communication in the presence of noise", *Proc. I.R.E.* **37**, 10-21.
68. R.A. Smith and R.A. Cass (1987) "Aliasing in the parafovea with incoherent light", *J. Opt. Soc. Am.* **A4**, 1530-1534.
69. A.W. Snyder, T.R.J. Bossomaier and A. Hughes (1986) "Optical image quality and the cone mosaic", *Science* **231**, 499-501.
70. A.W. Snyder, S.B. Laughlin and D.G. Stavenga (1977) "Information capacity of eyes", *Vision Res.* **17**, 1163-1175.
71. A.W. Snyder and W.H. Miller (1977) "Photoreceptor diameter and spacing for highest resolving power", *J. Opt. Soc. Amer.* **67**, 696-698.
72. R.E. Soodak, R.M. Shapley and E. Kaplan (1991) "Fine structure of receptive-field centers of X and Y cells of the cat", *Vis. Neurosci.* **6**, 621-628.
73. D.L. Still, *Optical Limits to Contrast Sensitivity in Human Peripheral Vision,* Ph. D. Thesis (Indiana University, 1989)
74. D.L. Still and L.N. Thibos (1989) "Peripheral image quality is almost as good as central image quality", *Invest. Ophthal. Vis. Sci.* **30** (suppl.), 219.
75. J. Ten Doesschate (1946) "Visual acuity and distribution of percipient elements on the retina.", *Ophthalmologica* **112**, 1-18.
76. L.N. Thibos, (1989). Image processing by the human eye. *Proc. SPIE Conf on Visual Communications and Image Processing IV,* **1199**, 1148-1153.
77. L.N. Thibos (1990) "Optical limitations of the Maxwellian-view interferometer", *Appl. Opt.* **29**, 1411-1419.
78. L.N. Thibos and A. Bradley (1992) "Use of interferometric visual stimulators in optometry", *Ophthalmic. Physiol. Opt.* **12**, 206-208.
79. L.N. Thibos, A. Bradley and D. Still (1991) "Interferometric measurement of visual acuity and the effect of ocular chromatic aberration", *Appl. Opt.* **30**, 2079-2087.
80. L.N. Thibos, F.E. Cheney and D.J. Walsh (1987) "Retinal limits to the detection and resolution of gratings", *J. Opt. Soc. Am. A* **4**, 1524-1529.
81. L.N. Thibos and W.R. Levick (1983) "Bimodal receptive fields of cat retinal ganglion cells", *Vision Res.* **23**, 1561-1572.
82. L.N. Thibos, D.J. Walsh and F.E. Cheney (1987) "Vision beyond the resolution limit: aliasing in the periphery", *Vision Res.* **27**, 2193-2197.
83. H. von Helmholtz, *Treatise on Physiological Optics* (1911), ed. J.P.C. Southall (The Optical Society of America, Washington, 1924).
84. J.J. Vos and A. van Meeteren (1991) "PHIND: an analytical model to predict acquisition distance with image intensifiers", *Appl. Opt.* **30**, 958-966.
85. G.L. Walls, *The Vertebrate Eye and its Adaptive Radiation,* (Cranbrook Institute of Science, Bloomfield Hills, Michigan, 1942).
86. Y. Wang, R.S. Anderson, L.N. Thibos and A. Bradley (1993) "Aliased frequencies enable the discrimination of compound gratings in peripheral vision", *Invest. Ophthal. Vis. Sci.* **34**, 777.

378

87. Y. Wang, A. Bradley and L.N. Thibos (1994) "Masking effect of supra-Nyquist gratings on sub-Nyquist gratings in peripheral vision", *Invest. Ophthal. Vis. Sci.* **35** (suppl.), 1954.

88. Y. Wang, L.N. Thibos, R. Anderson S., A. Bradley and K.M. Haggerty (1993) "Effect of sampling array irregularity on the perception of supra-Nyquist moving gratings", *Optom. Vis. Sci.* **70** (suppl.), 96.

89. Y. Wang, L.N. Thibos and A. Bradley (1993) "Masking effect of sub-Nyquist gratings on the detection of sub-and supra-Nyquist gratings in peripheral vision", *OSA Annual Meeting Technical Digest* **16**, 205.

90. H. Wassle and B.B. Boycott (1991) "Functional architecture of the mammalian retina", *Physiological Reviews* **71**, 447-480.

91. H. Wassle, U. Grunert, P. Martin and B.B. Boycott (1994) "Immunocytochemical characterization and spatial distribution of midget bipolar cells in the macaque monkey retina", *Vision Res.* **34**, 561-579.

92. H. Wassle, U. Grunert, J. Rohrenbeck and B.B. Boycott (1989) "Cortical magnification factor and the ganglion cell density of the primate retina", *Nature* **341**, 643-646.

93. H. Wassle, U. Grunert, J. Rohrenbeck and B.B. Boycott (1990) "Retinal ganglion cell density and cortical magnification factor in the primate", *Vision Res.* **30**, 1897-1911.

94. H. Wassle, L. Peichl and B.B. Boycott (1981) "Dendritic territories of cat retinal ganglion cells", *Nature* **292**, 344-345.

95. H. Wassle, L. Peichl and B.B. Boycott (1983) "Mosaics and territories of cat retinal ganglion cells", *Prog. Brain Res.* **58**, 183-190.

96. H. Wassle and H.J. Riemann (1978) "The mosaic of nerve cells in the mammalian retina", *Proc. R. Soc. Lond. B* **B 200**, 441-461.

97. R. Wehner (1987) "'Matched filters' - neural models of the external world", *J. Comp. Physiol. A* **161**, 511-531.

98. C.F.R. Weiman, (1988). 3-D sensing with polar exponential sensor arrays. *Proc. SPIE Conf. on Pattern Recognition and Signal Processing*, **938**, *Digital and Optical Shape Representation and Pattern Recognition*,

99. C.F.R. Weiman, (1988). Exponential sensor array geometry and simulation. *Proc. SPIE Conf. on Pattern Recognition and Signal Processing*, **938**, *Digital and Optical Shape Representation and Pattern Recognition*, 129-137.

100. C.F.R. Weiman, (1990). Video compression via log polar mapping. *Proc. SPIE Symp. on OE/Aerospace sensing*, *Digital and Optical Shape Representation and Pattern Recognition*,

101. C.F.R. Weiman and G. Chaikin (1979) "Logarithmic spiral grids for image processing and display", *Computer Graphics and Image Processing* **11**, 197-226.

102. T. Wertheim (1894) "Peripheral visual acuity", translated by I. Dunsky, *Am. J. Optom. Physiol. Optics* **57**, 919-924.

103. G. Westheimer (1959) "Retinal light distributions for circular apertures in Maxwellian view", *J. Opt. Soc. Am.* **49**, 41-44.

104. F.W. Weymouth (1958) "Visual sensory units and the minimal angle of resolution", *Am. J. Ophthalmol.* **46**, 102-113.

105. M.O. Wilkinson, *Neural Basis of Photopic and Scotopic Resolution Acuity Across the Human Retina,* Ph.D. Thesis (Indiana University, 1994)

106. D.R. Williams (1985) "Aliasing in human foveal vision", *Vision Res.* **25**, 195-205.

107. D.R. Williams and N.J. Coletta (1987) "Cone spacing and the visual resolution limit", *J. Opt. Soc. Am. A* **4**, 1514-1523.

108. H.R. Wilson, D. Levi, L. Maffei, J. Rovamo and R. DeValois, in *Visual perception: the neurophysiological foundations,* ed. L. Spillman and J.S. Werner (Academic Press, San Diego, 1990), 231-272.

109. J.I. Yellot (1982) "Spectral analysis of spatial sampling by photoreceptors: topological disorder prevents aliasing", *Vision Res.* **22**, 1205-1210.

110. A.I. Zayed, *Advances in Shannon's Sampling Theory,* (CRC Press, Boca Raton, 1993).

111. O. Zoth, in *Handbuch der Physiologie des Menschen,* ed. W. Nagel (Friedrich Vieweg und Sohn, Berlin, 1905), 353-356.

QUANTIFYING TARGET CONTRAST IN TARGET ACQUISITION RESEARCH

WILLIAM KOSNIK

The Analytic Sciences Corporation
750 E. Mulberry Avenue
San Antonio, TX, 78212-3159

Effective models of target acquisition must address issues of detecting targets against spatially structured backgrounds. This research focused on how acquisition performance is affected by backgrounds of varying complexity, target contrast, and motion. A metric was devised that allowed quantitative control of target contrast independently of the background. Observers searched for an aircraft embedded in backgrounds of differing complexity. The results showed that acquisition time increased as background complexity increased and target contrast decreased. Target motion facilitated acquisition performance. Although contrast had a systematic effect on acquisition performance, it was clear that factors other than contrast contributed to target visibility. Other factors that may have affected visibility included distracters and camouflaging effects introduced by the structured backgrounds.

1. Testing Acquisition Performance

1.1. Defining Target Contrast in Complex Scenes

There is much interest in developing quantitative models that can predict target acquisition performance.[1-5] Such models need to take into account the visual performance of the observer as well as the characteristics of the scene. Several current visual detection models developed primarily for air-to-air acquisition rely on simplified descriptions of target contrast.[2,6,7] These descriptions, which employ traditional contrast metrics such as the Weber or Michelson contrasts, are inadequate because they do not take into account the complex luminance distributions present in natural scenes.[8-10] In order to predict the visibility of complex targets in natural scenes, successful models must consider how the visual system processes complex images.

Recent approaches have attempted to characterize the contrast of complex scenes by filtering the scene with the human contrast sensitivity function.[8,11,12] These approaches advocate using the spatial frequency and orientation selectivity of the visual system to more accurately characterize the perceived scene contrast. It is argued that a spatially filtered contrast metric would characterize scene contrast better than traditional metrics that focus on physical scene contrast. Peli[8,13] has advocated the use of a spatially localized band-limited contrast metric that calculates a contrast value for every point in the scene. While this metric provides a highly precise measure of scene contrast, such an approach tends to be computationally intensive.

Other approaches have attempted to find an effective compromise between traditional descriptions of contrast and the computationally intensive point-for-point metrics.[5,10] A successful compromise would be computationally efficient, but would still adequately characterize the scene complexity to make accurate measurements of target visibility. The approach adopted here is similar to the one used by Moulden and co-workers[10] to characterize contrast in random dot patterns. They used the root mean square (*rms*) metric to describe the apparent contrast in random dot images. They found that this metric corresponded better to the perceived contrast of the image than several other candidate metrics. This measure, which specifies the luminance variation in the scene, has the advantage of being computationally efficient.

The *rms* metric could also be applied to certain air-to-surface and air-to-air acquisition situations. For reasonably small targets on natural terrain, visibility is mainly determined by the local luminance variation surrounding the target. (This approach assumes a relatively uniform luminance distribution of the target.) The *rms* metric might be a sufficient description of this luminance variation and, therefore, the perceived contrast. This method has the further advantage of controlling target contrast simply by varying its luminance. Because contrast is controlled independently of the background, task performance can be directly compared across different backgrounds.

The utility of the *rms* metric for predicting target visibility was evaluated in a realistic target acquisition context. The metric was used to define target contrast when aircraft targets were depicted in combination with simple and complex backgrounds and under static and dynamic conditions. These task conditions simulated air-to-air and air-to-surface target acquisition activities. Results of the experiment served as inputs to test three different visual search models. One model, the exponential model,[14] has been used to predict visual search performance using abstract search targets and backgrounds under the assumption of randomized scanning behavior. This model was tested to determine its appropriateness for modeling acquisition behavior employing complex natural scenes.

1.2. Stimulus Processing

The objective of the stimulus processing effort was to embed the targets into the backgrounds and manipulate the target contrast without changing the background. Target contrast could then be quantified and controlled independently of the background. This approach would permit comparisons of acquisition performance for targets on different backgrounds.

The target was a silhouette image of an aircraft, viewed from above and to the side. The aircraft subtended 0.6° from wing tip to wing tip. The backgrounds were a structureless (uniform) background, a natural terrain background, and a moving natural terrain (dynamic) background. The dynamic background was video footage of natural terrain shot from an over-flying aircraft. The target aircraft was stationary with respect to the viewer's frame of reference and the background moved behind it. This scheme simulated a low-flying aircraft viewed from another aircraft flying overhead at the same speed and direction. The mean luminance of the uniform and terrain backgrounds was 46.2 cd/m^2. The luminance of the dynamic background varied from frame to frame because of the changing scene, but its average luminance was close to the luminance of the other two backgrounds. Background images were displayed on a Video Monitors, Inc. 19" monochrome video display terminal. The background images subtended 23.9° by 23.3° at a distance of 1 m.

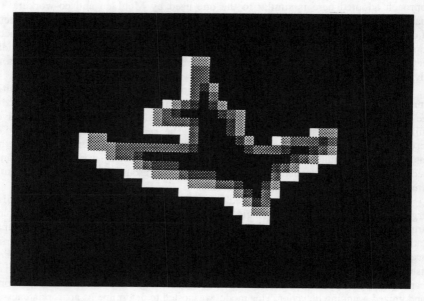

Figure 1. An illustration of the pixel areas selected for the aircraft, background, and blending operations. The aircraft is shown as the black central area, the background is shown as the white pixels, and the aircraft-background border selected for the blending operations is shown as the crosshatched area.

Target insertion and contrast manipulation procedures were performed with Precision Visuals, Inc., PV~WAVE^{TM} image-processing software. The target set was generated by first randomly selecting a location on a background. The aircraft was embedded in the background by substituting aircraft pixels for background pixels. Figure 1 shows an enlarged view of the aircraft and background pixel areas selected for the contrast manipulation operations. The aircraft is shown as the central black area. The background is shown as the area in white. The border between the aircraft and the background was smoothed by alpha blending, which is shown as the cross-hatched area. The blending process effectively low-pass filtered the aircraft edge to give the aircraft a more natural appearance against the terrain background.

Contrast calculations were performed on the aircraft and surround. The surround could be considered noise in which the signal (aircraft) was embedded. The number of background pixels involved in the contrast calculations was equal to the number of aircraft pixels. The background pixels were evenly distributed around the aircraft perimeter as shown in Figure 1. It seems clear that the background pixels in the immediate vicinity of the aircraft most directly determined its contrast; background features further away had less influence. Beyond this intuitive notion, however, selection of the size of the background area was arbitrary. The determination of the optimal size of the background remains for further study, but see Cannon's[15] chapter in this book and Peli[8,13] for further discussion of this topic.

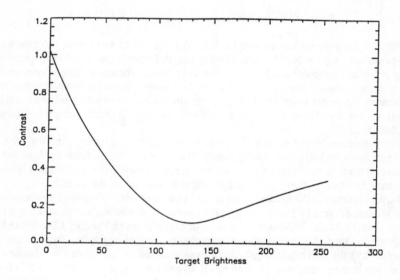

Figure 2. Target contrast as a function of target luminance on an arbitrarily selected location on the natural terrain background. The luminance distribution of the local background surrounding the target determines the contrast. As the target luminance approached the mean background luminance, target contrast falls to a minimum. The target contrast is maximized when the target luminance is at the extremes of its luminance range.

Target contrast was manipulated by varying target luminance. By adjusting the luminance of the aircraft pixels, the aircraft could be made to blend in with, or stand out from, the background. The relationship between target luminance and target contrast is shown in Figure 2 for one natural terrain location. The aircraft was least visible (lowest numerical contrast) when its pixels were set to the average luminance of the background pixels, thereby minimizing the variance of the combined aircraft and surround luminance distribution. Maximum visibility occurred when the aircraft pixels were set to the minimum or maximum of the available luminance range, thereby maximizing the luminance variance. The *rms* contrast was calculated by the expression:

$$rms = [(\sum(t_i\text{-m})^2 + \sum(b_i\text{-m})^2)/n]^{1/2} \qquad (1)$$

where t_i = the luminance of the ith target pixel, b_i = the luminance of the ith background pixel, $i = \{1,n/2\}$, the set of target (or background) pixels, m = the mean luminance of the target and background pixels, and n = the total number of target and background pixels. Because the mean luminance of the target and surround pixels varied from location to location, *rms* was normalized by dividing by the mean luminance or:

$$nrms = rms/m. \qquad (2)$$

Normalized contrast values of 0.15, 0.25, 0.35, and 0.45 *nrms* were selected and the above equations were solved for target luminance (t). Figure 3 shows enlarged views of the target at the four test contrasts. It can be seen that perceived contrast changes systematically with physical contrast. Thus, at face value, the *rms* metric appears to represent an adequate measure of the target contrast. Although the aircraft had only one luminance value, in principal, the technique could also be used for targets with complex luminance distributions.

The procedure for embedding targets in the natural terrain background was also used for the uniform and dynamic backgrounds. The pixels in the uniform background case constituted a single luminance value, so *nrms* contrasts were calculated from a two-value luminance distribution, one for the background and the other for the aircraft.

Target contrasts in the dynamic background condition were calculated by processing the video sequence frame by frame. A 30-s video sequence of moving terrain was played from a Sony U-matic Model VO-9600 video cassette recorder into a Parallax 1280 frame buffer one frame at a time. A target location was randomly selected on the first frame of the video sequence and the corresponding location was selected on all subsequent frames. The aircraft luminance value was adjusted to achieve the desired *nrms* contrast value for that particular frame. Aircraft luminance values were processed in the same way on subsequent frames. As the background image at the selected location varied from frame to frame, it was necessary to compute a new aircraft luminance value to achieve the same *nrms* contrast across all frames of the sequence. A set of 900 target luminance values corresponding to 900 frames in the 30-s sequence were calculated and stored in computer memory. Then the procedure was repeated on the next target location for the next trial until a complete set of trials had been constructed.

When the video sequence was played back at the time of testing, the stored target luminance values were overwritten onto the background image in real time. Some variation in the frame-to-frame *nrms* contrast could not be avoided, but this variation was always less than ±10% and usually less than ±5%. Because targets had to be embedded in the frames in real time, some compromise in video image quality had to be made for the sake of processing speed. To achieve the necessary processing speed the number of video lines

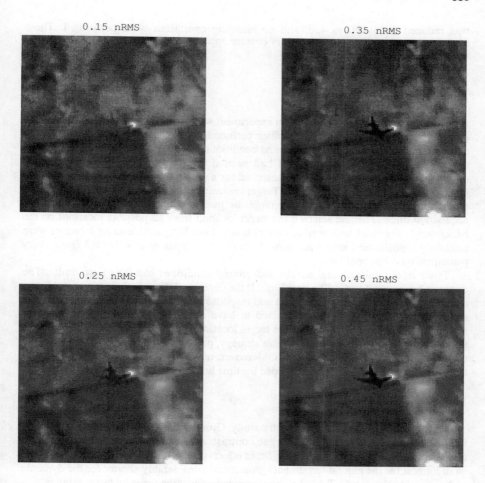

Figure 3. The four contrast levels of the aircraft target selected for use in the experiment. It can be seen that perceived contrast is a nonlinear function of physical contrast. (Reprinted with permission from *Huamn Factors*, Vol. 37, No. 3, 1995. Copyright 1995 by the Human Factors and Ergonomics Society. All rights reserved.)

was **reduced from** 480 to 450, and no blending operations were performed. These modifications gave the target a slightly coarser appearance and reduced the background image size to 23.9° by 21.8°.

1.3. Testing Procedure

The contrast metric was used in an experiment which tested the effect of background complexity and target motion on acquisition performance. Eight participants were randomly assigned to each of the three background conditions. Participants were male volunteers, ranging in age from 22 to 44. All had normal vision as assessed by a complete ophthalmological exam. Participants searched for a single target randomly positioned on one of the backgrounds on each trial. Target contrasts were randomly mixed from trial to trial. After the participant found the target he pushed a button which determined the acquisition time. Then he selected the target location from 12 possible locations on the background. Feedback was provided after his selection. The possible target locations were randomly repositioned after each trial. Data from 48 trials were collected from every participant on each condition.

Trials in the uniform and terrain background conditions had 90-s time limits. The dynamic background had a 30-s time limit. If the observer did not find the target within the allotted time, the trial was terminated and response time was scored as 90 s or 30 s, as appropriate. Participants were instructed to have a high level of confidence in their selections. If they were not sure of the target location, they were instructed to wait until time ran out and then guess. By using this strategy, participants always found the target on trials that did not exceed the time limits. Moreover, only a few trials—mostly in the natural terrain, low contrast conditions—exceeded the time limit.

1.4. Background Effects

Figure 4 shows the main results of the study. Group mean acquisition times are plotted in log seconds as a function of target contrast and background. Both background complexity and target contrast had significant effects on acquisition time. Acquisition times were longest for the natural terrain background and considerably shorter for the dynamic and uniform backgrounds. Table 1 shows the mean acquisition times by test condition.

Despite identical target contrasts, search performance differed markedly among the three backgrounds. These results indicated that acquisition performance was determined by more than just the target contrast. The large increases in acquisition time observed for the natural terrain background could be due to the additional structural features present in the background. It is likely that this background presented structure which had to be distinguished from the target. This structure effectively created distracters which had a marked effect on visual processing speed.

Background motion facilitated acquisition performance. Even though the dynamic background structure was more similar to the structure in the natural terrain background, the dynamic acquisition times more closely resembled the acquisition times of the uniform background. The addition of motion to the acquisition scene seemed to offset the distracting effects of background structure.

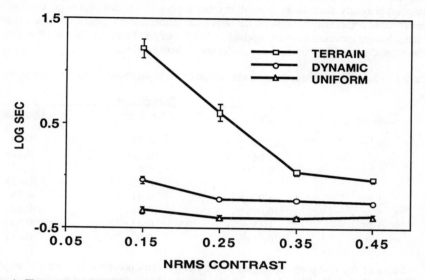

Figure 4. The mean acquisition times in log seconds by background and contrast condition. Acquisition times decreased as a function of background type and as target contrast increased. Error bars equal ±1 SEM. (Reprinted with permission from *Huamn Factors*, Vol. 37, No. 3, 1995. Copyright 1995 by the Human Factors and Ergonomics Society. All rights reserved.)

Motion enhancement of performance could be due to a number of different factors. It could be explained by the relatively greater sensitivity of the peripheral retina to motion, compared to its sensitivity to structure.[16,17] Because of its enhanced sensitivity to motion the peripheral retina probably played a greater role in the detection of moving targets than stationary targets. The motion effect could also be attributed to the greater sensitivity of the visual system to certain temporal frequencies.[18,19] Alternatively, figure-ground separation could have been enhanced from the parts of the scene that moved cohesively from those parts that did not[20]. In any case, motion appears to be a powerful search cue.

1.5. Contrast Effect

The contrast manipulation had a nonlinear effect on acquisition time. Figure 4 shows that acquisition times decreased as target contrast increased, but the rate of change slowed at higher contrast levels. It appeared that the acquisition times were approaching an asymptotic level at the highest contrast levels. Further increases in contrast probably would have resulted in a convergence of the three background curves at some optimal level of performance. The shortest average acquisition time was 0.41 s for the 0.35 *nrms* uniform background condition. On some trials the acquisition times were as low as 0.20 s, which may represent the minimum response time for this type of task, given the requirement to respond manually. Such short acquisition times suggest that under high target contrast, low background complexity conditions, the target was immediately visible anywhere within the scene. No eye movements were required to find the target. This result implies that virtually the entire display was processed in parallel under these conditions.

Table 1. Mean acquisition times (seconds) and standard errors (in parentheses) by background and contrast.

Contrast	Background		
	Terrain	*Uniform*	*Dynamic*
0.15	37.99	0.59	1.08
	(5.54)	(0.12)	(0.12)
0.25	9.91	0.42	0.61
	(2.49)	(0.03)	(0.03)
0.35	1.22	0.41	0.59
	(0.09)	(0.02)	(0.02)
0.45	1.18	0.43	0.55
	(0.16)	(0.02)	(0.01)

Some of the low-contrast targets in the natural terrain condition were not acquired within the time limit. One obvious question is if unlimited viewing time were allowed, would all of the targets have been found? An answer to this question might help establish an upper limit on expected acquisition times which could be very useful to target acquisition modelers. Upon closer examination, it was found that these targets blended in so well with the background that they could not be detected even when looking directly at them. In other words, they were below threshold. Therefore, it seems reasonable to conclude that the targets never would have been found no matter how long the observer searched. Thus, by examining the acquisition time distributions it may be possible to determine when further searching would not yield more targets.

1.6. Acquisition Variability

The variability associated with the mean acquisition times provided some additional insights into the acquisition process. Acquisition times varied widely among the different experimental conditions. In general, acquisition time variability increased as target contrast decreased and background complexity increased (see Table 3). Two sample distributions from the natural terrain condition are shown in Figure 5. The distribution for the low contrast condition is shown in the left panel and the high contrast condition is shown in the right panel. The standard deviations associated with these two distributions were 38.0 s and 1.1 s, respectively. The low variability observed for the high contrast condition suggested that acquisition performance could be predicted by target contrast alone. After target contrast exceeded some critical level, local background variation played little role in determining acquisition time.

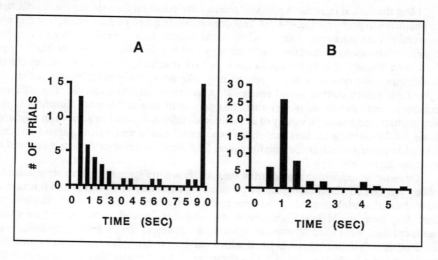

Figure 5. Two distributions from the natural terrain (A) low (0.15 *nrms*) and (B) high (0.45 *nrms*) target contrast conditions.

Acquisition times for the low contrast, natural terrain condition ranged from a high of 90 s to a low of 0.39 s. The wide range in acquisition time indicated that other factors besides contrast must be determining acquisition performance. One obvious factor is the probabilistic nature of the acquisition process itself, that is, the necessity of making eye movements to locate the targets. If initial eye movements bring the target near the fovea, then acquisition time is short. However, if eye movements do not bring the line of sight near the target until later in the search episode, acquisition time is correspondingly lengthened. Thus, the probabilistic nature of the search task accounts for some of the acquisition variability. But other factors may be responsible as well. It is also possible that factors not captured by the *nrms* metric could have had an impact on target visibility. One candidate is the structural content of the local background. Background structure might have affected target visibility by camouflaging or masking the target's shape, edge, or some other feature necessary for recognition. A contrast metric that takes into account only the luminance distribution of the background, and not its structural interaction with the target, may not completely describe the target's visibility. By constructing a metric that accounts for the spatial interaction between the target and background, the target contrast metric might better correspond to the visibility of the target.[8]

2. Modeling Acquisition Performance

Most theoretical treatments of visual search have relied on the exponential distribution to characterize performance.[14,21-23] This convention is based on the assumption that eye movements are randomly distributed in visual search. It is typically assumed that the observer follows no systematic search strategy and that fixations are just as likely to go back over already searched areas as areas not yet searched. However, when structured backgrounds are present, eye movements may take on a more orderly search pattern. A systematic search pattern would not result in an exponential distribution. The different conditions used in this study presented the opportunity to test the appropriateness of the exponential model under a variety of acquisition situations. In order to achieve an objective basis for determining the best model, the exponential model was tested against two other candidate models of acquisition performance. Statistical goodness-of-fit tests were used to evaluate the models.

Cumulative acquisition time distributions are shown in Figure 6 for three representative observers. The distributions depict the cumulative probability of detection as a function of time. Note that trials exceeding the time limits were not included in the distributions, as including them would have biased the model estimates. Instead, goodness-of-fit tests for censored data were used to provide unbiased estimates of the underlying distributions. Each observer's distribution was fitted with a cumulative Gaussian model, an exponential model,[14] and a Weibull model.[24] A two-parameter $\hat{D}$ test for normality was applied to the cumulative Gaussian model,[25] a one-parameter S^* statistic was used to test the exponential model,[26] and a two-parameter S statistic was used to evaluate the Weibull model.[27]

Because the goodness-of-fit tests tested the null hypothesis of no deviation between the data and the model, a good fit was indicated by a nonsignificant result. Thus, a $p > 0.20$ alpha level was chosen as the criterion for a good fit. The results are shown in Table 2. The Gaussian model fit 33% of the participants' distributions, compared to 15% for the exponential model, and 8% for the Weibull model.

The successful Gaussian fits were fairly evenly distributed across all of the participants and experimental conditions. The Gaussian model fit 25% of the natural terrain conditions, 31% of the uniform conditions, and 44% of the dynamic conditions. The exponential model fit 38% of the terrain background conditions, none of the uniform, and 6% of the dynamic background conditions. The exponential model fit 29% of the low contrast conditions and none of the high contrast conditions. The group means, standard deviations, and corresponding 95% confidence limits for the Gaussian model are reported in Table 3.

The results of the modeling analysis indicated that the cumulative Gaussian model fit more conditions than the exponential or Weibull models. Although the Gaussian model by no means adequately fit all of the acquisition distributions, it fit a wide variety of them. The number of successful cumulative Gaussian fits were fairly evenly distributed across nearly all of the experimental conditions. These results suggested that the Gaussian model could have wide applicability for predicting acquisition performance. Thus, the assumption of random eye movements during acquisition, as exemplified by the exponential model, was not supported for many of the search situations.

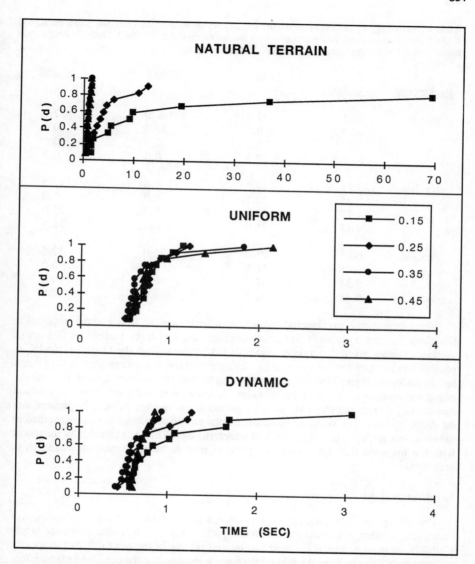

Figure 6. Cumulative probability of detection as a function of acquisition time for three representative observers. Note the differences in time scales. Some distributions did not reach unity because some acquisition times exceeded the time limit and were not included.

Table 2. Percentage of successful individual goodness-of-fit tests of the Gaussian, Exponential, and Weibull models. (Reprinted with permission from *Huamn Factors*, Vol. 37, No. 3, 1995. Copyright 1995 by the Human Factors and Ergonomics Society. All rights reserved.)

Background	Contrast	Gaussian	Exp	Weibull
Terrain	0.15	37.5	100.0	37.5
	0.25	0.0	50.0	0.0
	0.35	25.0	0.0	0.0
	0.45	37.5	0.0	0.0
Uniform	0.15	12.5	0.0	12.5
	0.25	12.5	0.0	0.0
	0.35	25.0	0.0	25.0
	0.45	75.0	0.0	12.5
Dynamic	0.15	25.0	25.0	12.5
	0.25	50.0	0.0	0.0
	0.35	37.5	0.0	0.0
	0.45	62.5	0.0	0.0

Nevertheless, the exponential model did a better job of fitting some acquisition situations than the cumulative Gaussian model. In fact, the exponential model fit more of the low contrast, natural terrain background distributions than the Gaussian model. A possible explanation for this unexpected finding is that the structure present in the natural terrain background provided few clues regarding the target's location. Indeed, because the target was randomly located in the background, an observer who tried to use background features to guide his search would not have gained any advantage. Instead, it appeared that the difficulty presented by the low contrast, natural terrain conditions may have resulted in the observers resorting to a more random search strategy. This interpretation is consistent with the proposal that eye movement patterns tend to be more random as search is prolonged.[28]

3. Conclusions

Predicting target acquisition performance under natural viewing conditions is a continuing challenge for researchers. Among the many variables that influence target visibility, contrast is one of the most crucial and yet one of the most difficult to specify quantitatively. Results from the foregoing research indicate that the combined visual effect of the target and background must be taken into account before a complete description of target visibility can be realized.

Table 3. Mean acquisition times (AT) in seconds, standard deviations (SD), and 95% confidence limits (CL) of the Gaussian model. (Reprinted with permission from *Huamn Factors*, Vol. 37, No. 3, 1995. Copyright 1995 by the Human Factors and Ergonomics Society. All rights reserved.)

Background	Contrast	AT	Lower CL	Upper CL	SD	Lower CL	Upper CL
Terrain	0.15	19.4*	13.4	25.4	17.2	12.3	22.1
	0.25	6.3*	4.9	7.7	9.6	5.9	13.3
	0.35	1.3	1.0	1.6	0.8	0.2	1.4
	0.45	1.2	0.8	1.6	0.8	0.3	1.3
Uniform	0.15	0.6	0.4	0.8	0.4	0.0	0.8
	0.25	0.5	0.4	0.6	0.2	0.1	0.3
	0.35	0.5	0.4	0.6	0.2	0.1	0.3
	0.45	0.5	0.4	0.6	0.2	0.1	0.3
Dynamic	0.15	1.7	1.3	2.1	1.3	0.7	1.9
	0.25	0.7	0.6	0.8	0,3	0.2	0.4
	0.35	0.7	0.6	0.8	0.2	0.2	0.2
	0.45	0.6	0.5	0.7	0.1	0.1	0.1

*Note: These values exclude truncated data.

Acknowledgments

The author gratefully acknowledges Anthony Catalano, James Brakefield, Gary Noojin, David Stolarski, William Rowe Elliott III, Michael Yochmowitz, and Marta Myers for their contributions to this project. This research was supported by the USAF Armstrong Laboratory, Occupational and Environmental Health Directorate, Optical Radiation Division, Contracts F33615-88-C-0631 to KRUG Life Sciences, Inc. and F33615-92-C-0017 to TASC, Inc.

References

1. H. E. Guttmann & R. G. Webster, "Determining the detectability range of camouflaged targets", *Human Factors* **14** (1972) 217-225.
2. A. Akerman III & R. E. Kinzly, "Predicting aircraft detectability", *Human Factors* **21** (1979) 277-291.
3. C. P. Greening, "Mathematical modeling of air-to-ground target acquisition", *Human Factors* **18** (1976) 111-148.
4. B. L. Sibernagel, "Using realistic sensor, target, and scene characteristics to develop a target acquisition model", *Human Factors* **24** (1982) 321-328.

5. A. van Meeteren, "Characterization of task performance with viewing instruments", *J. Opt. Soc. Am. [A]* **7(10)** (1990) 2016-2023.

6. I. Overington, "Towards a complete model of photopic visual threshold performance", *Opt. Eng.* **21** (1982) 2-13.

7. J. J Vos & A. van Meeteren, "PHIND: An analytical model to predict target acquisition distance with image intensifiers", *App. Opt.* **30** (1991) 958-966.

8. E. Peli, "Contrast in complex images", *J. Opt. Soc. Am. [A]* **7(10)** (1990) 2032-2040.

9. D. J. Field, "Relations between the statistics of natural images and the response properties of cortical cells", *J. Opt. Soc. Am. [A]* **4(12)** (1987) 2379-2394.

10. B. Moulden, F. Kingdom, & L. F. Gatley, "The standard deviation of luminance as a metric for contrast in random-dot images", *Perception* **19** (1990) 79-101.

11. T. J. Doll, S. W. McWhorter, & D. E. Schmieder, "Target and background characterization based on a simulation of human pattern perception", in *Characterization, Propagation, and Simulation of Sources and Backgrounds III, SPIE Proc. Vol. 1967* (1993) 432-454.

12. S. R. Thomas & N. Barsalou, see chapter 9 of this volume.

13. E. Peli, see chapter 3 of this volume.

14. E. S. Krendel & J. Wodinsky, "Search in an unstructured visual field", *J. Opt. Soc. Am.* **50** (1960) 562-568.

15. M. W. Cannon, see chapter 4 of this volume.

16. H. E. Petersen & D. J. Dugas, "The relative importance of contrast and motion in visual detection", *Human Factors* **14(3)** (1972) 207-216.

17. J. G. Rogers, "Peripheral contrast thresholds for moving images", *Human Factors* **14(3)** (1972) 199-205.

18. D. H. Kelly, "Motion and vision. II. Stabilized spatio-temporal threshold surface", *J. Opt. Soc. Am. [A]* **69(10)** (1979) 1340-1349.

19. R. Sekuler, A. Pantle, & E. Levinson, "Physiological basis of motion perception", in *Handbook of Sensory Physiology, Vol. III: Perception,* ed. R. Held, H.W. Leibowitz, and H.-L.Teuber (Springer-Verlag, New York, 1978), pp. 67-96.

20. P. McLeod, J. Driver, Z. Dienes, & J. Crisp, "Filtering by movement in visual search", *J. Exp. Psych.: Human Percept. Perf.* **17(1)** (1991) 55-64.

21. J. R. Bloomfield, "Visual search in complex fields: Size differences between target disc and surrounding discs", *Human Factors* **14** (1972) 139-148.

22. E. B. Davies, "Visual theory in target acquisition", in *AGARD Conf. Proc.* **41** (1968) 1-13.

23. L. G. Williams, "Target conspicuity and visual search", *Human Factors* **8** (1966) 80-92.

24. L. O. Harvey Jr., "Efficient estimation of sensory thresholds", *Beh. Res. Meth. Instr. Comp.* **18** (1986) 623-632.

25. H. W. Lilliefors, "On the Kolmogorov-Smirnov test for normality with mean and variance unknown", *J. Am. Stat. Assoc.* **62** (1967) 399-402.

26. J. M. Finkelstein & R. E. Schafer, "Improved goodness of fit tests", *Biometrik* **58** (1971) 641-645.

395

27. N. R. Mann, E. M. Scheuer, & K. W. Fertig, "A goodness of fit test for the two parameter Weibull or extreme value distribution with unknown parameters", *Comm. Stat.* **2** (1973) 383-400.
28. F. L. Engel, "Visual conspicuity, visual search and fixation tendencies of the eye", *Vision Res.* **17** (1977) 95-108.

SIMULATION OF SELECTIVE ATTENTION AND TRAINING EFFECTS IN VISUAL SEARCH AND DETECTION

THEODORE J. DOLL, SHANE W. MCWHORTER, DAVID E. SCHMIEDER, and ANTHONY A. WASILEWSKI

Georgia Tech Research Institute
Georgia Institute of Technology
Atlanta, GA 30332-0800, USA

The Georgia Tech Vision (GTV) model is a simulation of human visual search and detection based on research and models from the field of computational vision, including texture segregation and pop-out. The model is consistent with recent psychophysical and neurophysiological research on low-level visual processes. The model also incorporates findings from research on visual search, selective attention, and signal detection theory. A learning algorithm is used to simulate the effects of extended training on pop-out and visual search performance. The structure and algorithms of the model are described and the results of a validation test with human observers are presented.

1. Introduction

Over the past several years, we at Georgia Tech have been developing a simulation of the human visual system. The current implementation of the simulation is called the Georgia Tech Vision (GTV) model. The goal of this work is to develop a high-fidelity simulation that mimics as many functions of the human visual system as possible. In order to enable the GTV model to predict complex visual performance, it has been necessary to integrate findings from disparate areas of the vision and attention research literatures into a single comprehensive model of visual function. The GTV model incorporates findings from research on low-level visual processes, including texture segregation and pop-out, and from the visual search, selective attention, and signal detection theory literatures.

To date, the GTV model is able to predict where observers will focus their attention when searching for targets (typically vehicles) in cluttered terrain backgrounds, and accurately predicts the probability of detecting those targets. The current model accounts for the effects of motion and chromaticity on visual search and detection under both photopic and scotopic conditions, but is currently limited to monocular viewing. Of course, these capabilities are modest compared to those of the human visual system. It is anticipated that the GTV model will evolve over many years, gradually adding capabilities. Due to limited space available in this chapter and the fact that the model is continuously being improved, the current description is by no means a complete or final specification of the GTV model.

This chapter describes the structure and functioning of the GTV model as of October 1994, and focuses on three important, closely interrelated properties of the human visual system that are simulated by the model. These properties include: (1) the ability to process large amounts of stimulus information to a limited extent in parallel (preattentive processing), (2) the ability to select regions and/or features in the field of view for further processing (selective attention), and (3) the modification of selective attention and search performance with extended training.

Preattentive processing enables human observers to process objects of potential importance over the whole field in parallel. Perhaps the most widely studied example of preattentive processing is pop-out, the ability of persons with normal vision to perceive variations in pattern or texture in a single glimpse, without conscious effort. An object may pop out from its background even when there is no difference in the average intensities or chromaticities of the object and the background[3]. The term pop-out is reserved for pattern differences that are perceived effortlessly, in contrast to those that must be <u>discriminated</u>, i.e., require close inspection or focused attention. Preattentive processing also provides inputs that can be used to allocate processing resources for further, more detailed, analyses (attentive processing).

Preattentive processing is fundamental to visual search performance. There is substantial evidence that eye movements (saccades) during visual search are guided by preattentive processing of pattern information in peripheral vision. For example, recordings of eye movements over structured scenes reveal that the eye fixates on features such as edges and corners that are more likely to convey information than are plain surfaces[12]. In reading, the eyes of proficient readers search out larger words, which convey a high degree of meaning, rather than articles[29]. Visual search proficiency has even been used as a measure of peripheral visual acuity[2,10,19].

Thus it seems likely that preattentive processing of patterns outside the momentary area of focal attention plays an important role in determining where the observer will focus attention next. Several investigators have suggested that the "spotlight" of focal attention falls on locations in the visual field according to their *conspicuity*, which is a combination of features derived from early visual processing[21,31]. The GTV model uses a similar formulation. The probability that focal attention is directed to a given object or location is directly related to the extent to which it pops out, which is termed conspicuity.

In GTV, conspicuity depends on luminance contrast, chromatic contrast, temporal modulation, and texture differences. (A goal for the future is to add stereopsis to this list.) Perceptual segregation of textures is simulated using complex spatial frequency channels models, such as those developed by Graham and her colleagues[13,14] and by Wilson and Richards[44]. Since focal attention is closely related to fixation (though not necessarily identical), the probability that focal attention is directed to an object is called its probability of fixation (P_{fix}). In GTV, the simulation of preattentive processing and the prediction of conspicuities is one of several functions of the *search module*.

The second topic of this paper, selective attention, uses the inputs from the preattentive stage to focus processing resources for further analysis, such as object recognition, on a limited region of the visual field. A number of authors have argued that the complexity of the processing implied by tasks such as object recognition would make it prohibitive for a biological processor to perform such operations in parallel over the whole visual field[21,31,39]. Selective attention allows the observer to adaptively allocate the limited resources available for attentive processing to different parts of the visual field at different times.

But what rule is used to select one region of the visual field for further processing and exclude others? Koch and Ullman[21] have suggested that the outputs of the preattentive stage (low-level vision properties) are differentially weighted, and that the "spotlight" of attention is directed to the region of the visual field with the greatest weighted output, or *conspicuity*. In GTV, the computation of weights that predict conspicuity is performed by the *selective attention unit*.

The GTV representation of attentive processing is called the *discrimination module*. The results of target detection experiments with realistic targets and terrain background scenes show that observers are very conservative about reporting detections in cluttered images[9,26]. That is, they produce low false alarm rates, which indicates that they have performed enough analysis of the target shape to determine with high confidence that it is not a clutter object. Their performance in the "detection" task seems to be driven by the *discriminability* of the target from background clutter, rather than simply the detectability of the target pattern. Hence, the GTV representation of attentive processing is called the discrimination module rather than the detection module. Of course, attentive processing in humans is not limited to discrimination. Work is currently in progress to add additional capabilities, including object recognition and identification, to the GTV model.

Part of the adaptability of the human visual system derives from the third topic area mentioned earlier, i.e., the modification of selective attention through learning. Human observers learn "what to look for" and greatly improve their performance in the course of searching for particular targets in a given type of background[24,33]. Studies of visual search show that, after extensive practice, observers can learn to selectively attend to objects with particular combinations of features while ignoring objects with other features[32,33]. The results of such studies suggest that learning modifies the extent to which various low-level vision properties contribute to the conspicuity or salience of objects.

Many everyday search tasks, like military target acquisition and diagnostic inspection of medical imagery, involve extensive practice. Therefore, it is important to model the effects of learning on pop-out and visual search performance. One way of modeling the effects of learning is to change the relative weights of the low-level vision properties that contribute to conspicuity, as suggested by Koch and Ullman[21]. The GTV model includes a *learning algorithm*, in the form of a simple neural network, which automatically modifies the weighting of low-level properties in the computation of object conspicuities.

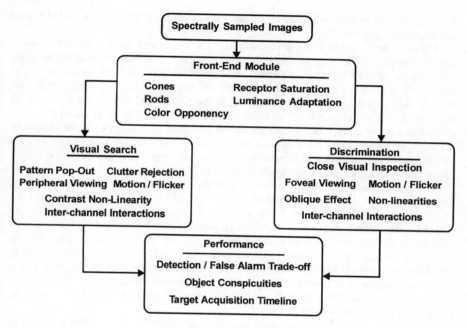

Figure 1. Major GTV modules.

2. Description of the GTV Model

The GTV model accepts either an individual image showing a static target in a background, or a series of images showing an animated sequence. Individual images are used when the goal is to evaluate the conspicuity or detectability of an object in a particular type of background. A series of images is used when the effects of object motion on search and detection are of interest. The animated sequences used to date typically represent a dynamic scenario in which one or more target vehicles move through a terrain background.

When the input to GTV is an animated sequence, a group of images is generated for the scenario every 0.33 sec. The 0.33 sec interval was chosen because it represents the approximate time between successive fixations (glimpses) as an observer searches a complex, cluttered image. Within each group, images are sampled at 60 Hz for a period of 0.125 sec, which is the approximate integration time of the visual system.

The input images may represent any image presented to human observers, i.e., visible band images seen with the unaided eye, images seen through a direct-view optical system (e.g., telescope), or images appearing on the display of an infrared sensor, night vision device, or image intensifier.

Figure 1 shows the four major modules of GTV: *Front-end, Search, Discrimination,* and *Performance*. The front-end module simulates the retinal receptors and initial processing stages of the human visual system. Its outputs are processed versions of the input image, which are the inputs for both the search and discrimination modules. The search module simulates the preattentive processing of the visual field that directs the focus of attention during visual search. The output of the search module is an image of the same dimensions as the input image which shows the locations and conspicuities of objects in the field of view. The discrimination module simulates attentive processing, and its output is also an image of the same dimensions as the input. The discrimination output image shows the detectability of objects in the field of view.

The performance module computes the probability of fixation and the probability of detection or false alarm for each object in the field of view. These computations are based on the output images of the search and discrimination modules. Objects are defined in the search output image, which is automatically segmented by the selective attention unit (described in greater detail below). Search performance is quantified in terms of a probability of fixation, P_{fix}, for each object. Discrimination performance is quantified in terms of the probability that the observer indicates "yes, the object is a target", given that it is fixated, $P_{yes/fix}$. The performance module also computes the observer's sensitivity (d') to the target, the overall (per glimpse) probability of detection, P_d, and the probability of false alarm, P_{fa}.

The four modules are run (iterated) once for each glimpse. In addition to its other functions, the performance module computes the cumulative P_d for each target and P_{fa} for each clutter object in the field of view over successive glimpses.

2.1. Front-End Module

The front-end module is shown in Fig. 2. As input, it requires up to four images of the same target/background scene for each glimpse. The individual images are calibrated to the spectral sensitivities of each of the four types of retinal receptors: short-, medium-, and long-wavelength cones, and rods[7,27,40]. Images with the required spectral distribution are generated by the Georgia Tech Sensor Model (GTSENSE)[34] from a spectral database that extends from 0.4 to 12.0 microns[35]. The model can be run using only the cone channels for photopic light levels, the rod channel alone for scotopic conditions, or all four channels for mesopic vision. Panchromatic images can also be input directly to the photopic luminance channel (marked "Lum" in Fig. 2).

One of the earliest operations in the human visual system and in the GTV front-end module is the calculation of color-opponent signals: red - green, blue - yellow, and red + green (luminance)[4,8,18]. Two important nonlinear processes also originate in this module. First, saturation of the rods is simulated by a compressive nonlinearity[1]. Second, the overall luminance of each input image is evaluated and the gains of the filters

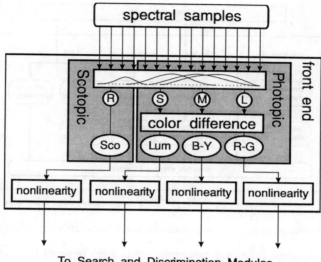

Figure 2. GTV front-end module.

in the pattern perception unit are adjusted for luminance adaptation, based on the findings of Kelly[20].

2.2. Search Module

The processed images from the front-end module, representing color-opponent and rod signals, serve as inputs to both the search and discrimination modules. The search module, shown in Fig. 3, is responsible for simulating preattentive processing. It provides predictions of the conspicuity of the most salient objects in the scene, from which P_{fix}'s are calculated.

The initial operations in the search module are: (a) temporal filtering and (b) temporal integration. The GTV temporal filter simulates the effects of motion and flicker on target conspicuity and discriminability, but does not currently simulate perception of direction or speed. A complete model of motion would require spatio-temporal filters, or temporal filtering on each channel prior spatial filtering.

The temporal filtering is done on separate channels from those that are spatially filtered, as shown in Fig. 3. Temporal and spatial filtering are separated out so that the outputs can be independently weighted. This allows the model to simulate selective attention to temporal modulation, independent of spatial variations in contrast.

Temporal filtering is done on only the photopic luminance and scotopic channels. This reflects the segregation of functions among higher visual pathways that carry

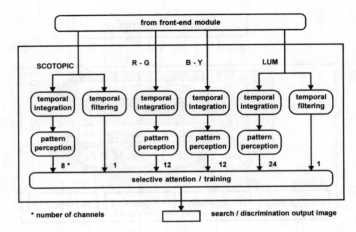

Figure 3. Structure of the GTV search and discrimination modules (see text for explanation).

information on form, color, and movement/stereo depth reported by Livingstone and Hubel[22,23]. The same temporal filter is applied to both the photopic luminance and scotopic channels.

Temporal filtering is accomplished by convolving the temporal impulse response function reported by Watson and Ahumada[42] with the time-sampled input images for each glimpse. The resulting images are then rectified, low-pass filtered, and fed to the selective attention unit. The images are also thresholded to remove any signal from stationary parts of the input image, since the temporal filter has a non-zero dc level.

The temporal integration unit simulates blurring of those parts of the image that move during a given fixation by averaging over the time-sampled images for each glimpse. The output of this unit is an image in which edges are blurred in proportion to their velocity or temporal modulation rate in the two-dimensional plane of the image.

The output of the temporal integration unit is input to the pattern perception unit (see Fig. 4). This unit is based on recently reported "complex" (two-stage) models of visual texture segregation[13,14,43]. The first stage involves filtering by oriented linear filters, followed by several nonlinear operations. The filters are generated by taking the Fourier transforms of difference of Gaussian (DOG) functions specified by Wilson and his colleagues[43]. Figure 5 shows examples of two DOG functions.

The next operation in the first stage is rectification of the images resulting from filtering, to provide measures of contrast energy in each channel. The rectified images are low-pass filtered to remove high-frequency artifacts introduced by rectification. This stage of the pattern perception unit also simulates important interactions between outputs of neighboring spatial frequency and orientation channels[17]. Finally, nonlinear effects of contrast level are simulated by a compressive nonlinearity. The first stage simulates the capability of the visual system to detect simple patterns and also accounts for masking and several other visual phenomena.

Since visual search depends heavily on peripheral vision, each of the DOG filters is shifted down in center frequency to simulate peripheral sensitivity. The amount of the shift is based on the cortical magnification factor[30]. In addition, the gains for the obliquely oriented filters are reduced to take into account the "oblique effect" (the fact that observers are more sensitive to vertical and horizontal than to oblique patterns)[5].

The number of filter channels processed in the pattern perception unit varies with the type of input, as indicated in Fig. 3. For the photopic luminance (red + green) input image, there are 24 filters (6 spatial frequency bands by 4 orientations). For red - green and blue - yellow images, there are 12 channels each (3 spatial frequency bands by 4 orientations). There is also a rod, or scotopic input image, which has 8 channels (2 spatial frequency bands by 4 orientations). Depending on the luminance of the input image, the scotopic channel is run alone, in combination with the photopic channels, or the photopic channels are run alone.

The second stage of the pattern perception unit, also shown in Fig. 4, simulates the capability of the visual system to segregate regions with different visual textures. Each channel of output from the first stage is band-pass filtered with a filter whose upper cutoff is approximately one octave lower than that of the first stage channel. The filters are

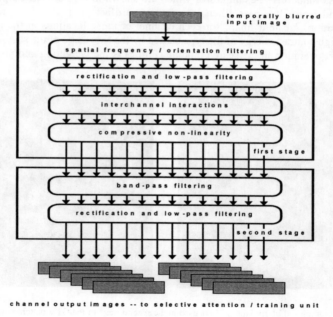

Figure 4. GTV pattern perception unit.

404

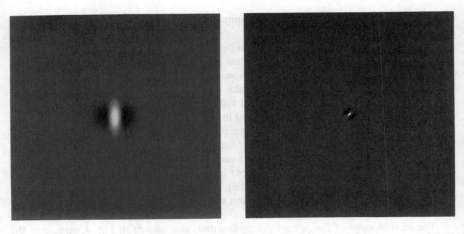

Figure 5. Examples of difference of Gaussian functions used in the first stage of the GTV pattern perception unit.

blurred mesa functions[41], examples of which are shown in Fig. 6. The outputs are then rectified and again low-pass filtered to remove artifacts introduced by rectification. These operations create a "map" for each channel of those locations in the input image that have high contrast energy of the type passed by the first stage of the same channel.

The next operation in the search module (Fig. 3) is the weighting and pooling of the

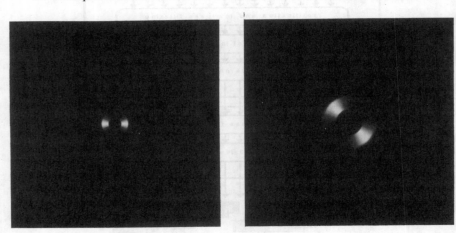

Figure 6. Examples of blurred mesa filters used in the second stage of the GTV pattern perception unit.

individual channel outputs. The weighting is done by the GTV selective attention unit, which is shown near the bottom of Fig. 3. As noted earlier, one way of modeling effects of learning on visual search is to postulate that human observers learn to weight certain of the outputs of low-level vision more heavily than others. For example, in searching for a tumor in an X-ray, the physician may pay special attention to objects with a particular range of shapes and sizes. This "top-down" aspect of visual search is modeled by differentially weighting the individual channel outputs. The channels are weighted to reflect the characteristics of the ensemble of targets that the observer sees in a given test condition. The weights are calculated by training a simple neural network, as described below. This allows the model to account for the fact that visual search tasks that initially require close, conscious inspection and serial search often become preattentive and parallel after extended practice (see earlier discussion).

The outputs of the pattern perception and temporal filtering units can be thought of as a multidimensional vector, R. In order to compute performance parameters (e.g., probabilities of fixation), the elements of the vector R must be weighted and pooled into a scalar value representing the perceived signal value, s, of each object in the scene.

The actual signal that any object generates in the observer's visual cortex will depend on where the image of the object falls on the retina. The major variable affecting R and s will be retinal eccentricity. The GTV model computes a number of different pairs of R and s values for each object, representing different intervals of retinal eccentricity. For images with relatively small fields of view, just two R and s values are computed for each object: one for foveal viewing and one for peripheral viewing. The foveal values are computed by the discrimination module, and the peripheral values are calculated by the search module.

A Hebbian learning/neural network approach is used to compute the weights and pool the channel outputs[11]. The network is trained to distinguish between targets and clutter objects typical of those in the scenes of interest. The neural network can be trained all at once, off-line, to simulate an experienced observer, or gradually and continuously over glimpses as the model is run, to simulate observer learning during the search and detection task. Training is conducted separately for peripheral and foveal vision (i.e., for search and discrimination).

The training procedure consists of presenting the network with the elements of the vector R as inputs. The network has one input node for each dimension of R. The same weights and neural network pooling operation are applied to every pixel in the input image. A standard neural network learning algorithm (simulated annealing) is iteratively applied to minimize the error function[11].

The neural network has certain features that allow it to find optimal weights. First, the network is self-calibrating. An error function is defined, and a learning algorithm automatically minimizes the error function. The learning algorithm is designed to find the absolute, as opposed to relative, minimum of the error function with a high confidence. Second, the neural network includes nonlinearities. The final output of the neural network is a sigmoid function of the weighted combination of the channel outputs. The sigmoid function is thresholded to zero when the weighted combination of the channel outputs is below a particular level. At the high end, the sigmoid function is also set to 1.0 when the weighted combination of channel outputs exceeds a specified value. The thresholded sigmoid function is consistent with the idea that human observers segment the field of view into dichotomous areas with and without objects.

The neural network learns by comparing its output (weighted channel outputs followed by the sigmoid function) to an ideal or desired output. The creation of the ideal image starts with an input image that shows the same target(s) in a background similar to that to be processed later. The target(s) need not be in the same position as they are in the images to be processed later. The target pixel values are then set to 1.0 and the background pixels are set to zero.

GTV is then run on an unmodified input image, and the outputs of each channel are saved. A linear combination of the output values (up to 58 values) at each pixel is computed and the result is transformed using the sigmoid function. The result of doing this at all pixels is a pooled search (or discrimination) output image array with values ranging from 0.0 to 1.0. The neural network learns by iteratively adjusting the channel weights in small, random increments, and comparing the pooled output image to the ideal image.

In several important respects, this learning algorithm simulates how an observer might be trained in a search task. The observer would be informed as to the actual locations of the targets in the scene. Some targets shown to the observer, however, may be undetectable or barely detectable. In a like manner, the GTV model is "shown" target locations in the ideal image. The neural network then determines how important each channel's information is in minimizing the error in detecting those targets. Specifically, when the weights are changed, it changes the output of the system. If that change is for the better (i.e., reduces the difference between the pooled, sigmoided output and the ideal image), then the new weights are retained. If the change increases the error beyond an allowable threshold, the weights are restored to their original values.

After a training period (currently a fixed number of iterations), the simulated observer is "on its own". The weights developed in the training process are used to compute target and clutter object conspicuities for the test image. Provided that the training set was representative of the test scenes, knowledge of the weights alone will be adequate to predict target conspicuities (search) or detectabilities (discrimination). However, if the targets in the test images are not detectable, or the training set was not representative of the test set, then performance will be poor. This result also holds under these conditions for human observers.

The output of the neural network is a pooled search (or discrimination) output image in which each pixel value is a weighted combination of the corresponding pixel values in the individual channel outputs. Two versions of the pooled search (or discrimination) output image are saved—one sigmoided and one consisting of the weighted combination before the sigmoid function is applied (i.e., an "unsigmoided" output image). Figure 7b shows the unsigmoided search output image for the input image shown in Fig. 7a.

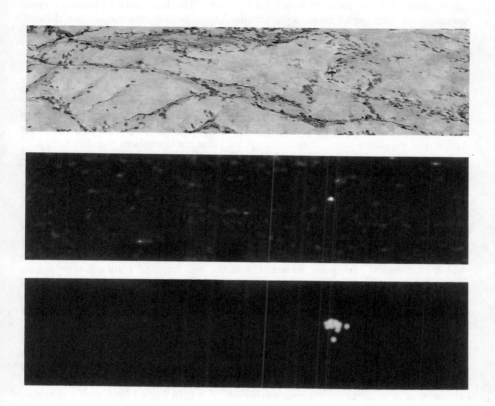

Figure 7. a) (top) Example input image. b) (middle) GTV output for image in Fig. 7a with selective attention simulated. c) (bottom) Observer-indicated locations in Fig. 7a after 0.33 sec exposure.

2.3. Discrimination Module

The structure of the discrimination module is the same as that of the search module (Fig. 3). The major difference between the discrimination and search modules is that discrimination simulates attentive rather than preattentive processing. It therefore uses filters tuned for foveal rather than peripheral viewing. The discrimination module outputs an image for each spatial frequency/orientation/chromatic/temporal modulation channel. As noted earlier, the neural network is trained separately for search and discrimination.

2.4. Performance Module

This module computes P_{fix}'s for each of the bright spots (called "blobs") in the pooled search output image (see example in Fig. 7b). It also computes the probability that the observer (mistakenly or correctly) designates each blob as a target. If the blob in question is in fact a target, then the computed value is a detection probability, P_d. If the bright spot is a clutter object, then the computed value is a false alarm probability, P_{fa}.

Conspicuities for each blob are calculated by pooling pixel values of the unsigmoided search output image over the area of each blob. Blob boundaries are defined by the sigmoided search output image. Recall that the sigmoided output segments the field of view into discrete objects. Blobs are defined as contiguous pixels with non-zero values. The pooling is done by using the Quick formula[28].

The fixation process is modeled as a noisy decision process. The extreme detector model[15] is used to quantify the P_{fix} for the target in the presence of background clutter blobs. "Noise" sources include quantum noise, neural noise, and clutter (i.e., the extent to which clutter blob luminance, texture, chromatic, and temporal contrasts approximate those of the target). An additional source of noise is the influence on the conspicuity of each blob of spatial variations in contrast energy outside the area of that blob. For example, the spatial conspicuity of a target in a cluttered terrain background will be influenced by the placement of the target relative to clutter objects, such as trees and rocks.

A probabilistic model is used to describe sequential dependencies between fixations on successive glimpses. The model assumes search without replacement. Once a blob is fixated, it is evaluated to determine whether it is a target, and one of two outcomes occurs. The simulated observer responds "yes, the object is a target" if its detectability is greater than or equal to the observer's criterion. If it is in fact a target, then a detection has occurred and the simulation terminates. If it is a clutter blob, then a false alarm has occurred and the simulation again terminates. The other possible outcome is that its detectability is less than the observer's criterion. In this case, the blob is rejected as a possible target (whether or not it really is) and it is not fixated again during the simulation. This model produces P_{fix}'s for each blob that converge to values determined by the probability that the blob is determined to be a target ($P_{yes/fix}$). The speed with which the P_{fix}'s converge is directly related to the number of blobs in the field of view.

The process of computing the probability of saying "yes" given fixation, $P_{yes/fix}$, starts with the computation of a signal value for each blob. The signal value is calculated by integrating the pooled discrimination output over the blob area, defined by the sigmoided search output, using the Quick formula[28]. A predicted signal-to-clutter ratio (SCR) is then computed for each blob (both targets and clutter). The SCR is defined as the blob signal value minus the mean value of the clutter blobs, the quantity divided by the standard deviation of clutter blobs. A power function is used to scale SCR's to measured d' values from visual search and detection experiments with human observers using the same images. The scaled SCR values are called estimated sensitivities, d'_{est}. The Theory of Signal Detectability (TSD) is then used to predict the $P_{yes/fix}$ for each blob, based on the d'_{est} values for each blob and an assumed or measured decision criterion. Depending on the target and background characteristics, either an equal variance TSD model is used, or it is assumed that the variance of the signal + noise distribution increases with the difference between the means of the distributions according to the ratio $\Delta\mu/\Delta\sigma \approx 4$[16]. The P_d (P_{fa}) for each target (clutter object) on a given glimpse is the product of its $P_{yes/fix}$ and P_{fix}.

The performance module also calculates the overall probabilities of detection, P_d, and false alarm, P_{fa}, for each glimpse by summing over all targets and clutter objects, respectively. Cumulative P_d's and P_{fa}'s are also tabulated for the series of glimpses.

3. Validation Test Results

Preliminary tests of the model demonstrated a need for the selective attention unit. Figures 8a and b show examples of an input image and the corresponding *unweighted* search output generated before the selective attention unit was implemented. In this case, the search output was generated by pooling the channel outputs using the Quick[28] formula with an exponent of 2.0. Note that the target (lower right-center of image) produced a prominent bright spot in the search output, indicating that it has a high conspicuity. However, there are many other bright spots produced by clutter objects. Since the search output represents a single glimpse, the sum of the P_{fix}'s over all the objects in the image must equal 1.0. Therefore, even though the target's conspicuity is high in this case, its predicted P_{fix} is relatively low due to the presence of distracting clutter.

The selective attention unit was implemented because validation tests revealed that experienced observers are much less distracted by clutter than the search output image in Fig. 8b suggests. Naturally, observers initially had difficulty detecting the targets in images like Fig. 8a. However, after three or four hours of practice on similar images, the target popped out for most observers, even though they were given only a short time to search the image (from 0.33 to 1.33 sec). That is, the observers were able to preattentively reject most of the clutter. This was true even though the test procedure was designed so that it was unlikely that observers became familiar with any particular background scene (32 different backgrounds were used).

Figure 7a shows one of the input images used in the first validation test of the model. The input image contains a single target, located on the middle-right side, roughly centered vertically. The image was exposed for 0.33 sec and was followed by a noise mask.

Part of the observer's task in this test was to place a cursor on the location in the noise mask corresponding to the location in the input image that looked most like a target. Figure 7c shows the search performance of experienced observers for the input image in Fig. 7a. The white dots in Fig. 7c mark the locations indicated by the observers. Note that almost all of the observers placed the cursor on or near the target. Observers were able to search much more efficiently than an unweighted search output, like that in Fig. 8b, indicates. This result suggests that observers learned to selectively attend to certain cues while ignoring or rejecting others.

Figure 7b shows the weighted search output image produced by the selective attention unit. This output contains many fewer bright spots than does Fig. 8b, showing that the weighting by the selective attention unit reduces the predicted conspicuity of clutter objects. In Fig. 7b, the target is by far the brightest spot, which ensures that its P_{fix} will be

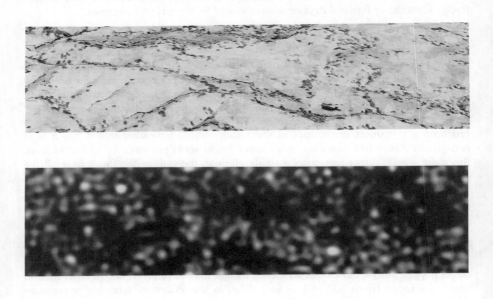

Figure 8. a) (top) Example input image. b) (bottom) GTV output for image in Fig. 8a with no selective attention unit.

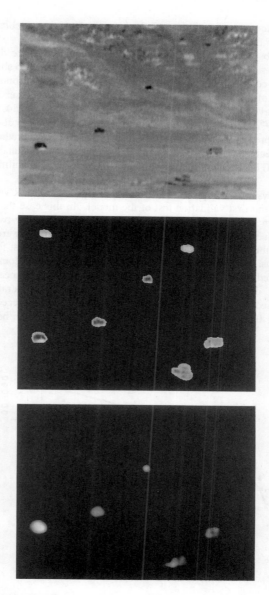

Figure 9. a) (top) Simulated infrared input image. b) (middle) "Ideal" image used to train GTV showing location of targets. c) (bottom) GTV output for image in Fig. 9a.

412

close to 1.0 when the image is put through the extreme detector model in the performance module (see earlier discussion).

Like human observers, GTV occasionally misses targets that are difficult to detect. Figure 9a shows a simulated infrared image with 7 targets. Figure 9b shows the locations of the targets. By comparing Figs. 9a and b, one can see that the second and sixth targets from the left edge of the image are difficult to detect. In a recent observer test, the measured P_d's for the seven targets were 0.974, 0.0, 1.0, 0.923, 0.564, 0.154, and 0.974, left to right, respectively[25]. The image in Fig. 9a was submitted to GTV to determine how well the model would predict the P_d's of human observers. The GTV prediction is shown in Fig. 9c. GTV detected targets 1, 3, 4, 5, and 7, but missed targets 2 and 6. These results demonstrate that GTV predicts the limitations as well as the capabilities of the human visual system.

Figure 10 shows a best-fit power function relating predicted SCR values to measured observer d's from the first validation test of the model. In this case the target was a stationary tank shown in a monochromatic terrain background. Thirty-two different backgrounds based on aerial photography were used. The backgrounds were of either of two clutter levels and the target appeared at one of four simulated ranges, for a total of eight stimulus conditions. Within each condition, the target appeared randomly at one of eight positions distributed horizontally across the image, and the target aspect angle presented to the observer (45 deg left side, 45 deg right side, and front-on) was randomized. Seven observers performed a yes/no detection task. Test images were preceded by a fixation cross, exposed for 0.67 sec, and followed by a noise mask. As can be seen in Fig. 10,

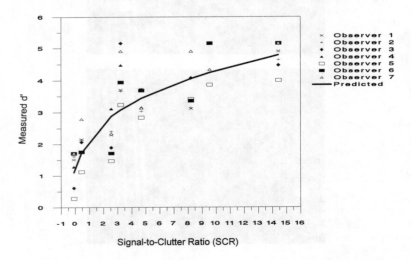

Figure 10. Model predictions versus observer data from first validation test of GTV.

there was considerable inter- and intra-observer variability in performance, which limits the goodness of fit that the model can achieve to the data of individual subjects. However, the predicted d's accounted for 83 percent of the variance in the mean measured d's over the eight conditions. A second validation test is currently underway to validate the model for full color images with moving targets.

4. Summary and Conclusions

Visual search is a necessary precursor to detection in most real-world situations. Therefore, in order to simulate or predict detection performance in real world tasks, it is necessary to simulate visual search. Although there are many models of visual search, most are restricted to simple, highly artificial stimuli[6,45,36,37,38]. Such models have more to say about selective attention than vision *per se*. GTV, on the other hand, is able to predict search and detection performance for realistic targets in real terrain backgrounds. GTV is unique in that it relates low-level vision properties to object conspicuities and visual search performance. Since it has the low-level vision "front-end", it is able to handle virtually any input scene and target. It is not limited, as are many other visual search models, to targets and distracters with highly constrained features.

One of the lessons learned in developing GTV is that a low-level vision front-end is necessary, but not sufficient. Accurate prediction of object conspicuities and visual search performance for experienced observers viewing realistic scenes requires (at least) the simulation of the three processes of human vision mentioned earlier. These processes include: (1) preattentive processing, (2) selective attention, and (3) the modification of selective attention with experience.

The results of the initial test of the GTV model show that a model of preattentive processing consisting of complex spatial frequency channels (i.e., two filtering stages, including nonlinear processes) is necessary to predict the location of the focus of attention during visual search. This test was limited to static, monochromatic imagery. The current version of GTV includes algorithms for processing chromatic and temporal contrast as well as luminance contrast. Tests are currently underway to test these algorithms with full color imagery and moving targets with moving parts (e.g., helicopter rotor blades).

The results of the validation tests conducted at Georgia Tech also show that a two-stage pattern perception model, while necessary to predict pop-out and conspicuity, is not sufficient. Two-stage pattern perception models identify all the regions in the input image that have high texture or contrast energy. But experienced human observers are not affected by all the patterns—they are able to selectively attend to some pattern elements and reject others. They are therefore much less distracted by clutter than an unmodified two-stage model would predict. Said another way, once observers have gained experience with a given set of targets in a specified type of background, those targets are much more conspicuous than a two-stage pattern perception routine would predict. GTV predicts the selective attention performance of experienced observers by differentially weighting the properties of the stimulus generated by low-level vision

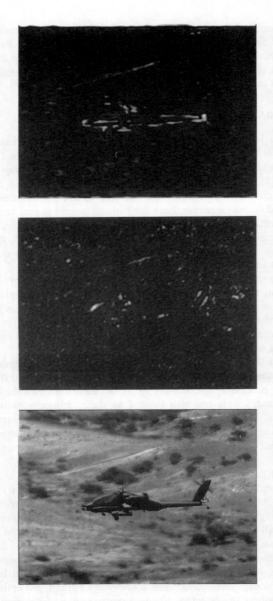

Figure 11. a) (top) GTV search output for a high spatial frequency, horizontal channel. b) (middle) Search output for high frequency, 45 deg channel. c) (bottom) Input image for outputs shown in Figs. 11a and b.

processes. In addition, GTV uses a simple neural network to model the effects of experience and learning on the weights applied to low-level vision properties.

The goal in the development of GTV has been to build a general model of human visual performance. We have endeavored to keep the model's structure and algorithms as close to the neurophysiology of the visual system as possible. Because of this, we believe that the GTV model will find a wide variety of applications.

One such application is to use the outputs of the individual channels of GTV as a tool for diagnosing which features of a target contribute most to its conspicuity, and for designing treatments that increase or reduce conspicuity. Reducing conspicuity would be useful if one wished to disguise the target. Conversely, one might want to increase the conspicuity of vehicles to enhance safety. By processing images of a given target at a variety of viewing angles and in a variety of illumination conditions, one can identify target features that pop-out, or have high (or low) conspicuity generally.

For example, Figs. 11a and b show the search module outputs for individual channels produced by the luminance (red + green) component of the input image shown in Fig. 11c. Figure 11a is the search output for a high-spatial-frequency, horizontally-oriented filter channel, while Fig. 11b is the search output for the same spatial frequency, oriented at 45 deg. In Fig. 11a, the edges along the underside, nose, and tail of the aircraft, which contrast sharply with the background, appear as prominent cues. In Fig. 11b, the front edge of the canopy and the leading and trailing edges of the tail appear as significant cues. The conspicuity of these areas could be reduced by repainting them to make their luminances, chromaticities, and/or patterns more similar to those of the background. Conversely, areas that show low output in Figs. 11a and b could be made more conspicuous. This example illustrates the potential utility of GTV as a tool for altering the conspicuity and detectability of targets.

The results obtained to date show that GTV is a valuable tool for predicting object conspicuities and detectabilities, especially in complex, cluttered backgrounds. However, it is anticipated that it will take many years of refinement and testing until the model begins to approach the complexity and capabilities of the human visual system. Some areas for further development of GTV include the addition of target recognition and identification capabilities, simulation of depth perception, including stereopsis and monocular depth cues, and enhancement of the GTV motion perception algorithms, including perception of motion-in-depth.

Acknowledgments

The development of the GTV model has been supported by the Army Aviation and Troop Command, Aviation Applied Technology Directorate (ATCOM/AATD) at Ft. Eustis, VA, the Air Force Special Operations Command (AFSOC) through the Air Force Warner Robins Air Logistics Center (WRALC/LNXEA) at Robins Air Force Base, GA, and the Army Aviation and Troop Command (ATCOM/AMSAT-B-Y) at St. Louis, MO. The authors express their appreciation to Mr. Ray Wall, Mr. Mac Dinning, and Mr. Hal Reddick of ATCOM/AATD, Mr. James Smith and Mr. Mark Scott of WRALC, and Mr.

Russell Stanton of ATCOM/AMSAT-B-Y. Thanks are due to Dr. Hugh Wilson of the University of Chicago, who served as a scientific consultant to the project, and to Dr. Robert Hyde, Director of the Electro-Optics, Environment, and Materials Laboratory of the Georgia Tech Research Institute, for his administrative support. The authors are also grateful to the graduate students who supported this research over the past three years, including Ms. Gisele Welch, Mr. Matthew Mazurczyk, Mr. Charles McDowell, and Ms. Elizabeth Rhodes.

References

1. Aguilar, M. and Stiles, W. S., "Saturation of the rod mechanism of the retina at high levels of stimulation," *Optica Acta* **1** (1954) 59-65.
2. Bellamy, L. J. and Courtney, A. J., "Development of a search task for the measurement of peripheral visual acuity," *Ergonomics* **24** (1981) 497-509.
3. Bergen, J. R., "Theories of visual texture perception," in *Vision and Visual Dysfunction, Vol. 10B: Spatial Vision* ed. D. Regan (MacMillan, New York, 1991), pp. 114-134.
4. Boynton, R. M., *Human Color Vision* (Holt, Rinehart & Winston, New York, 1979).
5. Campbell, F. W., Kulikowski, J. J., and Levinson J., "The effect of orientation on the visual resolution of gratings," *Journal of Physiology* **187** (1966) 427-436.
6. Cave, K. R. and Wolfe, J. M., "Modeling the role of parallel processing in visual search," *Cognitive Psychology* **22** (1990) 225-271.
7. Crawford, B. H., "The scotopic visibility function," *Physics Society Proceedings* **62** (1949) 321-334.
8. De Valois, R. L. and De Valois, K. K., "Neural coding of color," in *Handbook of perception: Vol. 5E.* eds. C. Carterette and M. P. Friedman. (Academic Press, New York, 1975), pp. 117-166.
9. Doll, T. J. and Schmieder, D. E., "Observer false alarm effects on detection in clutter," *Optical Engineering* **32** (1993) 1675-1684.
10. Erikson, R. A., "Relation between visual search time and visual acuity," *Human Factors* **6** (1964) 165-178.
11. Freeman, J. A. and Skapura, D. M., *Neural Networks: Algorithms, Applications, and Programming Techniques* (Addison-Welsly, Reading, MA, 1992).
12. Gould, J. D., "Looking at pictures," in *Eye Movements and Psychological Processes*, eds. R. A. Monty and J. W. Senders (Lawrence Erlbaum Associates, Hillsdale, NJ, 1976), pp. 323-346.
13. Graham, N., "Complex channels, early local nonlinearities, and normalization in texture segregation," in *Computational Models of Visual Processing* eds. M. S. Landy and J. A. Movshon (MIT Press, Cambridge, MA, 1991), pp. 273-290.
14. Graham, N., Beck, J., and Sutter, A., "Nonlinear processes in spatial-frequency channel models of perceived texture segregation: Effects of sign and amount of contrast," *Vision Research* **32** (1992) 719-743.

15. Green, D. A. and Dai, H., "Probability of being correct with 1 of M orthogonal signals," *Perception & Psychophysics* **49** (1991) 100-101.
16. Green, D. A. and Swets, J. A., *Signal Detection Theory and Psychophysics* (Wiley, New York, 1966).
17. Greenlee, M. W. and Magnussen, S., "Interactions among spatial frequency and orientation channels adapted concurrently," *Vision Research* **28** (1988) 1303-1310.
18. Hurvich, L. M., *Color Vision* (Sinauer Associates, Sunderlan, MA, 1981).
19. Johnston, D. M., "Search performance as a function of peripheral acuity," *Human Factors* **7** (1965) 528-535.
20. Kelly, D. H., "Adaptation effects on spatio-temporal sine-wave thresholds," *Vision Research* **12** (1972) 89-101.
21. Koch, C. and Ullman, S., "Shifts in selective visual attention: Towards the underlying neural circuitry," *Human Neurobiology* **4** (1985) 219-227.
22. Livingstone, M. S. and Hubel, D. H., "Psychophysical evidence for separate channels for the perception of form, color, movement, and depth," *The Journal of Neuroscience* **7** (1987) 3416-3468.
23. Livingstone, M. and Hubel, D., "Segregation of form, color, movement, and depth: Anatomy, physiology, and perception," *Science* **240** (1988) 740-749.
24. Neisser, U., Novick, R., and Lazar, R., "Searching for ten targets simultaneously," *Perceptual and Motor Skills* **17** (1963) 955-961.
25. O'Kane, B. (March, 1994). Personal communication to the authors.
26. O'Kane, B. L., Walters, C. P., and D'Agostino, J. D., *Report on Perception Experiments in Support of Low-Observables Thermal Performance Models* (U. S. Army CECOM Night Vision and Electronic Sensors Directorate, Ft. Belvoir, VA, 1993).
27. Pokorny, J. and Smith, V. C., "Colorimetry and color discrimination," in *Handbook of Perception and Human Performance. Vol. 1: Sensory Processes and Perception* eds. K. Boff, L. Kaufman, and J. P. Thomas (Wiley, New York, 1986), pp. 8:1-8:51.
28. Quick, R. F., Jr., "A vector-magnitude model of contrast detection," *Kybernetic* **16** (1974) 65-67.
29. Rayner, K., "Foveal and parafoveal cues in reading," in *Attention and Performance VII* ed. J. Requin (Lawrence Erlbaum and Associates, Hillsdale, NJ, 1978), pp. 141-161.
30. Rovamo, J. and Virsu, V., "An estimation and application of the human cortical magnification factor," *Experimental Brain Research* **37** (1979) 495-510.
31. Sandon, P. A., "Simulating visual attention," *Journal of Cognitive Neuroscience* **2** (1989) 213-231.
32. Schneider, W., Dumais, S. T., and Shiffrin, R. M., "Automatic and controlled processing and attention," in *Varieties of Attention* eds. R. Parasuraman and D. R. Davies (Academic Press, Orlando, FL, 1984), pp. 1-27.
33. Schneider, W. and Shiffrin, R., "Controlled and automatic human information processing I: Detection, search, and attention," *Psychological Review* **84** (1977) 1-66.

34. Stewart, J. M., *GTSENSE User's/Analyst's Manual* (Georgia Tech Research Institute, Atlanta, GA, 1994).

35. Stewart, J. M. and Hetzler, M. C., *VISEO Data Collection User's/Analyst's Manual* (Georgia Tech Research Institute, Atlanta, GA, 1994).

36. Treisman, A., "Features and objects in visual processing," *Scientific American* **255** (1986) 114-124.

37. Treisman, A., Cavanagh, P., Fischer, B., Ramachandran, V. S., and Von der Heydt, R., "Form perception and attention: Striate cortex and beyond," in *Visual Perception: The Neurophysiological Foundations* eds. L. Spillmann and J. Werner (Academic Press, New York, 1991), pp. 273-316.

38. Treisman, A. and Gelade, G., "A feature-integration theory of attention," *Cognitive Psychology* **12** (1980) 97-136.

39. Tsotsos, J. K., "Analyzing vision at the complexity level," *Behavioral and Brain Sciences* **13** (1990) 423-469.

40. Wald, G., "Human vision and the spectrum," *Science* **101** (1945) 653-658.

41. Watson, A. B., "The cortex transform: Rapid computation of simulated neural images," *Computer Vision, Graphics, and Image Processing* **39** (1987) 311-327.

42. Watson, A. B. and Ahumada, A. J., "Model of human visual-motion sensing," *Journal of the Optical Society of America A* **2** (1985) 322-341.

43. Wilson, H. R., McFarlane, D. K., and Phillips, G. C., "Spatial frequency tuning of orientation selective units estimated by oblique masking," *Vision Research* **23** (1983) 873-882.

44. Wilson, H. R. and Richards, W. A., "Curvature and separation discrimination at texture boundaries," *Journal of the Optical Society of America A* **9** (1992) 1653-1662.

45. Wolfe, J. M., Cave, K. R., and Franzel, S. L., "Guided search: An alternative to the feature integration model for visual search," *Journal of Experimental Psychology: Human Perception and Performance* **15** (1989) 419-433.